TRENDS IN CHILD NEUROLOGY

A Festschrift for Jean Aicardi

ISBN 2-7420-0111-5

Éditions John Libbey Eurotext
127, avenue de la République, 92120 Montrouge, France.
Tél : (1) 46.73.06.60

John Libbey and Company Ltd
13, Smiths Yard, Summerley Street, London SW18 4HR, England.
Tel : (1) 947.27.77

John Libbey CIC
Via L. Spallanzani, 11, 00161 Rome, Italy.
Tel : (06) 862.289

© John Libbey Eurotext, 1996, Paris.

Il est interdit de reproduire intégralement ou partiellement le présent ouvrage — loi du 11 mars 1957 — sans autorisation de l'éditeur ou du Centre français du Copyright, 6 *bis*, rue Gabriel-Laumain, 75010 Paris.

TRENDS IN CHILD NEUROLOGY

A Festschrift for Jean Aicardi

Editors
Alexis Arzimanoglou
Françoise Goutières

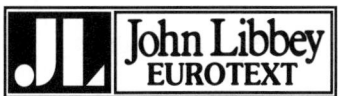

Foreword

The last decade has seen dramatic developments in the field of Child Neurology. A large amount of the pioneering work was carried out by Jean Aicardi, our teacher and friend, as well as by many of his disciples or colleagues.

The mere fact that neuropediatricians, from every corner of the planet, gathered together in Paris to honor him is yet again an indication that Jean Aicardi is certainly a world recognized authority in Child Neurology. This Festschrift took place at the Lutetia Hotel the 13-14 October 1995, in the same place where, 23 years earlier, Jean Aicardi participated in the first meeting of the *Société Européenne de Neurologie Pédiatrique*.

The following collection of authoritative reviews on a wide range of topics, each so different and yet relevant, reflects the interest that Jean Aicardi has generated amongst us all. His pioneering work in the field of epilepsies inspired today's acquired knowledge on the evolution of epilepsies with age, medical and surgical treatment, epilepsy and language disorders or epilepsy and abnormalities of cortical development. His contribution also opened the gateway for further research in a great variety of other pathologies such as degenerative diseases, muscular and metabolic disorders. Today's revolution in neurogenetics was made possible because of the meticulous clinical work of doctors like Jean Aicardi.

We would like to thank Jean Aicardi for being our collaborator and mentor. We would like to thank all the authors for putting together this collection of valuable works which represents the state of the art in Child Neurology. We would also like to thank all the participants for their valuable contribution and presence at the meeting. We feel privileged to have taken part in this process.

The meeting and this publication were made possible by a grant from Hoechst Marion Roussel, which we gratefully acknowledge. John Libbey Eurotext and its collaborators have been of a great help in collecting and reviewing all contributions.

Alexis Arzimanoglou
Françoise Goutières

A Festschrift for Jean Aicardi

Organizing and Scientific Committee

Alexis Arzimanoglou
Marie-Anne Barthez
Marie Bourgeois
Françoise Goutières
Jean-Marc Pinard
Marc Tardieu
Josefa Tabacs
Brigitte Tricot

Association Bibliographie Recherche En Neurologie

Caroline Dumas, Valery Labonne, John Mumford
and Hoechst Marion Roussel Laboratories

Chairpersons

J. Roger
G. Erba
C. Chevrie-Muller
P.G. Barth
D. Gardner-Medwin
E. Brett
M.T. Vanier

M. Revol
O. Eeg-Olofsson
H. Szliwowski
P. Landrieu
G. Ponsot
M. de Negri
M. Tardieu

List of participants

Pr AICARDI Jean
Pr ANDERMANN Frederick
Dr ANDRE Monique
Pr ARTHUIS Michel
Dr ARTIGAS Josep
Dr ARZIMANOGLOU Alexis
Pr AUBOURG Patrick
Dr BABINET J.M.
Dr BARBOSA Célia
Dr BARBOT Clara
Pr BARTH P.G.
Dr BARTHEZ Marie-Anne
Dr BELPAIRE M.C.
Dr BERTERROTTIERE Dominique
Dr BILLARD Catherine
Dr BOEL Marc
Dr BOESPFLUG Odile
Dr BOGICEVIC Dragana
Dr BOON Martha
Dr BORDARIER Cécile
Dr BORMANS Jeannie
Dr BOULLOCHE Jacques
Dr BOURGEOIS Marie
Pr BRETT Edward
Pr CAILLE Bernard
Dr CHABROL Brigitte
Dr CHEDAL Jacques
Dr CHEVRIE-MULLER Claude
Dr CHIRON Catherine
Dr COLAMARIA Vito
Dr CONTI Danièle
Dr COUVREUR Jacques
Dr CRUZ Romeu
Dr DE MEURON Gilles
Pr DE NEGRI Maurizio
Dr DE SAINT MARTIN Anne

Dr DELAVELLE Jacqueline
Pr DEONNA Thierry
Dr DIAS Karine
Dr DIEBLER Claude
Dr DRAVET Charlotte
Pr DUBOWITZ Victor
Dr DUBRU J.M.
Pr DUCHOWNY Michael
Pr DULAC Olivier
Dr DUMAS Caroline
Dr DUSSER Anne
Dr DWORZAK Patricia
Dr EEG-OLOFSSON Orvar
Pr ERBA Guiseppe
Dr ESCOFET SOTERAS Conxita
Pr EVRARD Philippe
Pr FARDEAU Michel
Dr FARKAS Edith
Pr FEJERMAN Natalio
Pr FERNANDEZ Emilio
Dr FERRANDO LUCAS Maria Teresa
Dr FLURIN
Dr FRENKEL Anne-Laure
Pr FUKUYAMA Yukio
Dr GARDNER-MEDWIN David
Dr GAUTIER Marthe
Dr GENTON Pierre
Dr GOBBI Guiseppe
Dr GOUTIERES Françoise
Dr GRASSET E.
Dr GREEN Stweart
Dr GRUYER Michel
Dr GUERRINI Renzo
Dr GUITET Montserrat
Pr GUZZETTA Francesco
Dr HAENGGELI Charles-Antoine

Pr HAGBERG Bengt
Dr HANAOKA Shigeru
Pr HANEFELD F.
Pr HAREL Shaul
Dr HERON Bénédicte
Dr HERON Delphine
Dr HIRSCH Edouard
Pr HIRSCH Jean-François
Pr HOLGUIN Jorge
Pr HOPKINS Ian
Dr IANNETTI Paola
Pr JACKSON Graeme
Dr JUIF J. Georges
Dr KAHN BENSAUDE Irène
Pr KRÄGELOH Ingeborg
Dr KULAKOWSKI Sophie
Dr LABONNE Valery
Pr LANDRIEU Pierre
Dr LE BERRE Claude
Dr LEROY Patricia
Dr LEVEAU Jacques
Dr LEVY GOMEZ Antonio
Dr LIVET Marie-Odile
Dr LIVINGSTON John
Dr LOMBES Anne
Dr LOPEZ-CASAS Jesus
Dr LORENTE Isabel
Pr LYON Gilles
Pr MANCINI Josette
Dr MAROTEAUX Pierre
Dr MEDINA M. Angeles
Dr MELKI Judith
Dr MISSON Jean-Paul
Pr MOTTE Jacques
Dr MOUTARD Marie-Laure
Dr MUMFORD John
Pr MUNNICH Arnold
Pr NEVILLE Brian
Dr NEWTON Richard
Dr NUTTIN Christian
Dr OGIER de BAULNY Hélène
Dr PARAIN Dominique
Dr PAVONE Laurenzo
Dr PEDESPAN Jean-Michel

Dr PEUDENIER Sylviane
Dr PINARD Jean-Marc
Pr PINSARD Nicole
Pr POLL-THE Bwee Tien
Pr PONSOT Gérard
Mme PORA
Pr POSER Charles
Dr PRUDENT Muriel
Pr RAPIN Isabelle
Dr RAVNIK Igor
Dr REJOU Franck
Dr RENIER W.O.
Dr REVOL Michel
Pr ROBINSON R.O.
Dr ROGER Joseph
Pr RONDOT Pierre
Dr ROPERT J.C.
Dr ROSSI Livia
Dr ROULET PEREZ Eliane
Dr ROY Claude
Dr RUGGIERI Victor
Dr SAINT MARTIN Jacques
Pr SAINTE ROSE Christian
Dr SALEFRANQUE Françoise
Dr SANS Anna
Dr SAUVIER Jacques
Dr SEBIRE Guillaume
Dr SPEGEL Milan
Pr SZLIWOWSKI Henri
Mme TABACS Joséfa
Pr TARDIEU Marc
Pr TAYLOR David
Dr TESTARD Hervé
Dr TOUATI Guy
Melle TRICOT Brigitte
Dr TRUSCELLI Danièle
Dr URTIZBEREA Jon Andoni
Dr VANHULLE C.
Dr VANIER Marie-Thérèse
Melle VIAUD-DELMON Isabelle
Dr WACHTER Henri
Dr WALLACE Sheila
Dr WESTZBURGER Catherine
Pr WILSON John

A message from the President of the International Child Neurology Association

October 12, 1995

Dear Jean,

On behalf of all members of the International Child Neurology Association (ICNA), I address a few words of appreciation to your excellent achievements in the field of child neurology during your untiring years of work. I got to know you through the activities of ICNA, and have always been impressed by your vast knowledge and experience, not only on science and medicine but also on art, culture, history, linguistics, etc, etc, whenever we started talking on either business or other general topics.

You started your official business as President of ICNA with launching of the Decade of the Brain, and we took advantage of your strong leadership for promotion of an important medical speciality, CHILD NEUROLOGY. Owing to your deep insight and clear judgment, the Association became more prosperous and attracted more colleagues to join international activities toward our common destination: HEALTH OF THE CHILD'S BRAIN. Even if you officially retire from your clinical activities, we expect your continuous support and help to us in future as well, in medical, scientific, and social aspects of child neurology.

To my regret, I cannot attend this important "Réunion en l'Honneur de Jean Aicardi" for personal reasons, but I hope it will be a big success to memorize your incomparable contribution to our Association as well as to the speciality of child neurology. Finally, I wish health of both you and your wife for long years to come. Thank you again, and with my best personal regards.

Sincerely,

Yoshiyuki Suzuki

A message from the President of the Société Européenne de Neurologie Pédiatrique

J'ai le plaisir et l'honneur de saluer Jean Aicardi au nom de la Société Européenne de Neurologie Pédiatrique, dont il est un membre important d'après sa constitution à Oxford en 1971. Il peut être suggestif de rappeler que la première réunion de la Société, organisée par Gilles Lyon en 1972, a eu lieu dans ce même Hôtel Lutétia.

Jean Aicardi a contribué considérablement à former l'esprit de la Société, en ses deux aspects fondamentaux : la rigueur scientifique et le sentiment authentique d'amitié ; et la Société lui est reconnaissante pour ce qu'il lui a donné en termes de participation, contribution scientifique et enseignement.

Jean Aicardi a augmenté de plus en plus son prestige international, mais nous pensons et espérons que notre Société restera pour lui toujours un point de repère important, ainsi que la Société le considérera toujours comme l'un des membres les plus prestigieux et les plus aimés.

Maurizio De Negri

An address of thanks by Jean Aicardi

Retirement is an appropriate time to look back on one's career and to try, privately, to assess what has been and has not been achieved. Its public celebration is a unique opportunity to get together old and more recent friends, disciples and colleagues and I am deeply moved that so many of them, from so many parts of the world, have wished to participate and to give me such a testimony of their esteem and sympathy at this final point of my professional life. I am particularly grateful to those who have had the courage to dedicate their time and skills to the writing of chapters of such an outstanding quality. I am proud to have contributed to the education of some of the writers and participants. One of my weaknesses is to believe that they may owe a part of their professional skills to my teaching, even though I am well aware that it is through opposition, rather than through imitation, that teaching is ultimately fruitful.

Retirement is also the right moment to acknowledge the enormous debt that I owe to all my past collaborators, from the oldest and most faithful friends who have helped and supported me for more than twenty-five years, to the most recent and youngest ones, whose enthusiasm, activity and abilities constitute for me an enormous encouragement.

It is both a pleasure and a great honour that so many distinguished colleagues — some my former pupils — from many countries all over the world, have accepted to contribute to this homage by their presence and their writings. Their esteem and moral support have been of tremendous importance throughout my career and for this, I am deeply indebted.

Finally, I wish to express my special gratitude to the members of the Organizing Committee who have taken great pains to set up the meeting and to publish this book, and to those who have made them possible by their generous support.

Jean Aicardi

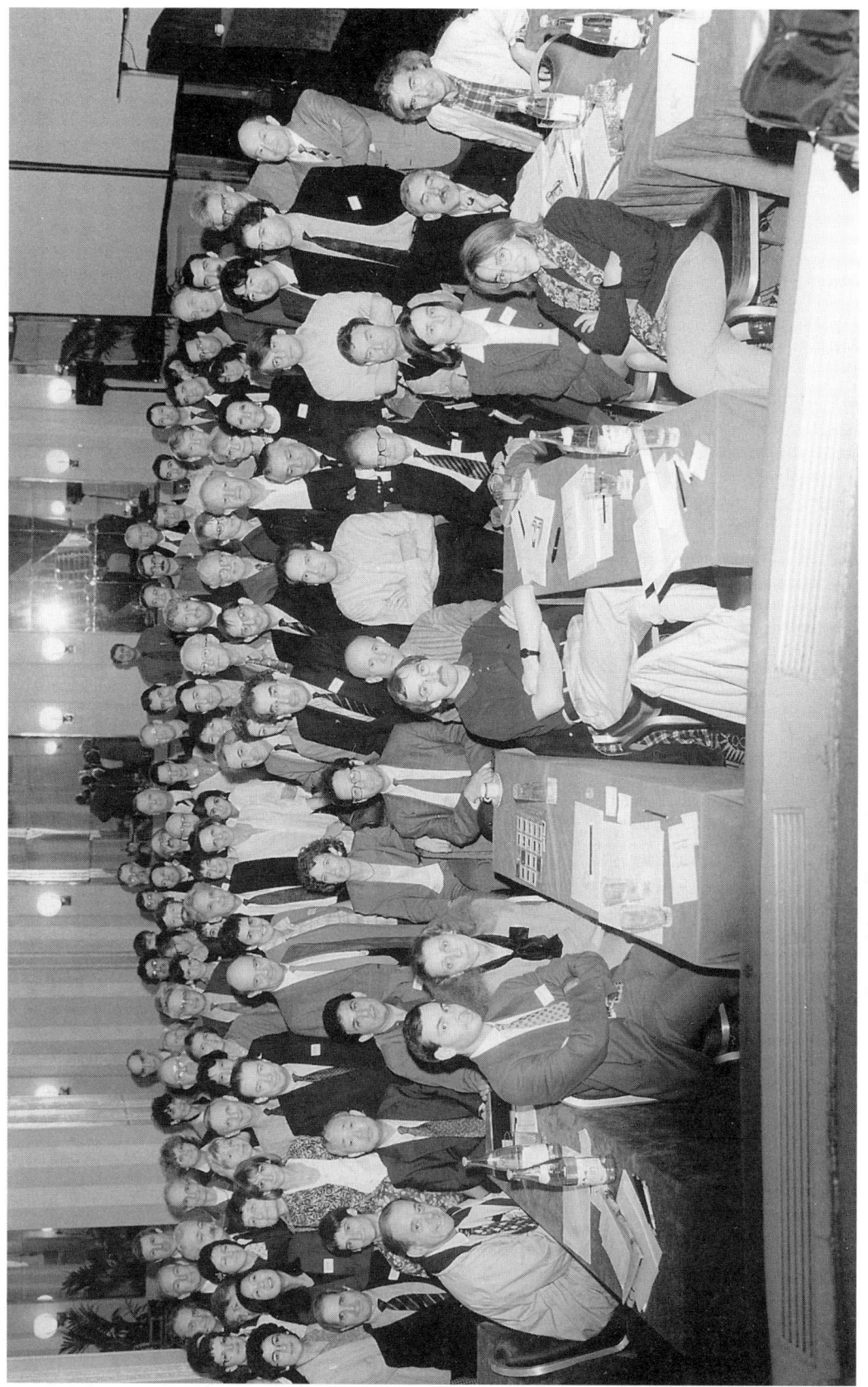

Jean Aicardi meeting. Hôtel Lutetia, Paris, 13 October 1995.

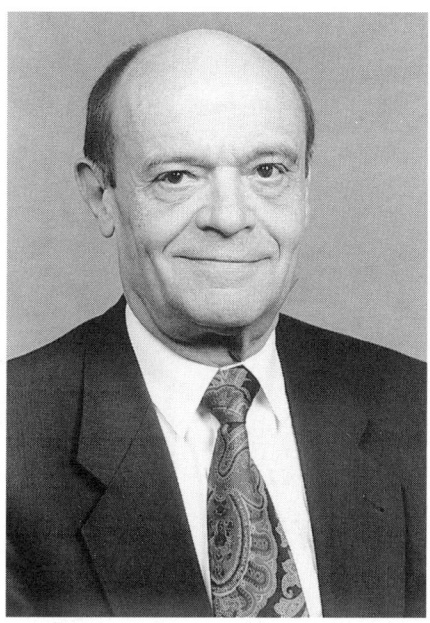

Jean Aicardi

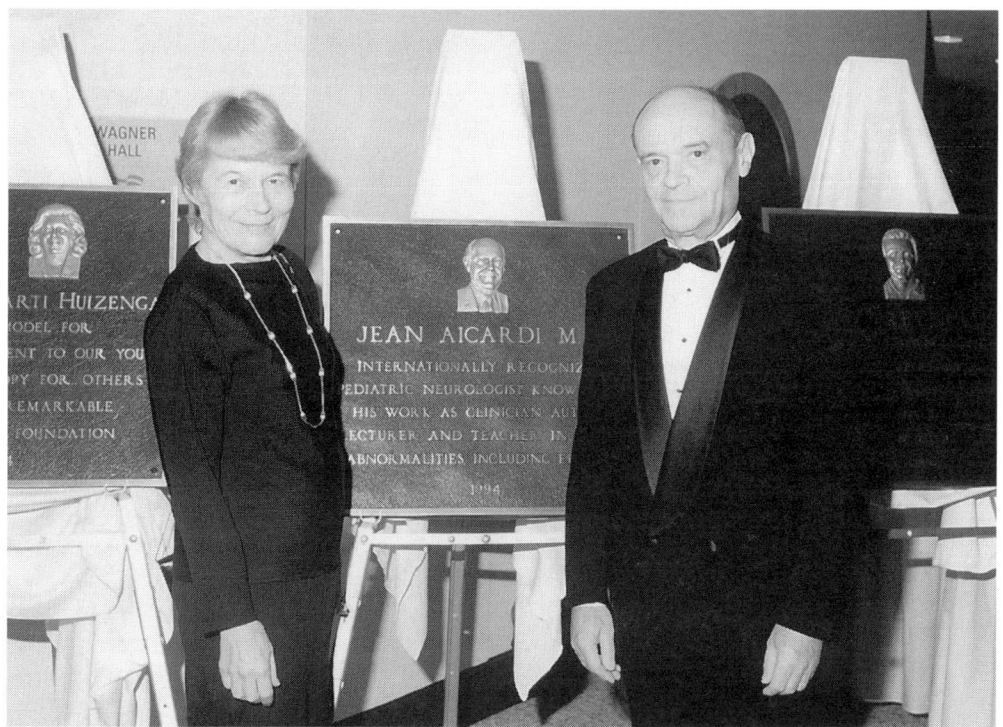

Miami, Children's Hospital, 5 November 1994.
Induction into the Ambassador David M. Walters Hall of Frame.

Boulevard Beaumarchais, Paris,
22 December 1991.
With Dr. Claude Chevrie-Muller
and Dr. Alexis Arzimanoglou.

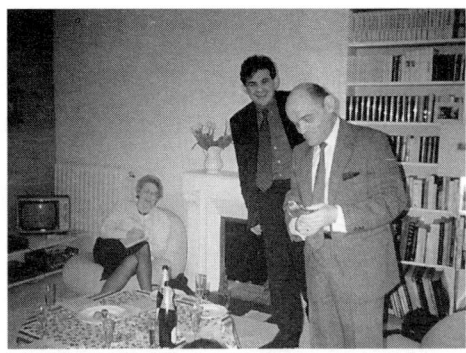

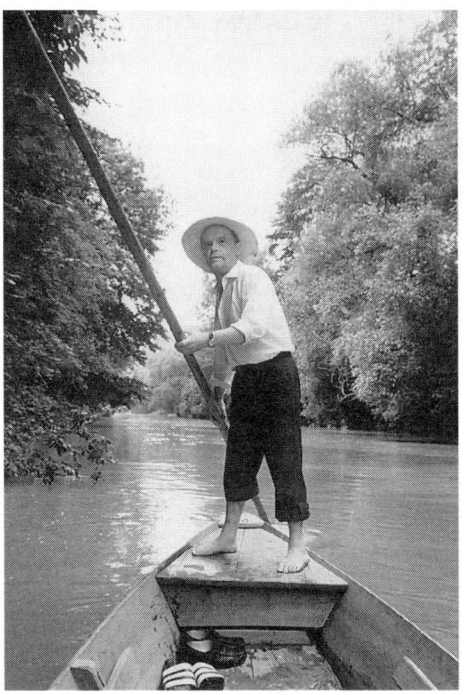

Tübingen, June 1986.
Punting on the Neckar.

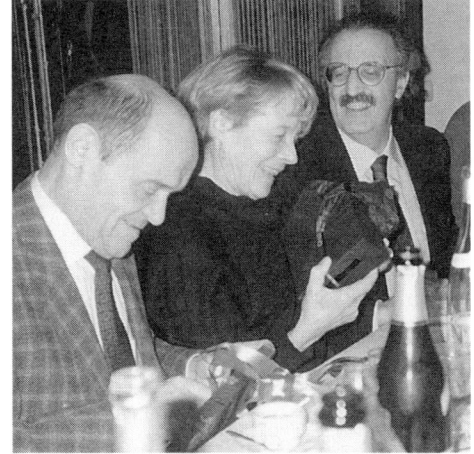

Jean and Jeanne Aicardi
with Emilio Fernandez in Barcelona.

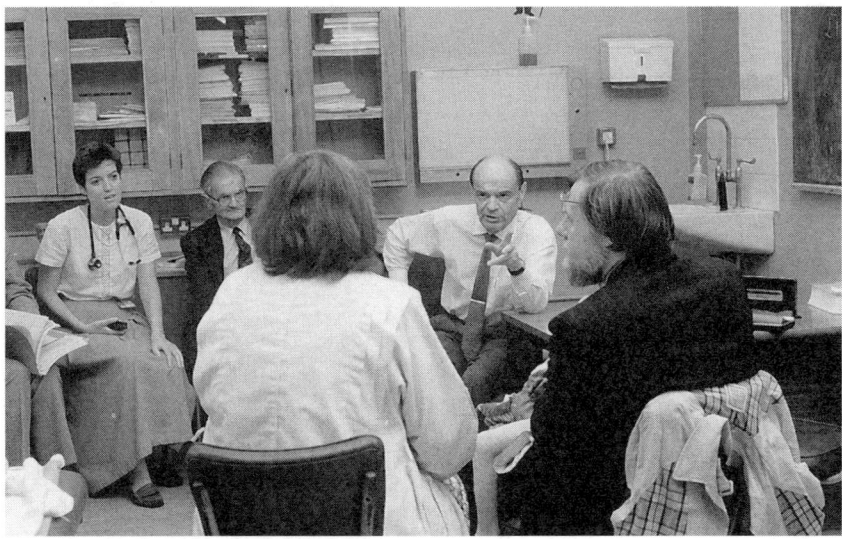

Birmingham, Autumn 1992.
With Neil Gordon talking with parents at Stewart Green's Clinic.

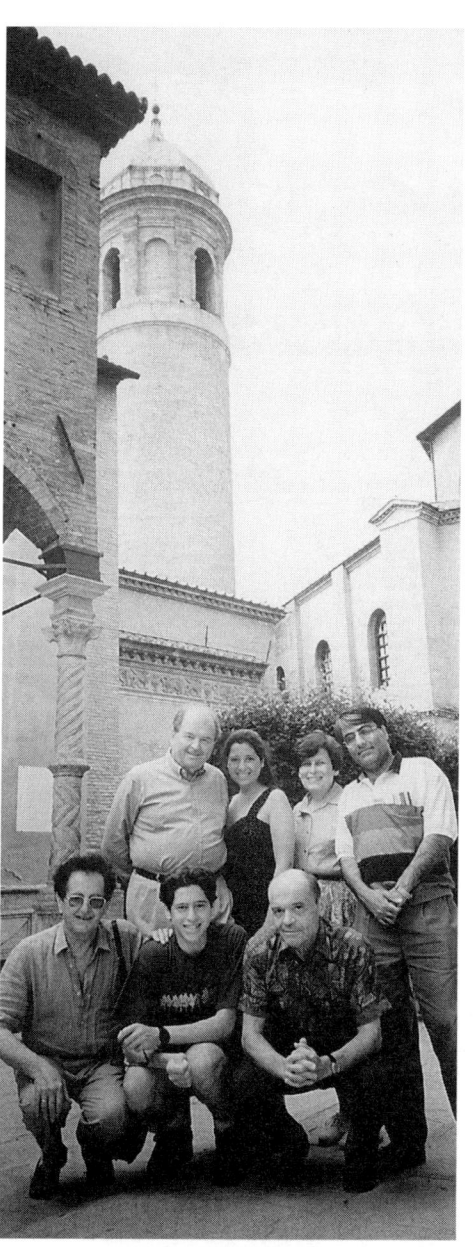

Pise, June 1993.
With Fred, Annie,
Eva Andermann, Harry Chugani,
Jo Roger, Marc Andermann.

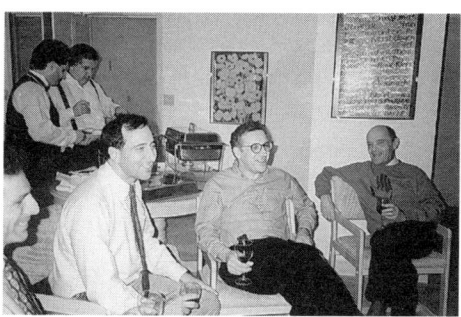

Miami, December 1994.
Farewell Party. With Trevor Resnick,
Mike Duchowny, Marcel Deray.

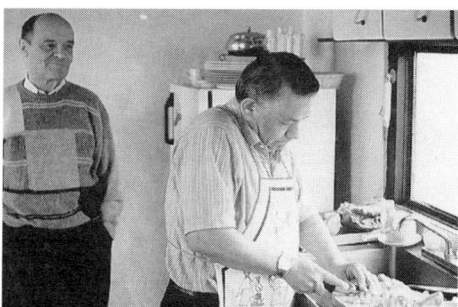

Bogota, March 1994.
With Jorge Holguin at work.

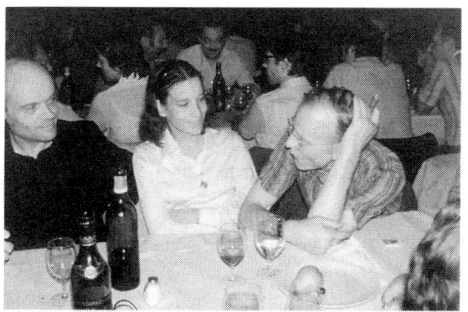

Jean Aicardi, Françoise Goutières,
Ronald Mac Keith.

Contents

Foreword V
Organizing and scientific committee VI
List of participants VII
A message from the President of the
International Child Neurology Association IX
A message from the President of the
Société Européenne de Neurologie Pédiatrique XI
An address of thanks by Jean Aicardi XIII
List of contributors XXIII

1. Jean Aicardi
   F. Goutières 1

2. Epilepsies during the first year of life
   N. Fejerman 7

3. Migraine and epilepsy
   J. Holguin 15

4. The paediatric issues in epilepsy surgery. The Great Ormond
   Street, Institute of Child Health London experience
   B. Neville 21

5. Developmental influences on the electrophysiologic investigation of
   pediatric epilepsy surgery candidates
   M. Duchowny, P. Jayakar, R. Resnick, A.S. Harvey 29

6. Hemifacial spasm or subcortical (infratentorial) epilepsy: a case report of a child with Goldenhar's syndrome and a pontomedullary junction lesion
   A.A. Arzimanoglou 43

7. Epilepsy, autistic regression and disintegrative disorder
   I. Rapin 53

8. Cognitive disorders in childhood epilepsy
   O. Dulac 59

9. Comments about the assessment and treatment of some dysphasic children
   D. Truscelli 63

10. Developmental defects of the corpus callosum
    G. Lyon 69

11. Aicardi syndrome with normal developmental progress, remission of epilepsy and bilateral intraventricular tumours
    I.J. Hopkins 77

12. Subcortical laminar heterotopia and other X-linked cerebral cortical dysgenesis
    J.-M. Pinard 81

13. Magnetic resonance in temporal lobe epilepsy
    G.D. Jackson 89

14. Congenital muscular dystrophies : an overview
    Y. Fukuyama, M. Osawa, K. Saito 107

15. Molecular genetics of spinal muscular atrophy
    J. Melki, A. Munnich 137

16. Rett syndrome: recent clinical and biological aspects
    B. Hagberg 143

17. Essential tremor in childhood
    E. Fernandez-Alvarez, J. Lopez-Casas 147

18. Dopa-sensitive progressive childhood dystonia (Segawa's syndrome). From symptom to gene. A 20 years history
    T. Deonna 157

19. **Alternating hemiplegia of childhood. A report of 29 cases and a review of the literature**
    M. Bourgeois 163

20. **Peroxisomal disorders**
    B.T. Poll-The 169

21. **Diagnosis of basal ganglia lesions; additional aspects from proton spectroscopy**
    I. Krägeloh-Mann, W. Grodd, D. Auer, P. Toft 181

22. **Pelizaeus Merzbacher disease and X-linked dysmyelinating diseases**
    O. Boespflug-Tanguy, C. Mimault, G. Giraud, F. Cailloux, D. Pham Dinh, B. Dastugue, A. Dautigny 189

23. **Schilder's myelinoclastic diffuse sclerosis and other multifocal leukoencephalopathies**
    A. Levy-Gomes 195

24. **Schilder's myelinoclastic diffuse sclerosis**
    C.M. Poser 199

25. **X-linked adrenoleukodystrophy**
    P. Aubourg 205

26. **Genetic and environmental determinants of neocortical development**
    P. Evrard 221

List of contributors

Aubourg P., Medical School University of Paris V-René Descartes, INSERM U 342 and Hôpital Saint-Vincent-de-Paul, 82, avenue Denfert-Rochereau, 75014 Paris, France.
Arzimanoglou A.A., Child Neurology Unit and Epilepsy Research Group, Hôpital Salpêtrière, 47, boulevard de l'Hôpital, 75013 Paris, France.
Auer D., Max Planck Institute for Psychiatry, München, Germany.

Boespflug-Tanguy O., INSERM U 384, Faculté de Médecine, 28, place Henri-Dunant, BP 38, 63001 Clermont-Ferrand Cedex, France.
Bourgeois M., Neurological Unit, Department of Pediatrics, Hôpital des Enfants Malades, 149, rue de Sèvres, 75743 Paris Cedex 15, France.

Cailloux F., INSERM U 384, Faculté de Médecine, 28, place Henri-Dunant, BP 38, 63001 Clermont-Ferrand Cedex, France.

Dautigny A., URA CNRS 1488, Université Paris VI, 9, quai Saint-Bernard, 75252 Paris Cedex 05, France.
Dastugue B., INSERM U 384, Faculté de Médecine, 28, place Henri-Dunant, BP 38, 63001 Clermont-Ferrand Cedex, France.
Deonna T., Pediatric Department, Neuropediatric Unit, CHUV, Lausanne, Switzerland.
Duchowny M., Neuroscience Program, Miami Children's Hospital, 3200 S.W. 60th Court, Miami, FL 33156, USA.
Dulac O., Neuropediatrics Department, Hôpital Saint-Vincent-de-Paul, 82, avenue Denfert-Rochereau, 75014 Paris, France.

Evrard P., Service de Neurologie Pédiatrique et Laboratoire de Neurologie du Développement, Faculté de Médecine Xavier-Bichat, Hôpital Robert-Debré, 48, boulevard Sérurier, 75019 Paris, France.

Fejerman N., Department of Neurology, Hospital de Pediatría Juan P Garrahan, Vidt 2052-2°C, Buenos Aires 1425, Argentina.
Fernandez-Alvarez E., Department of Child Neurology, Hospital San Juan de Dios, Barcelona, Spain.
Fukuyama Y,. Department of Pediatrics, Tokyo Women's Medical College, and Child Neurology Institute, Tokyo, Japan.

Giraud G., INSERM U 384, Faculté de Médecine, 28, place Henri-Dunant, BP 38, 63001 Clermont-Ferrand Cedex, France.
Goutières F., Neurological Unit, Hôpital des Enfants Malades, 149, rue de Sèvres, 75743 Paris Cedex 15, France.
Grodd W., Department of Neuroradiology, University of Tübingen, Germany.

Hagberg B., Department of Pediatrics, East Hospital, S-416 85 Gothenburg, Sweden.
Harvey A.S., Neuroscience Program, Miami Children's Hospital, 3200 S.W. 60th Court, Miami, FL 33156, USA.
Holguin J., Hospital de Pediatría, Medelin, Colombia.
Hopkins I.J., Royal Children's Hospital, Melbourne, Australia.

Jackson G.D., University of Melbourne, Austin Hospital, Victoria, Australia.
Jayakar P., Neuroscience Program, Miami Children's Hospital, 3200 S.W. 60th Court, Miami, FL 33156, USA.

Krägeloh-Mann I., Division of Child Neurology, Pediatric Hospital, University of München (TU), Germany.

Levy-Gomes A., Pediatric Neurology Unit, Hospital Santa Maria, University of Lisbon, Portugal.
Lopez-Casas J., Department of Child Neurology, Hospital San Juan de Dios, Barcelona, Spain.
Lyon G., 50, rue d'Assas, 75006 Paris, France.

Melki J., Unité de Recherches sur les Handicaps Génétiques de l'Enfant, INSERM U 393, IFREM Hôpital Necker-Enfants Malades, rue de Sèvres, 75015 Paris, France.
Mimault C., INSERM U 384, Faculté de Médecine, 28, place Henri-Dunant, BP 38, 63001 Clermont-Ferrand Cedex, France.
Munnich A., Unité de Recherches sur les Handicaps Génétiques de l'Enfant, INSERM U 393, IFREM Hôpital Necker-Enfants Malades, rue de Sèvres, 75015 Paris, France.

Neville B., Institute of Child Health, Great Ormond Street Hospital for Children NHS Trust, University of London, The Wolfson Centre, Mecklenburgh Square, London WC1N 2AP, UK.

Osawa M., Department of Pediatrics, Tokyo Women's Medical College, Tokyo, Japan.

Pham Dinh D., URA CNRS 1488, Université Paris VI, 9, quai Saint-Bernard, 75252 Paris Cedex 05, France.
Pinard J.-M., Service de Neuropédiatrie, Hôpital R. Poincaré, 92380 Garches, France.
Poll-The B.T., University Children's Hospital "Wilhelmina Kinderziekenhuis", Nieuwegracht 137, 3512 LK Utrecht, The Netherlands.

Poser C.M., Harvard Neurological Unit, Beth Israel Hospital, 330 Brookline Ave, Boston, Ma 02215, USA.

Rapin I., Saul R. Korey Department of Neurology, Department of Pediatrics, and Rose F. Kennedy Center for Research in Mental Retardation and Human Development, Albert Einstein College of Medicine, Bronx, NY, USA.

Resnick T., Neuroscience Program, Miami Children's Hospital, 3200 S.W. 60th Court, Miami, FL 33156, USA.

Saito K., Department of Pediatrics, Tokyo Women's Medical College, Tokyo, Japan.

Toft P., Magnetic Resonance Research Center, Hvidovre Hospital, Copenhagen, Denmark.

Truscelli D., Service de Rééducation Neurologique, Centre Hospitalier de Bicêtre, 94275 Le Kremlin-Bicêtre, France.

1

Jean Aicardi

F. GOUTIÈRES

Neurological Unit, Hôpital des Enfants Malades, Paris, France.

Nous sommes réunis ici aujourd'hui en l'honneur de Jean Aicardi, pour lui témoigner notre amitié, et le remercier pour son œuvre accomplie en neurologie pédiatrique. Étant avec J.J.Chevrie sa plus ancienne collaboratrice, il m'est donc échu le délicat privilège de lui exprimer notre gratitude au nom de vous tous et d'ouvrir cette journée en retraçant pour vous les principales étapes de sa carrière.

Jean Aicardi est né le 8 novembre 1926, à Rambouillet, dans une famille de lointaine ascendance italienne, de la région de Gênes. Il est le septième de neuf frères et sœurs, ce qui lui donne ainsi l'occasion de connaître très tôt les joies et les difficultés de la vie en communauté et de développer précocement les facultés d'échange et de communication qu'il montrera plus tard.

Rien dans sa famille ne le prédisposait à la médecine et c'est après des études secondaires littéraires classiques au lycée d'Aix-en-Provence puis au lycée Hoche de Versailles qu'il décide d'être médecin et s'inscrit en 1945 comme étudiant à la Faculté de Médecine de Paris. La carrière hospitalière parisienne, qui se déroulait alors parallèlement aux études à la Faculté, impliquait que l'on passe le concours d'externat, puis d'internat, ce qu'il fait avec succès en 1951, année où il est nommé interne des Hôpitaux de Paris.

C'est alors que se décide son orientation future de pédiatre et de neuropédiatre, auprès de deux patrons d'internat qui suscitent son admiration : Robert Debré qui, à l'Hôpital des Enfants Malades, va donner l'essor que l'on sait à la pédiatrie, et Raymond Garcin à la Salpêtrière, dont le sens aigu de l'observation clinique et la rigueur du raisonnement neurologique resteront ses guides tout au long de sa carrière.

En 1955, à la fin de son internat, il soutient sa thèse de Docteur en Médecine à la Faculté de Médecine de Paris. Le sujet de sa thèse qui porte sur "200 observations de convulsions dans la 1re année de vie", confirme sa vocation de neuropédiatre et révèle son intérêt précoce pour l'épilepsie de l'enfant.

Dès sa thèse soutenue, conseillé par Robert Debré, il quitte le milieu pédiatrique parisien et, en précurseur, part aux États-Unis où il séjournera de 1955 à 1956, comme Research Fellow d'abord à Harvard Medical School auprès de Janneway, puis à Cincinnati auprès de Fred Silverman, en compagnie de Jacques Couvreur qui restera un de ses meilleurs amis. C'est là le début de liens professionnels et amicaux avec de nombreux collègues américains.

De retour à Paris, il retrouve l'Hôpital des Enfants Malades, où il est nommé en 1957 chef de clinique à la Faculté, puis en 1961, à l'âge de 35 ans, médecin assistant des Hôpitaux.

Aux Enfants Malades, règne toujours Robert Debré entouré de ses élèves, chacun responsable d'une branche particulière de la pédiatrie, la neuropédiatrie étant confiée à Stéphane Thieffry.

Ce n'est cependant pas immédiatement dans le service de Stéphane Thieffry qu'il sera affecté à son retour des États-Unis, mais dans celui de chirurgie infantile du Professeur Marcel Fèvre, où il sera attaché médical jusqu'en 1964, et c'est pendant ces années médico-chirurgicales qu'il acquiert une connaissance approfondie des problèmes plus généraux de la pédiatrie qu'il montrera plus tard.

Toutefois le bâtiment de chirurgie pédiatrique des Enfants Malades est situé en face du pavillon Duchêne de Boulogne affecté à la neuropédiatrie, et il va y passer de nombreuses heures, y prendre des gardes auprès des enfants atteints de poliomyélite et commencer sa longue collaboration avec Stéphane Thieffry dont il restera l'assistant pendant 22 ans, jusqu'au départ de ce dernier à la retraite en 1979.

Dans ce pavillon Duchêne de Boulogne, où sont également assistants Gilles Lyon, Michel Arthuis et Mme Martin, il sera l'un des fondateurs de la neuropédiatrie naissante.

Sa première publication sur un sujet neurologique : "Les spasmes en flexion du nourrisson, 36 observations - étude critique", qui sera signée, tradition oblige, Stéphane Thieffry et Jean Aicardi, paraît dans *La Semaine des Hôpitaux de Paris* en 1958.

Mais 1958 est pour une autre raison, beaucoup plus personnelle, une année très importante pour lui : c'est celle de son mariage avec Jeanne, que la plupart d'entre vous connaissent et à qui nous sommes tous reconnaissants pour le soutien qu'elle a apporté à son mari et aussi pour sa disponibilité permanente et la gentillesse de son accueil dont nous avons souvent profité, boulevard Beaumarchais, adresse de renom international.

En 1964, Stéphane Thieffry succède au Professeur Marcel Lelong dans la chaire de pédiatrie et puériculture et son service se déplace en bloc à l'Hôpital Saint-Vincent-de-Paul.

Là, Jean Aicardi est responsable pour la première fois d'une unité de 24 lits de nourrissons dans la salle Billard, aidé au début par J.J. Chevrie, son premier chef de clinique, puis par moi-même, qui succède à Chevrie en 1968. C'est dans cette salle Billard, régentée par une redoutable et méticuleuse surveillante au voile amidonné, Mme Séguin, qu'il va dispenser son enseignement au cours des visites du lundi et du vendredi matin et de sa consultation du jeudi, auxquelles nombreux d'entre vous ont participé comme externe, interne, chef de clinique ou visiteur étranger.

Les lundi après-midi, dans le laboratoire de neuropathologie d'Edith Farkas, ont lieu des séances de coupe de cerveaux où l'analyse critique de l'observation clinique est confrontée avec sa solution. Ces confrontations clinicopathologiques donneront lieu à plusieurs publications sur des sujets aussi divers que le rôle de la gémellité et des perturbations circulatoires au cours de la grossesse dans les encéphalomalacies multikystiques, les encéphalites subaiguës de la rougeole au cours des immuno-suppressions, l'atrophie olivopontocérébelleuse avec atteinte de la corne antérieure.

Mais c'est dans le petit bureau du 3e étage qu'il partage avec J.J. Chevrie, sa secrétaire Florence et moi-même, qu'il va, imperturbable malgré la sonnerie du téléphone et le bruit de la machine à écrire, rédiger des articles qui, pour beaucoup, sont encore d'actualité.

En 1965 paraît, dans la revue *Electroencephalography and Clinical Neurophysiology*, en collaboration avec Jacques Lefevre et Antoinette Lerique : "A new syndrome: spasms in flexion, callosal agenesis, ocular abnormalities", travail qu'il reprendra quatre ans plus tard en français avec J.J. Chevrie et Françoise Rousselie, syndrome depuis universellement connu sous le nom de syndrome d'Aicardi.

Pendant les quinze ans qu'il passe à Saint-Vincent-de-Paul, de 1964 à 1979, il fait paraître 75 articles originaux, dont 23 sur l'épilepsie de l'enfant. Plusieurs de ces articles sur les spasmes infantiles, les séquelles d'état de mal convulsifs ou les convulsions de la première année, sont encore d'actualité et cités dans les travaux récents sur ces sujets. A cela s'ajoutent 20 chapitres de livres, sans compter les conférences et communications dans les congrès, car commence à cette époque, parallèlement à sa carrière d'écrivain, celle de *visiting professor* et de grand voyageur.

C'est également pendant ces années passées à Saint-Vincent-de-Paul que vont naître et se développer ses liens amicaux et professionnels avec Henri Gastaut et son équipe de Marseille, et aussi avec plusieurs collègues européens, notamment anglais, et en particulier Ronald Mc Keith avec qui il aimera discuter de délicats problèmes cliniques au cours des réunions scientifiques de l'*European Federation of Child Neurology Societies*.

N'ayant pas été nommé médecin des Hôpitaux, la carrière hospitalo-universitaire parisienne lui est fermée, et c'est en tant que chercheur de l'Institut national de la santé et de la recherche médicale, où il est nommé en 1969 Maître de recherche, puis en 1986 Directeur de recherche, qu'il poursuivra son activité de neuropédiatre et développera en précurseur la recherche clinique à une époque où l'expérimentation animale est beaucoup mieux appréciée que le travail d'observation clinique.

Mais en 1979, Stéphane Thieffry atteint l'âge de la retraite. Un an plus tôt, Gilles Lyon avait déjà quitté le service pour Bruxelles. N'étant pas médecin des Hôpitaux, Jean Aicardi ne peut pas prendre la direction du service de Saint-Vincent-de-Paul et il est appelé par Jean Frezal aux Enfants Malades afin d'y mettre sur pied dans son service une unité de neurologie pédiatrique.

Le 1er octobre 1979, à l'âge de 53 ans, accompagné de J.J. Chevrie et de moi-même, il s'installe donc aux Enfants Malades, où il restera jusqu'en 1991.

Après quinze ans d'abandon depuis le départ de Stéphane Thieffry, la neurologie pédiatrique renaît aux Enfants Malades et s'organise dans des conditions difficiles, au prix de longues journées de travail, y compris les week-ends, de consultations surchargées et de longues et fatigantes visites en salle. Il ne connaît pas les vacances et ne s'absente du service que pour répondre à des invitations à l'étranger, participer à des congrès internationaux où il se montre un intervenant très actif et un auditeur très attentif et très assidu de toutes les sessions scientifiques.

Pendant ces douze dernières années passées aux Enfants Malades, il publiera d'autres travaux importants : avec Hagberg et Karin Dias, il va redécouvrir le syndrome de Rett qui était resté méconnu depuis la publication originale de Rett et qui, à partir du travail qu'ils publient en commun dans les *Annals of Neurology*, va prendre l'essor que l'on sait. Le syndrome ataxie-apraxie oculomotrice, les hémiplégies alternantes du nourrisson sont d'autres exemples de pathologie qu'il révélera aux neuropédiatres. Mais l'épilepsie restera un point central de son activité et pendant ces douze ans, il écrira en français, anglais ou espagnol, pas moins de 56 articles ou chapitres de livres sur divers aspects de l'épilepsie de l'enfant. Il rédigera surtout la 1re édition de son livre *Epilepsy in children* qui paraît en 1986 et sera suivie, huit ans plus tard, d'une seconde édition.

Mais là ne se limite pas son activité d'écrivain : pendant deux ans, les deux dernières années qu'il passera aux Enfants Malades, il les consacrera à rédiger l'ensemble de son énorme expérience clinique qu'il condensera dans le gros petit livre rouge *Diseases of the nervous system in childhood* que vous connaissez tous.

Cependant va arriver le 8 novembre 1991, jour de ses 65 ans. Pour l'Assistance publique des hôpitaux de Paris, atteint par l'âge de la retraite, il doit quitter les Enfants Malades et c'est là que prennent fin, à ma grande tristesse, nos 23 ans de collaboration. Nos collègues anglais sont beaucoup plus heureux car il va continuer son activité clinique à Londres comme *Honorary Professor* à l'*Institute of Child Health* et *Honorary Consultant* à *Great Ormond Street*.

Son travail de clinicien et de chercheur, internationalement reconnu, a été récompensé par l'attribution de nombreuses distinctions honorifiques. Il est membre de 17 sociétés françaises et étrangères de neurologie, neuropédiatrie et épilepsie, parmi lesquelles je ne citerai que la Société européenne de neurologie pédiatrique, l'European society of child neurology, et l'International child neurology association dont il a été le Président.

Il a été Professeur invité dans de nombreux hôpitaux ou universités, de Tokyo à Cincinatti, en passant par Buenos-Aires, Madras, Sydney, Sherbrooke, Vancouver, et Miami où son portrait et son nom sont inscrits sur the *Hall of Fame*, le hall de la Célébrité de l'hôpital.

Enfin il est l'invité de prestigieuses *memorial lectures* parmi lesquelles la *Ronald Mc Keith lecture*, la *Hower Award lecture* devant la Child neurology society et la *William Lennox lecture* devant l'American epilepsy society.

Avant de terminer cette évocation de la carrière professionnelle de Jean Aicardi, permettez-moi de profiter quelques instants de la place que j'occupe en ce moment pour m'adresser directement à lui et évoquer quelques souvenirs personnels.

Cher Jean, vous ne vous souvenez certainement pas de cette matinée de février 1964 où, jeune externe, je vous présentais au premier étage du Pavillon Duchêne de Boulogne, une petite fille avec une hémiplégie congénitale. Ce matin-là, où je vous voyais pour la première fois, vous m'aviez impressionnée par la façon dont vous aviez analysé le handicap de l'enfant en la regardant simplement marcher et jouer avec le marteau à réflexes, en l'examinant sans presque y toucher, technique d'examen que vous ne cesserez d'inculquer à tous vos élèves successifs et qui privilégie l'étude du comportement naturel plutôt que la recherche acharnée des réflexes dans les pleurs et l'opposition.

Je voudrais évoquer vos visites en salle auprès des enfants hospitalisés. Ces visites étaient longues et fatigantes mais toujours enrichissantes et source de plaisir pour vos internes car vous les agrémentiez de réflexions philosophiques, ou de citations littéraires de vos auteurs favoris : Shakespeare, Hippocrate dont les aphorismes avaient votre prédilection, ou Molière dont la modernité vous paraissait frappante et dont vous déploriez qu'il ne soit plus de ce monde pour stigmatiser certaines analyses psychanalytiques.

Vous demandiez beaucoup à vos collaborateurs. L'activité du service était très importante et le roulement des malades très rapide, mais vous ne vouliez pas connaître les problèmes d'intendance : vous désiriez un scanner, il fallait obtenir un scanner même si l'appareil était en panne ; vous vouliez hospitaliser un consultant, il fallait trouver un lit même si le service était complet. Il y avait des moments où, je vous l'avoue aujourd'hui, j'étais exaspérée. Mais vous aviez raison car on obtenait le scanner et on trouvait un lit.

Vous demandiez à chacun d'entre nous de fournir le maximum de travail, d'énergie, de temps et chacun s'efforçait de répondre à votre demande car tous avaient à cœur de ne pas vous décevoir, ce qui est le meilleur témoignage d'admiration et de respect que des élèves puissent avoir envers leur maître.

A cette admiration et ce respect, il faut ajouter l'affection que beaucoup de ceux qui sont ici vous portent et qui nous a tous fait trembler quand une grave maladie enfantine vous a frappé sur le tard.

C'est pour vous témoigner ces sentiments que ces deux journées ont été organisées.

Faute de temps, seuls vos élèves directs ou vos meilleurs amis prendront la parole, mais tous les participants vous sont unanimement reconnaissants.

2

Epilepsies during the first year of life

N. FEJERMAN

Department of Neurology, Hospital de Pediatría Juan P. Garrahan, Buenos Aires, Argentina.

I would first add to the title "excluding neonatal seizures". Seizures in the neonatal period are subject of special concern. A group of specialists gathered by the Classification and Terminology Commission and by the Pediatric Epileptology Commission of the International League against Epilepsy (ILAE) has been working on its classification on account of video-EEG record analysis, and the main goal is to differentiate epileptic from non epileptic fits [1]. The well defined idiopathic epileptic syndrome appearing only during the first weeks of life is "benign familial neonatal convulsions" in which a linkage with markers on chromosome 20 has been demonstrated [2]. There is a second idiopathic neonatal syndrome included in ILAE's Classification, called "benign idiopathic neonatal convulsions" or "fifth day fits" [3] but its incidence may have fallen significantly in the last decade and it is even questioned as being a real epileptic syndrome [4]. Seizures in small infants are "atypical" when compared with seizures in childhood. Their clinical expression may be limited to mild changes in muscle tone, staring, flushing, pallor or cyanosis of face, clonic jerking of eyes or eyelids, eye deviation, mouthing phenomena, etc. Generalized seizures are usually either clonic or tonic and sometimes unilateral hemispheric predominance is interpreted as a lack of organization in an immature brain. Partial seizures are quite frequent, but differentiation between simple and complex partial seizures is not easy, since consciousness is difficult to judge from cribside observation [5]. Myoclonus is more readily recognized, and absences are very rarely registered in babies except the staring and motion arrest seen in complex partial seizures [6]. Anyhow, video-EEG monitoring provides a more objective mean to assess not only clinical features of seizures but also their correlation to epileptic discharges [7].

Due to the space limitations, I will not deal here with differential diagnosis between epileptic and non epileptic episodic symptoms in infants. Nevertheless, enough challenge is to delineate the epileptic syndromes prevalent in this age. It has been stated that a high proportion of epilepsies with onset in the first years of life do not belong to recognized epileptic syndromes [4]. In fact there are only a few series of well studied patients and their nosologic placement was a common methodologic problem [8-14].

In the Tables I, II, III, some of the results found in these series are compared. As can be seen, in two series patients were grouped by type of seizures [9, 13] in another, by epileptic syndromes [14] and in the fourth one with a mixture of both criteria [12]. In all these series neonatal seizures were excluded and febrile convulsions were disclosed as a different group.

What would be the way to present the same subject at this moment ? Are there new tools to identify better epileptic seizures or syndromes ?

In Table IV, the experience of our service with 471 patients below a year of age seen in the last five years is summarized.

Table I. Epilepsies in the first year of life (excluding neonatal and febrile seizures) follow-up in large series.

Authors	N° of cases	Length of follow-up
Chevrie and Aicardi [9]	334	1 year or more
Matsumoto et al. [12]	278	until age 6 years
Cavazzuti et al. [13]	387	> 5 years

Table II. Epilepsies in the first year of life (patients with normal mental outcome).

	Infantile spasms		Status		Other			
					Generalized		Partial	
	Total: 157		Total: 35		Total: 81		Total: 40	
Chevrie and Aicardi [9]	Crypto	Sympto	Crypto	Sympto	Crypto	Sympto	Crypto	Sympto
	26/66	5/91	5/15	1/20	17/45	3/36	6/14	2/26
	(39%)	(6%)	(33%)	(5%)	(38%)	(8%)	(43%)	(8%)
	Total: 183		Total: 66		Total: 138 (Generalized + partial)			
Cavazzuti et al. [13]	Crypto	Sympto	Crypto	Sympto	Crypto		Sympto	
	31/73	0/110	14/31	9/35	49/81 (60%)		15/57 (26%)	
	(42%)		(45%)	(26%)				
	Total: 113		Not specified		Generalized(*)		Partial	
Matsumoto et al. [12]	Crypto + Sympto				Total: 98		Total: 28	
	13 (11.5%)				Crypto + Sympto		Crypto + Sympto	
					79 (80.6%)		13 (46.4%)	

(*)secondary generalized epilepsies are not included

Table III. Epilepsies in the first year of life. Different criteria of classification.

Matsumoto et al. [12]	Infantile spasms	113 cases	
	Generalized motor seizures	98 cases	
	Secondary generalized epilepsy	35 cases	
	Partial seizures	28 cases	
	Hemiconvulsions	4 cases	
	Total	278 cases	
Dalla Bernardina et al. [14]	Epileptic encephalopathies	141 cases	(45%)
	Partial organic epilepsies	83 cases	(26%)
	Partial epilepsies without deficits	5 cases	(2%)
	Benign partial epilepsies	3 cases	(1 %)
	Generalized cryptogenic epilepsy	8 cases	(2.5%)
	Benign myoclonic epilepsy	2 cases	(0.5%)
	Severe myoclonic epilepsy of infancy	32 cases	(10 %)
	Unclassifiable epilepsies	42 cases	(13%)
	Total	316 cases	(100%)

Table IV. First year epilepsies (excluding neonatal seizures and febrile convulsions) in 471 patients. According to ILAE's last classification [15].

	Number of patients	
Partial		
Idiopathic		
Benign infantile familial convusions	12	2.5%
Symptomatic	130	28%
Cryptogenic	25	5.3%
Generalized		
Idiopathic		
Benign myoclonic epilepsy in infancy	6	1.3%
Cryptogenic or symptomatic		
Symptomatic West syndrome	155	33%
Cryptogenic West syndrome	65	14%
Cryptogenic myoclonic epilepsy	6	1.3%
Other not classified criptogenic epilepsies	10	2%
Early myoclonic encephalopathy	4	0.8%
Early infantile epilectic encephalopathy	8	1.6%
Other not classified symptomatic epilepsies	14	3%
Undetermined wether focal or generalized		
Severe myoclonic epilepsy in infancy	15	3.2%
Symptomatic epilepsy with MISF	3	0.6%
Other not classified epilepsies	3	0.6%
Special syndromes		
Occasional seizures	15	3%

What is new or what could be changed or added at present ?

Localization-related epilepsies and syndromes (item 1 of ILAE's classification)

Japanese authors had reported cases of infants with benign cryptogenic afebrile convulsions [12]. In 1987, Watanabe et al. [16] presented 9 infants — 8 of whom were 3 to 9 months old — with clinical and ictal EEG features of complex partial seizures: clusters of seizures appearing in wakefulness or sleep with initial motion arrest, decreased responsiveness, staring, head rotation, and mild convulsive movements. Six of them also showed automatisms. Ictal EEG showed focal discharges starting in temporal regions in 5 patients and in centroparietal areas in 3 cases. Four patients had close relatives with history of benign infantile convulsions. All patients responded well to antiepileptic drugs and remained seizure-free for more than 3 years. They proposed the term "benign complex partial epilepsies in infancy" [16]. A few years later Vigevano et al. [17, 18] presented 5 infants with clusters of seizures lasting 1 to several minutes characterized by: "psychomotor arrest, slow deviation of the head and eyes to one side, diffuse hypertonia, cyanosis, and unilateral limb jerks..." These 5 children had 13 close relatives with history of benign convulsions with onset between 4 and 8 months of age. Interictal EEG were normal and ictal records showed "recruiting rythm beginning in the left or right central occipital areas". Patients were followed-up from 24 to 32 months with complete control of seizures, and normal psychomotor development. They proposed to call them "benign infantile familial convulsions" [17, 18]. As can be seen, there is a significant overlap between these two series of patients. More recently the same authors reported about a multicenter study collecting data on 18 families with 34 first and second-degree relatives with history of BIFC [19]. Autosomal dominant inheritance seems to be proved [20]. In a review of 17 cases of benign epilepsy with partial seizures in patients between 8 days and 3 years of life, onset of seizures was between 17 and 45 days in 6 cases, fulfilling features of benign idiopathic neonatal convulsions. No case of partial epilepsy with favorable outcome started with seizures between 1,5 and 14 months of age [21]. The same group studied 23 infants with cryptogenic partial epilepsies and curiously enough there was no case starting between 4 and 8 months [22]. In another series of 40 patients beginning before 3 years of age, 9 might have been considered as cryptogenic [23]. According to selection bias, other centers may show different experiences. From 14 infants with complex partial seizures, 13 manifested intractable seizures and profound global delay [2, 24].

Generalized epilepsies and syndromes (item 2 of ILAE's classification)

Quite recently 6 neurologically normal infants were reported with myoclonic jerks resembling the seizures of benign myoclonic epilepsy of infancy but occurring as reflex responses to unexpected auditory and tactile stimuli. Five of them had also rare spontaneous attacks. Onset took place between 6 and 21 months and seizures disappeared in 4-14 months, either spontaneously or under treatment with valproate. Myoclonic jerks were single or in clusters, dominant over upper limbs. Most attacks were brief and were elicitable both in wakefulness and in sleep. Waking interictal EEGs were normal. Sleep EEGs were characterized by brief polyspike and wave discharges. The authors proposed it as a distinct age-related idiopathic epileptic syndrome related to startle reaction [25].

If we go to item 2.2 of ILAE's classification some new criteria must be discussed concerning West syndrome (WS). Idiopathic WS was proposed as an alternative group when fulfilling several clinical and EEG criteria (Table V). This diagnosis would make more clear the choice of therapeutic schedules and the development of prospective studies to evaluate prognosis [26] and even to think about differential diagnosis [27]. It was also striking to find that an apparently symptomatic group of WS patients — as are the cases of WS in babies with type 1 neurofibromatosis — behaved as idiopathic or cryptogenic in terms of their excellent response to treatment and good evolution [28].

Table V. Idiopathic West syndrome.

Normal development until onset of symmetric infantile spasms with no other types of seizures
Normal neurological examination
Normal MRI
Symmetrical hypsarrhythmia reappearing between consecutive spasms in each cluster
Disappearance of spikes after intravenous diazepam

Finally, WS being an age-dependent epileptic encephalopathy [29], it will appear associated to any new brain pathology encountered in children below one year of age. An example is PEHO syndrome, name given to the association of progressive pncephalopathy with edema, hypsarrhythmia and optic atrophy. This is a new autosomal recessive disorder with WS, progressive visual failure and severe psychomotor retardation [30, 31]. Among the symptomatic generalized epilepsies, a peculiar "myoclonic status" in non-progressive encephalopathies has been reported in 22 cases [32]. The initial ictal manifestations were often subcontinuous absences accompanied by jerks of eye-lids and distal muscles appearing during the first year of life. All patients had severe encephalopathies with a picture of hypotonic-ataxic cerebral palsy with dystonic-dyskinetic movements, EEG abnormalities were found in interictal and ictal records and the most typical pattern was a sequence of slow waves with superimposed spikes forming particular spike-wave complexes. Curiously enough a couple of cases of Angelman's syndrome were recognized among these patients and the peculiar EEG in this syndrome has already been shown [33].

This leads us to item 2.3 of ILAE's classification which can give rise to discussions, not only considering nosologic interpretations about early myoclonic encephalopathy and early infantile epileptic encephalopathy (Table VI), but also in reference to several new etiologic alternatives among the so-called specific syndromes, either in the field of neuronal migration disorders or of proven or suspected inborn errors of metabolism. But we have no time or room here to enter in this subject.

Table VI. EME vs early infantile epileptic encephalopathy (EIEE).

	EME	EIEE
Onset	1st month	1st trimester
Dominant	Erratic	Tonic
Seizures	Myoclonia	Spasms
EEG	"B-S" pattern without differences in awake and sleep tracings	"B-S" pattern enhanced by sleep
Etiology	Metabolic or cryptogenic	Congenital brain malformations

Finally, a word about "severe myoclonic (or polymorphic) epilepsy in infancy" (SMEI) included in item 3. It is without doubt an epileptic syndrome with onset during the first year of life, but it is seldom recognized at this age. The occurrence of repeated and prolonged uni or bilateral febrile seizures in a normally developping baby does not seem to be enough to diagnose SMEI. Only through evolution, showing afebrile seizures, slowing of neuropsychic development and EEG abnormalities we can arrive to this diagnosis [34].

References

1. Mizrahi EM. Neonatal seizures: problems in diagnosis and classification. *Epilepsia* 1987 ; 28 (suppl. 1) : S46-55.
2. Leppert M, Anderson VE, Quattelbaum T, Stauffer D, O'Connell P, Nakamura Y, Lalouel JM, White R. Benign familial neonatal convulsions linked to genetic markers on chromosome 20. *Nature* 1989 ; 337 : 647-8.
3. Plouin P. Benign idiopathic neonatal convulsions (familial and non familial) In : Roger J. et al., eds. *Epileptic syndromes in infancy, childhood and adolescence* (2nd edition). London : John Libbey, 1992 : 3-12.
4. Aicardi J. *Epilepsy in children* (2nd edition). New York : Raven Press, 1994 : 244-52.
5. Duchowny M. The syndrome of partial seizures in infancy. *J Child Neurol* 1992 ; 7, 1 : 66-9.
6. Cavazzuti GB, Ferrari F, Galli V, Benatti A. Epilepsy with typical absence seizures with onset during the first year of life. *Epilepsia* 1989 ; 30,6 : 802-6.
7. Foley CM, Legido A, Miles DK, Grover WD. Diagnostic value of pediatric outpatient video-EEG. *Pediatr Neurol* 1995 ; 12, 2 : 120-8.
8. Chevrie JJ, Aicardi J. Convulsive disorders in the first year of life: etiologic factors. *Epilepsia* 1977 ; 18,4 : 489-98.
9. Chevrie JJ, Aicardi J. Convulsive disorders in the first year of life: neurological and mental outcome and mortality. *Epilepsia* 1978 ; 19,1 : 67-74.
10. Chevrie JJ, Aicardi J. Convulsive disorders in the first year of life: persistence of epileptic seizures. *Epilepsia* 1979 ; 20, 6 : 643-9.
11. Aicardi J, Chevrie JJ. Les épilepsies de nourrison en dehors des syndromes de West et de Lennox-Gastaut. *Rev EEG Neurophysiol* 1981 ; 11 : 412-8.

12. Matsumoto A, Watanabe K, Sugiura M, Negoro T, Takaesu E, Iwase K. Long-term prognosis of convulsive disorders in the first year of life: mental and physical development and seizure persistence. *Epilepsia* 1983 ; 24, 3 : 321-9.
13. Cavazuti GB, Ferrari P, Lalla M. Follow-up study of 482 cases with convulsive disorders in the first year of life. *Dev Med Child Neurol* 1984 ; 26 : 425-37.
14. Dalla Bernardina B, Colamaria V, Capovilla G, Bondavalli S. Nosological classification of epilepsies in the first three years of life. In : *Epilepsy: an update on research and therapy*. New York : Alan R. Liss, Inc., 1983 : 165-83.
15. Commission on classification and terminology of the International League against Epilepsy. Proposal for revised classification of epilepsies and epilepctic syndromes. *Epilepsia* 1989 ; 30, 4 : 389-99.
16. Watanabe K, Yamamoto N, Negoro T, Takaesu E, Aso K, Furune S, Takahashi I. Benign complex partial epilepsies in infancy. *Pediatr Neurol* 1987 ; 3, 4 : 208-17.
17. Vigevano F, DiCapua M, Fusco L, Ricci S, Sebastianelli R, Lucchini P. Six-month benign familial convulsions. *Epilepsia* 1990 ; 31 : 613.
18. Vigevano F, Fusco L, DiCapua M, Ricci S, Sebastianelli R, Lucchini P. Benign infantile familial convulsions. *Eur J Pediatr* 1992 ; 151 : 608-12.
19. Vigevano F, Fusco L, DiCapua M, Ricci S, Sebastianelli R, Lucchini P, Dordi B, Chindemi A, Dulac O, Malafosse A. Benign familial convulsions: clinical aspects (abstract from the European Congress of Epileptology). *Epilepsia* 1994 ; 35 (suppl 7) : 9.
20. Echenne B, Humbertclaude V, Rivier F, *et al*. Benign infantile epilepsy with autosomal dominant inheritance. *Brain Dev* 1994 ; 16, 2 : 108-11.
21. Dulac O, Cusmai R, de Oliveira K. Is there a partial benign epilepsy in infancy? *Epilepsia* 1989 ; 30, 6 : 798-801.
22. Luna D, Dulac O, Plouin P. Ictal characteristics of cryptogenic partial epilepsies in infancy. *Epilepsia* 1989 ; 30, 6 : 827-32.
23. Dravet C, Catani C, Bureau M, Roger J. Partial epilepsies in infancy: a study of 40 cases. *Epilepsia* 1989 ; 30, 6 : 807-12.
24. Duchowny M. Complex partial seizures of infancy. *Arch Neurol* 1987 ; 44 : 911-4.
25. Ricci S, Cusmai R, Fusco L, Vigevano F. Reflex myoclonic epilepsy in infancy: a new age-dependent idiopathic epileptic syndrome related to startle reaction. *Epilepsia* 1995 ; 36, 4 : 342-8.
26. Dulac O, Plouin P. Cryptogenic/idioipathic West syndrome. In : Dulac O, *et al.*, eds. *Infantile spasms and West syndrome*. London : W.B. Saunders, 1994 : 232-43.
27. Fejerman N. Differential diagnosis. In : Dulac O, *et al.*, eds. *Infantile spasms and West syndrome*. London : W.B. Saunders, 1994 : 88-98.
28. Motte J, Billard C, Fejerman N, Sfaello Z, Arroyo H, Dulac O. Neurofibromatosis type one and West syndrome: a relatively benign association. *Epilepsia* 1993 ; 34, 4 : 723-6.
29. Ohtsuka Y, Ogino T, Murakami N, Nimaki N, Kobayashi K, Ohtahara S. Developmental aspects of epilepsy with special reference to age dependent epileptic encephalopathy. *Jap J Psychiatr Neurol* 1986 ; 40, 3 : 307-13.
30. Salonen R, Somer M, Haltia M, Lorentz M, Norio R. Progressive encephalopathy with edema, hypsarrhythmia, and optic atrophy (PEHO syndrome). *Clin Genet* 1991 ; 39 : 287-93.
31. Caraballo R, Carignani M, Chamoles N, Fejerman N. PEHO syndrome in 3 non-finnish patients. Abstracts of 7th congress of the international child neurology association. San Francisco USA ; 1994 : Abs 326.

32. Dalla Bernardina B, Fontana E, Sgro V, Colamaria V, Elia M. Myoclonic epilepsy (myoclonic status) in non progressive encephalopathies. In : Roger J, *et al.,* eds. *Epileptic syndromes in infancy, childhood and adolescence* 2nd edition. London : John Libbey, 1992 : 89-96.
33. Van Lierde A, Atza MG, Giardino D, Viani F. Angelman's syndrome in the first year of life. *Dev Med Child Neurol* 1990 ; 32, 11 : 1011-6.
34. Fejerman N. Severe myoclonic epilepsy in infancy. In : Wallace S, ed. *Epilepsy in children.* London : Chapman and Hall, 1995 (in press).

3

Migraine and epilepsy

J. HOLGUIN

Medelin, Colombia.

Migraine and epilepsy share many similar clinical and laboratory manifestations: episodic character, changes in mood, behaviour and consciousness, focal sensory and motor symptoms, hallucination, and ressembling electroencephalographic patterns. This makes sometimes their differential diagnosis very difficult. Some children suffer from both disorders; it is then essential to identify the two conditions, since they have different course and prognosis and respond to particular forms of treatment.

At this meeting we would like to present our experience over the past thirty years and to review some of our work on the association of the two pathologies. We will also review some of the theories on the nature of this puzzling relationship, in an effort to point out elements for differential diagnosis, and give some examples of the cases we had to handle in our neurology clinics held at the University Paediatric Hospital as well as at the Centre for private neuropaediatric consultation. The distribution of the 1,270 cases of migraine of our register, aged 1 to 21 years, is shown in Table I.

As our "migraine register" existed before the publication by the International Headache Society (IHS) in 1985 of the cephalalgia classification, the terminology we initially used was the one recommended by the US National Institute of Health (NIH). During the last ten years we have been using the categories proposed by the IHS.

Types of seizures and epilepsies have been grouped according to the categories suggested by the European Leagues Against Epilepsy in 1964. We later started using the ILAE classification of 1981 and we recently started updating our terminology to conform to current usage.

Table I.

"Common" migraine	680 cases
"Classic" migraine	540
Basilar	6
Hemiplegic	6
Vestibular	6
Confusional	4
Ophthalmoplegic	3
Alice in Wonderland Syndrome	2
Migrainous "equivalents"	2
Alternating hemiplegia	2
"Cluster"	3
"Convulsive"	3
Post-traumatic	10
Total	1,270

(F:1,174 ; M: 646)

Among our 1,270 migraine sufferers, 46 boys and 68 girls (114 cases) also showed epileptic symptoms, in the following distribution (Table II).

Table II.

Partial benign	63 cases
With centro-temporal spikes	22
With occipital spikes	41
Partial	36
Simple	16
Simple post-traumatic	4
Complex	20
Complex post-traumatic	6
Generalized	12
Vertigo	1
Convulsions	4
Clonic spasms	3
Convulsive-clonic	3
Generalized myoclonic spasms	1
Unclassified	3
Total	114

Different authors report varying degrees of association between migraine and epilepsy (Table III). In our series, 8.9% of migraine sufferers were also epileptic, but this frequency is certainly due to the special sample studied by the observer, as many headache patients were sent to his clinic.

Table III.

Ely [1]	8.6%
Lennox & Lennox [2]	24.0%
Lees & Watkins [3]	2.1%
Lance & Anthony [4]	2.0%
Basser [5]	5.9%

A recent study carried out at Columbia University, using a strictly epidemiological methodology, showed that patients with epilepsy were 2.4 times more likely to suffer from migraine than other non-epileptic family members.

The relationship between migraine and epilepsy

The question of a possible relationship between migraine and the epilepsies has arisen mainly from cases of migraine associated with, followed by, or interposed with epileptic seizures. The problem remains largely unresolved and complex. Very often a partial or generalized seizure leaves an intense headache and some children present post-ictal migraine symptoms. The syndrome of benign epilepsy of childhood with occipital spike and wave complexes often presents with such an intense headache that clinical differentiation of the two pathologies becomes very difficult. Other syndromes share a post-ictal deficit, as happens in some forms of migrainous hemiplegia (hereditary or not) and some post-convulsive hemiplegias. Some pathologies may initially present with symptoms compatible with the diagnosis of isolated migraine attacks to develop, sometimes after a rather long period of time, a more serious symptomatology, as happens with some vascular malformations, mostly arteriovenous but occasionally aneurysmal.

The following examples of clinical cases illustrate the problem of this complex relationship:

C.J.M., now aged 34, daughter of a colleague, was sent to our clinic by her pediatrician in March 1972 because of a classic left-sided migraine, characterized by intense and increasing in frequency episodes. Clinical examination evidenced a moderate paresis of the upper right arm with homolateral pyramidal signs. Auscultation revealed a generalized venous hum, stronger over the left eye. Arteriography showed a massive arteriovenous malformation concerning the middle and posterior left hemisphere. Advice was sought at the Massachusetts General Hospital (Pr. Debrun) and surgery was considered as dangerous. The girl later presented focal right-sided seizures, controlled by carbamazepine, and progressively developed hemiparesis and atrophy of the right side. She works as a teacher, got married and has two children.

Basilar migraine symptoms are alternating hemiparesis, episodes of fainting, vertigo, ataxia and sensory manifestations of one side of the body. Although electroencephalographic abnormalities are rather spectacular, it is considered as a benign syndrome more often affecting adolescent girls.

C.D.V., a country girl aged six years, experienced an episode of "cold" with a temperature of 37.8°C associated to drowsiness, ataxia and speech difficulties. Screening was done at a provincial hospital to rule out encephalitis or poisoning. Three days later she was in perfect health. Similar episodes reoccured when she was nine, eleven and 14 years old. She is now 23 and, like her father and mother, she occasionally suffers from migraine episodes with aura of moderate intensity.

J.P.G., a nine-year-old boy, has suffered from migraine episodes with aura since the age of four. In recent years, when the aura appears he may have a short (1 to 3 minutes) generalized attack, sometimes convulsive, sometimes convulsive-clonic, followed by a migrainous headache that can last several hours.

F.T.V., a 14-year-old girl, presented with common migraine for the past four years. During the 18 months prior to the onset of the headaches she experienced episodes of fainting, falls and convulsive spasms that could last two to four minutes.

D.P.T., a boy of eleven years, has had migraines with aura for the past 3 years. The headache affects the left side and always triggers a right-sided seizure lasting 3 to 5 minutes. A post-ictal hemiparesis that can last from a few minutes to several hours is then observed. During the period between attacks the EEG evidences spikes and sharp waves of medium voltage in the left hemisphere. Simple NMR and angular resonance tests were normal.

The relationships of migraine to epilepsy have been the subject of considerable controversy [1-5]. Hughlings Jackson, in 1875, considered them to be related entities produced by abnormal neuronic discharges, but with different types of neuronal alteration. Gowers [6] justified the inclusion of migraine in *The borderland of Epilepsy* because the two disorders have many similarities and are often "mistaken for each other and their distinction may sometimes be difficult". More recent authors, such as Livingstone [7], regarded migraine as " aconvulsive equivalent" and Jonas [8] as "an autonomic convulsio". Lennox and Lennox shared Jackson's opinion.

Many modern authors think of migraine and epilepsy as separate but related entities, as they both originate from neuronal hyperactivity. They both appear episodically. Migraine may also produce symptoms of confusion, stupor or even coma and can sometimes be accompanied by deficits in one or both hemispheres. The EEG can show focal or generalized abnormalities, paroxysmal discharges, spike-waves, etc. In some cases, especially those with a long history of migraine, MRI can reveal focal alterations in the substantia alba [9].

Furthermore, migraine may be at the origin of cerebral infarcts which may become epileptogenic. Antiepileptic drugs can control migraine and some authors [10-12] recommend their regular use. The two pathologies may coexist in 1% to 17% of the cases (according to the different series), a fact which underlines the need to identify, differentiate and treat them accordingly.

A group of patients with migraneous headaches, cerebral infarcts, lactic acidosis and hemiplegias occurring in recurrent bouts, suffer a familial form of mitochondrial encephalopathy [12]. Table IV gives additional clues for differential diagnosis of the two conditions.

Table IV. Differential diagnosis of epilepsy and migraine.

Migraine	Epilepsy
History (prospective event diary)	Sudden onset - sleep seizures
Recurrent, spontaneous headaches of gradual onset, scotoma, simple visual hallucinations	Recurrent - spontaneous Generalized or focal tonic Tonic-clonic convulsions sensible to protic stimulation
Diet triggers	
Sensible to migraine medication	EEG: interictal spikes, sharp waves, spikes and waves
	Positive response to anticonvulsants

References

1. Ely FA. The migraine-epilepsy syndrome: a statistical study of heredity. *Arch Neurol Psychiatr* 1930 ; 24 : 943-9.
2. Lennox GW, Lennox MA. *Epilepsy and related disorders*. Boston : Little Brown, 1960.
3. Lees F, Watkins SM. Loss of consciousness in migraine. *Lancet* 1963 ; 2 : 647-50.
4. Lance JW, Anthony M. Some clinical aspects of migraine. A prospective survey of 500 patients. *Arch Neurol* 1966 ; 15 : 356-61.
5. Basser LS. The relation of migraine and epilepsy. *Brain* 1969 ; 92 : 285-300.
6. Gowers WR. *The borderland of epilepsy*. London : J. & A. Churchill, 1907.
7. Livingstone S. *The diagnosis and treatment of convulsive disorders in children*. Springfiels Ill : Charles C. Thomas, 1954.
8. Jonas AD. Headaches as seizures equivalents. *Headache* 1966 ; 6 : 78-87.
9. De Benedettis O, Lorenzetti A, Sina C, Bernasconi V. Magnetic resonance imaging in migraine and tension-type headache. *Headache* 1994 ; 35 : 264-8.
10. Prensky AL, Sommer D. Diagnosis and treatment of migraine in children. *Neurology* 1979 ; 29 : 506-10.
11. Fernandez F. Cefaleas en niños. Diagnóstico y tratamiento. XV Congresso Colombiano de Pediatría. 1985, Bucaramanga.
12. Anderman F, Lugaresi E. *Migraine and epilepsy*. Boston : Butterworths, 1987.
13. Holguin J, Diaz H, Morales LF. *Migraña "simple" y "acompañada"*. XIV Congreso Colombiano de Pediat, Bucaramanga 1984. Memorias : 139-43.
14. Holguin J. *Migraña comatosa. Presentación de tres casos familiares*. I Congreso Nacional Asociación Colombiana de Neurologia, Bogotá 1993. Memorias : 73-5.
15. Fisher RS. *Imitators of epilepsy*. New York : Demos, 1994.

4

The paediatric issues in epilepsy surgery. The Great Ormond Street, Institute of Child Health London experience

B.G.R. NEVILLE

Institute of Child Health, The Wolfson Centre, London, UK.

The surgical treatment of epilepsy has been practiced for a hundred years in various forms but it is only more recently that specific attention has been given to children. Although the model for surgical treatment in adults applies reasonably well to older children with mesial temporal sclerosis I hope to illustrate that this model is quite inappropriate for the majority of children who are being considered for surgical treatment. In paediatric patients not one model but many different strategies are required through which we may however discern a number of common issues.

The epilepsy program at Great Ormond Street has been greatly helped by the presence of Jean Aicardi for the past two years. He has contributed an encyclopedic knowledge of the literature and a unique ability to recall patients with specific problems related to the child in question. I believe Jean's memory gets better as he gets older! The decisive therapy of surgery in childhood epilepsy has been built on a background of well classified clinical syndromes with an agreed natural history and Jean Aicardi has made many of the critical contributions to this field. Clearly the practice of such surgery will also raise and clarify issues within this large and difficult field. The program that I will describe is research led with a specific emphasis on clinical symptomatology in young children with epilepsy and on imaging and neuropsychological and neuropsychiatric aspects of the subject.

If we start with what is taken as the most straight forward model from the adult and adolescent experience in which the technical aspects of assessment and surgery most closely resemble adult practice several important paediatric issues nevertheless emerge. It has been clear that an accumulating burden of disability occurs within intractable temporal lobe epilepsy which continues through childhood and adolescence. The seminal 30 year study of 100 patients by Kit Ounsted et al. at Oxford indicated a high psychosocial morbidity and very significant mortality for those with continuing epilepsy. In a pre-imaging situation they were nevertheless able to define adverse factors which were identifiable early enough in childhood to allow early surgical treatment [1]. The broad conclusion from our point of view is that intractable temporal lobe epilepsy is in effect a progressive disease which precludes many of the cognitive psychological and social gains of adolescence and severely restricts adult life in many patients. Since surgery is in the majority of cases reasonably straight forward the issue becomes "why leave the lesion?" rather than "have we tried every possible combination of anti-epileptic drugs?" before recommending definitive surgical treatment.

In adults epilepsy surgery requires accurate localization of epileptogenesis, a lesion, intractability, natural history information that gives strong support to the condition not being benign and that the surgical solution is a technical possibility at a risk that is acceptable on the basis of the predicted untreated natural history.

In all areas of paediatric practice an intervention strategy is tested to its limit by approaching younger and younger children. One of our main contentions is that modern imaging has allowed early detection of many more lesions than was previously possible. However the issues of intractability and natural history are more difficult amongst a heterogeneous group of conditions and it is essential that our assumptions about nonsurgical outcome are explicit and subject to at the very least audit but also where possible case controlled comparative studies.

The paediatric dimensions to epilepsy surgery

Up to 60% of epilepsy starts in childhood and many epilepsy syndromes have their main effects or sometimes their total natural history is contained within the childhood period. Developing children appear to have sensitive periods in early life for both language and social development which can be severely disturbed by early onset epilepsy. We also need to make constant reference to normal development if we are to identify the child whose development, although showing some improvement, is falling progressively further from the expected normal rate of acquisition of skills.

A wide range of pathologies occur and our first 51 cases operated on contained the following pathologies:

- 16 tumors, mainly dysembryoplastic,
- 15 developmental defects,
- 7 hippocampal sclerosis,
- 6 arachnoid, porencephalic, and extradural cysts,
- 3 Rasmussen syndrome,
- 3 Sturge-Weber syndrome,
- 1 gliosis.

Amongst the most problematic of epilepsy syndromes are ones of massive regression of language and social functioning which in early life require very careful developmental behavioral assessments to identify the changes early and to separate fixed early developmental deviation from that which is being driven by active epilepsy. I think one should err on the side of being concerned that epilepsy may be a significant contributor to early developmental deviation and regression since it raises the possibility of intervention at an early stage. We can no longer work on the "well-known fact" that children with early onset epilepsy inevitably do badly. There are also situations in which seizure control by drugs like phenobarbitone may be at the cost of poor developmental progress. Rasmussen's encephalitis lacks a definitive pharmacological treatment and the Sturge-Weber syndrome which combines ischaemic and epileptic mechanisms each require disease specific tactics.

It is intrinsically more difficult to manage children through investigation procedures and well trained paediatric staff and the appropriate use of a sedative and anaesthetic procedures are required much more commonly than in adults. Often children have yet to achieve testable levels of function particularly in cognitive areas. Nevertheless because many syndromes of epilepsy allow a short and early window of opportunity for treatment and it is our task to identify this opportunity and to use modern technology to clarify the discreet issues and test the value of modern methods of assessment.

The epilepsy surgery team at Great Ormond Street and the Institute of Child Health in London contains the disciplines of paediatric neurology, neurosurgery, neurophysiology, neuropsychiatry, neuroimaging, and magnetic resonance (MR) physics, neuropsychology, neuropathology, and nursing. In our view it is not possible to deal adequately with the range of problems presented without this multidisciplinary group and without diagnostic and management support of a major multi-specialist children's unit. I will briefly summarize the development and use of specific image modes and the early indications of their localizing value and predictive capacity.

The patients

Of the patients we have considered as candidates for epilepsy surgery, over half have proved to be eligible. The age range of the children is from under 1 year old, and half of the children operated on are under 6 years old (Figure 1). Nearly half the resective procedures are hemispherectomies. This discussion focuses on resective procedures and does not address in detail section of the corpus callosum and sub-pial transections.

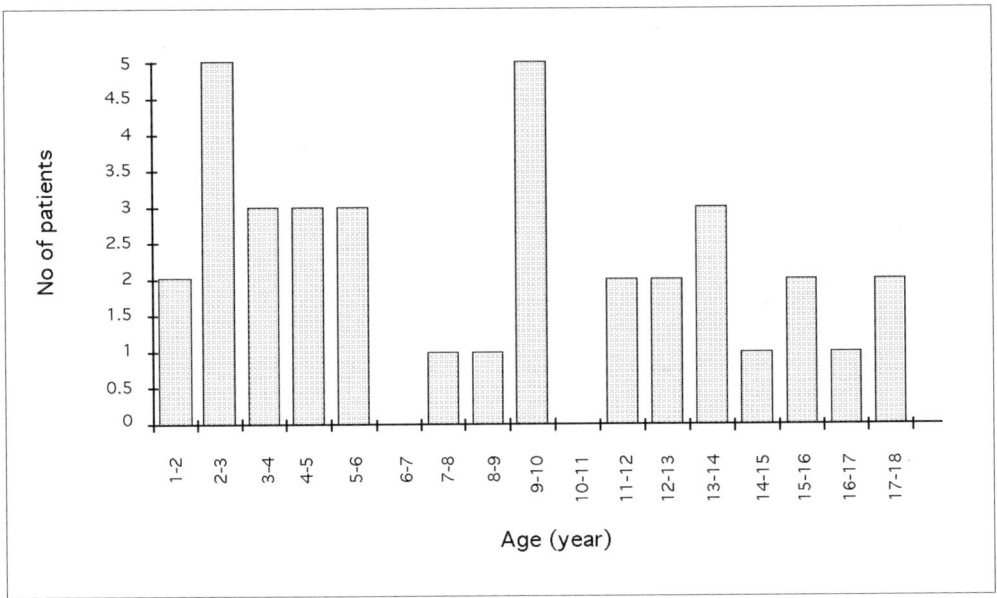

Figure 1. Age at surgery.

Magnetic resonance studies

When magnetic resonance imaging is optimized for a specific purpose, its repertoire and sensitivity is now considerable. In our study of intractable temporal lobe epilepsy with optimized MR, the positive rate in those with clinical diagnosis of temporal lobe epilepsy was over 90%. A similar rate was found in those with clinically unlocalized epilepsy [2]. The use of T2 mapping has greatly enhanced precise information on damage to mesial temporal structures [3]. One child with a biphasic encephalitic-like illness with two bursts of seizures a few months apart showed abnormalities appearing successively in the hippocampus of first one side and then the other, and he became amnesiac after the second episode. By looking at the T2 relaxation times [4] in this patient, abnormally high figures were found in both hippocampi. This subject has been investigated in detail in our temporal lobe epilepsy patients. We have found a high rate of abnormality and a significant rate of bilateral abnormality in children with temporal lobe epilepsy in whom the imaging suggested unilateral disease. If we turn to the use of MR as a chemical mode using proton spectroscopy, it is possible to look at the volume within a 2 cm cube in the medical temporal structures that, although including some of the hippocampus, contains more neocortex. Using this mode with a Siemens' Clinical 1.5 Tesla MR System in a children's hospital with strong academic physics support, it has been possible to obtain proton spectra in a large number of children with epilepsy. The specific findings are of a high rate of reduction of the substance N-acetylspartate for which there is good evidence of it being localized in neurons. There is also a relative or absolute increase in creatine- and choline-containing compounds that are predominately glial in origin [5]. Once again a significant rate of bilateral abnormality was found. We have nevertheless been operating on such children with bilateral abnormalities, and there is provisional evidence that these measures may relate to hemisphere-specific cognitive functions but not to their epileptogenicity. MR can also be used as a functional imaging mode, and we have studied in detail one child with epilepsia partialis continua in which a clear cortical abnormality was switched on and off by the occurrence of seizures [6].

Single photon emission computerized tomography (SPECT)

Dr. Helen Cross has worked specifically in the area of SPECT. Adult studies have suggested a high rate of abnormality in ictal recordings. Continuous EEG monitoring usually with drug withdrawal allows the administration of the radioactive-labeled lipophyllic substance HMPAO during a seizure and the demonstration of focal timelocked hyperperfusion has been successfully developed. This has shown a high yield in both temporal lobe and whole hemisphere pathologies [7]. It has some value in extratemporal epilepsy, but this has not yet been assessed in detail. There has also been a high rate of interictal hypoperfusion which seems to correlate with a reduced N-acetylspartate to choline plus creatine-containing compounds ratio. We have been impressed by SPECT as a functional mode in this context. It is important to emphasize that this is true functional imaging of a seizure as was the imaging of a child with epilepsia partialis continua using MR. The studies reporting the use of positron emission tomography (PET) interictally are using a functional imaging mode for a largely structural purpose.

A non invasive package for the preoperative assessment of children for epilepsy surgery

The above investigations with a detailed neuropsychology, where it is possible, has greatly reduced the need for invasive monitoring. It is clear, however, that invasive monitoring is sometimes required, particularly in extratemporal epilepsies. One is likely to be at the lower end of the cost/benefit range, however, with more invasive investigations being used for relatively lower yield. To date, this package of noninvasive investigations has been used on approximately 50 children who have received surgery. The early results indicate a high localizing and lateralizing yield for MR and SPECT. The outcome time is short at present but David Taylor, the neuropsychiatrist within the team, has developed a scheme of categorization of the aims of surgery that will allow comparability of results from different centers. Simple seizure remission data does not do justice to the quality-of-life aims of surgery and the wide variations in type and distribution of pathology.

Some of the most difficult issues that we have faced have been disease specific. In some young children with lateralized developmental defects, for example hemimegalencephaly, good or complete control of seizures may be obtained with drugs such as phenobarbitone and phenytoin. Some children suffer relative or complete developmental arrest associated with this process, which is only overcome when seizures break through and hemispherectomy is thought justifiable. How early should such children be operated on? On several occasions we have seen children who are globally very delayed but with evidence of purely unilateral pathology and have seen useful if partial recovery with surgery at a later age than we would now feel was ideal. It is also clear that a number of children regress massively with unilateral temporal lesions and these require very early intervention, but whether that should be limited to a lesionectomy is not yet agreed. The relatively early diagnosis of Rasmussen disease, either by biopsy or by highly suspicious clinical and radiological findings, is a considerable problem. It has been difficult to offer hemispherectomy when the child still has useful hand function, but that is the logic when the epilepsy syndrome is destroying their life. Clearly, we all hope there will be a medical treatment for this condition in the near future.

Autistic regression

We have identified two situations in which severe autistic regression occurs and may be surgically remediable. The first is the severe end of the Landau-Kleffner syndrome: the reason for including this condition within this general rubric is that the children begin with characteristic seizures, EEG abnormalities and language regression but develop loss of social functioning and very often extremely difficult behaviour as a later phase. This aspect of the syndrome appears to be similarly partially responsive to subpial transections but a large series is required perhaps from several centers in order to be clearer about this. The other situation has been the regression which has occurred in children with "congenital tumors" mostly dysembryoplastic neuroepitheliomas with epilepsy starting in the first year of life. We have now seen six children with this pattern and all have had right temporal lesions involving neocortex and surgery has only been partially effective though it has sometimes been done late and on the basis of the presence of a tumor rather than as an epilepsy surgery procedure. These two situations may well amount to an emergency indication for surgical intervention and our current techniques of excision or disconnection may need to be rethought in this context.

The use of surgery in childhood epilepsy occurs within a large multidisciplinary team. It involves intervention in many different clinical syndromes with a wide range of pathologies and with significant problems in predicting outcomes. We must categorize the clinical situations in a way which will allow comparison between centers. Our provisional assessment of our results, in terms of seizure relief using this noninvasive package for the investigation of children, suggests that in a difficult younger group of patients, the results are at least comparable with other series of patients managed on more traditional grounds.

References

1. Ounsted C, Lindsay J, Richards P. *Temporal lobe epilepsy. A biographical study.* London : MacKeith Press, 1987.
2. Aicardi J. *Epilepsy in children.* New York : Raven Press, 1994.
3. Cross JH, Jackson GD, Neville BGR, Connelly A, Kirkham FJ, Boyd SG, Pitt MC, Gadian DG. Magnetic resonance imaging in intractable epilepsy of childhood. *Arch Dis Child.* 1993 ; 69 : 104-9.
4. Jackson GD, Connelly A, Duncan JS, Gadian DG, Grunewald R. MRI detection of hippocampal pathology in temporal lobe epilepsy: increased sensitivity using quantitative T2 relaxometry. *Neurology* 1993 ; 43 : 1793-9.
5. Gadian DG, Connelly A, Duncan JS, Cross JH, Kirkham FJ, Johnson CL, Vargha-Khadem F, Neville BGR, Jackson GD. IH magnetic resonance spectroscopy in the investigation of intractable epilepsy. *Acta Neurol Scand* 1994 ; 89 : 116-22.
6. Jackson GD, Connelly A, Cross JH, Gordon I, Gadian DG. Functional magnetic resonance imaging of focal seizures. *Neurology* 1994 ; 44 : 850-6.
7. Cross JH, Gordon I, Jackson GD, Boyd SG, Todd-Pokropek A, Anderson PJ, Neville BGR. Children with intractable focal epilepsy; ictal and interictal 99mTc HMPAO single photon emission computed tomography. *Dev Med Child Neurol* 1995 ; 37 : 673-81.

5

Developmental influences on the electrophysiologic investigation of pediatric epilepsy surgery candidates

M. DUCHOWNY, P. JAYAKAR, T. RESNICK, A.S. HARVEY

Comprehensive Epilepsy Center and Neuroscience Program, Miami Children's Hospital, Miami, Florida, USA.

The referral of children with intractable epilepsy for surgery is now widely accepted by the medical community. The endorsement of surgical therapy is the result of growing recognition that successful surgery is a viable option to treat medically resistant epilepsy [1-3]. Much of the progress in surgical therapy has followed advances in the interpretation of electroclinical seizure semiology, improvements in surgical methodology and the revolutionary progress in functional and anatomical brain imaging [4, 5], facilitating more accurate identification of the epileptogenic region [5, 6].

The favorable experience with surgery has further increased the pool of potential surgical candidates and created an even more pressing need to effectively and accurately define cortical regions responsible for seizure generation [7, 8]. While surgical candidates are routinely screened for evidence of medical intractability, a precise defininion and resection of the epileptogenic zone, defined as an area of cortex which includes the zone of electrophysiologic seizure origin and associated structural abnormality, will ultimately determine case selection and outcome. If localization cannot be accomplished, surgery may be imprecise leading to an increased risk of postoperative failure.

Electrophysiologic studies continue to provide definitive localizing information while at the same time facilitating mapping of cortical regions critical for language and movement [9]. This information is particularly vital in the workup of pediatric epilepsy surgery candidates who must be understood in the context of unique developmental factors. Whereas adults are often evaluated for surgery on the basis of their seizure semiology, scalp EEG and neuroimaging data, similar studies in the pre-adolescent child are less often definitive [10]. Furthermore, adults present with partial seizures of temporo-limbic origin, whereas children are more prone to extra-temporal epilepsy or temporal lobe seizures with wider and more variable epileptogenic zones [11-14]. Planning seizure surgery in very young children with epilepsy therefore presents unique and complex challenges, particularly in patients with normal MRI or functional neuroimaging studies.

It has been our experience that developmental factors heavily influence the clinical and electrophysiologic evaluation of pediatric epilepsy surgery candidates [12]. Developmental variables modify the preoperative electrophysiological evaluation of young surgical candidates in several ways. Many children with developmental pathology and intractable seizures are also neurologically impaired in other domains including cognition, coordination and behavior. Their neurological deficits may be extremely severe and limit their ability to complete investigational protocols. Testing therefore needs to be scaled to mental status as well as the chronolological age. The influence of developmental factors on the EEG and electroclinical seizure semiology is well known and has been reported in several excellent reviews [15, 16]. Lastly, the range of developmental errors in morphogenesis and cellular migration underlying chronic epilepsy is diverse [17] and impacts on epileptogenesis in ways that are not fully understood. Thus, the term "developmental" as it applies to pediatric epilepsy surgery patients connotes a broad spectrum of normal and abnormal influences on the clinical, neurophysiologic and pathological expression of intractable partial seizures. These influences have major implications for the interpretation of electrophysiologic investigations as well.

Developmental influences on the scalp EEG evaluation

The rapidly changing EEG features of infants and young children are recognized to reflect dynamic postnatal processes including maturation of myelination, synaptic connectivity and neuronal dropout. The relatively immature neonatal cortex, for example, cannot support sustained and widespread hypersynchronized cortical discharges, even in the presence of diffuse pathological changes. As a consequence, clinical seizures in very early life tend to be focal rather than generalized, and are temporally and spatially dissociated from electrographic seizure patterns. With advancing chronologic age, the EEG and clinical semiology of partial seizures becomes more robust and seizures propagate rapidly [18]. The spasms in some cases of West syndrome, for example, are now regarded as a generalized manifestation of focal regions of dysplastic cortex which may be amenable to excisional procedures [19]. The task of defining consistent focality is particularly challenging for focal epileptiform activity that propagates rapidly. Not uncommonly, focal epileptiform patterns are identified interictally prior to the phase of generalization [20]. The appearance of generalized epileptiform patterns may also be restricted to a finite window of time, thus constituting a phase in an overall developmental progression (Figure 1). Focality may also be defined by alterations of EEG background such as polymorphic slowing or attenuation of fast frequencies. In some cases, focal intermittent fast activity (Figure 2) may provide the only clue to a primarily localized epileptogenic dysfunction [21, 22].

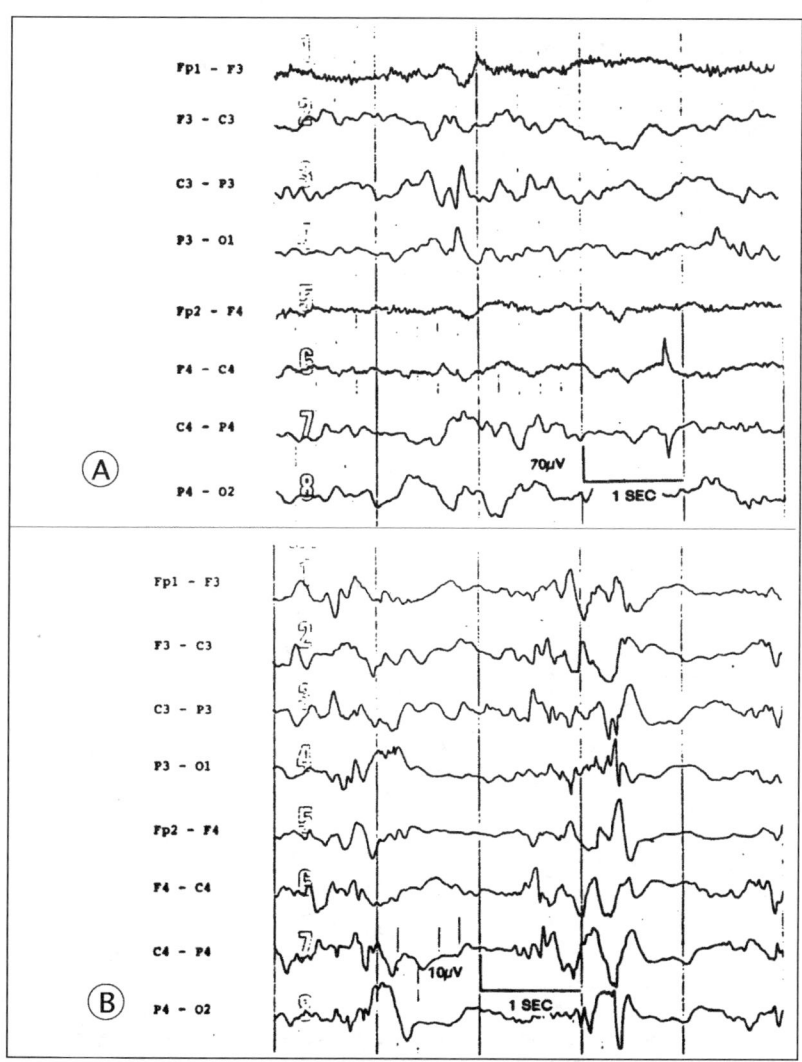

Figure 1. A. Interictal EEG in a 3 month old infant with a focal dysplastic lesion in parietal cortex and partial seizures. Left parietal spikes and sharp waves are frequent throughout the recording and correlate with the structural lesion. **B.** Interictal EEG in the same patient recorded at age 4 1/2 months following onset of infantile spasms. The EEG now demonstrates a burst-suppression pattern. Interestingly : phase reversal of the spike focus can still be observed within the generalized burst.

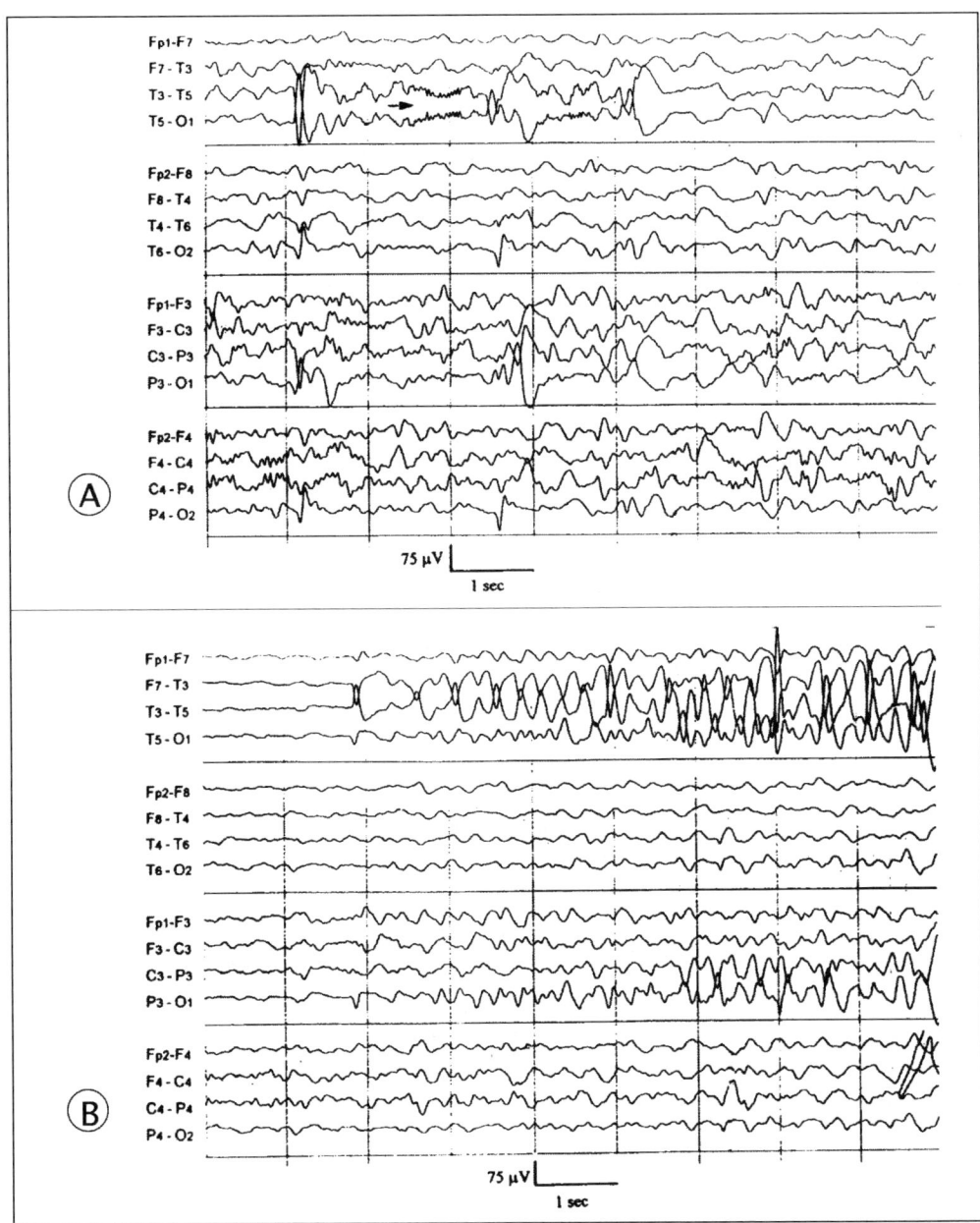

Figure 2. Scalp EEG recordings in a patient with cortical dysplasia. **A.** Multifocal spikes were observed over both hemispheres interictally with focal intermittent fast activity (arrow) over the left temporal region. **B.** Ictal EEG recording confirmed left temporal seizure origin.

When undertaking epilepsy surgery, it is critical to exclude benign epilepsy syndromes and progressive degenerative diseases. While these conditions should be evident from review of the history, patients occasionally present diagnostic uncertainty. Cases of resistant partial epilepsy arising in rolandic or occipital cortex may display EEG patterns resembling benign syndromes. Benign occipital epilepsy of childhood, for example, may manifest prominent EEG discharges localized to one occipital lobe which are similar to the electrographic features of lesional occipital epilepsy [23, 24]. A benign familial disorder may be suspected in the presence of a family history, activation with photic stimulation and when MRI scans are normal.

The scalp EEG has historically served to evaluate temporal lobe seizure foci in adults. Ictal and interictal scalp EEG patterns are often highly localizing, but bitemporal discharges are a frequent source of localization failure [25]. Adult temporal lobectomy patients are more likely to harbor postnatally acquired lesions such as hippocampal sclerosis (HS) which is typically the sole pathological finding in over half of temporal lobectomy specimens [26]. Brain tumors including indolent gliomas and gangliogliomas are also common [27].

By contrast, highly localized scalp EEG patterns as occur in the adult are less common in children whose partial epilepsy is also less frequently associated with acquired lesions [28-30]. Developmental abnormalities of cortex including dysplasias, glial neuronal hamartomas, and developmental tumors (glial-neuronal and dysembryoplastic) are the most characteristic pathologies in younger patients and may be remarkably widespread, usually either multilobar or hemispheric in extent (Figure 3) [31, 32]. Consequently, multifocal interictal abnormalities and widespread ictal discharges are frequent findings on the preoperative evaluation. Although HS is now recognized to occur in childhood, it is more typically found in association with developmental lesions rather than an isolated finding following postnatal events such as febrile status epilepticus or meningitis [33, 34].

The predominance of developmental pathology in children with intractable partial epilepsy is particularly striking in very young surgical candidates. Table I presents clinico-pathologic data in 26 infants under age 3 years undergoing surgery at Miami Children's Hospital for medically resistant and often catastrophic partial seizures. Developmental pathology was identified in most cases, whereas acquired (*i.e.* atrophic/sclerotic) lesions were unusual. Extensive resections (hemispherectomy or multilobar excision) were performed in approximately half the cases, consistent with the more widespread anatomic and functional derangement of developmental lesions that produce epilepsy in early life. Less than 20% underwent temporal lobectomy, a proportion that is considerably less than adults for whom this procedure is the predominant form of surgical therapy [35]. Direct comparisons of children and adults with cortical dysplasia and epilepsy also reveal a higher incidence of extratemporal seizures and catastrophic presentations in younger patients [36].

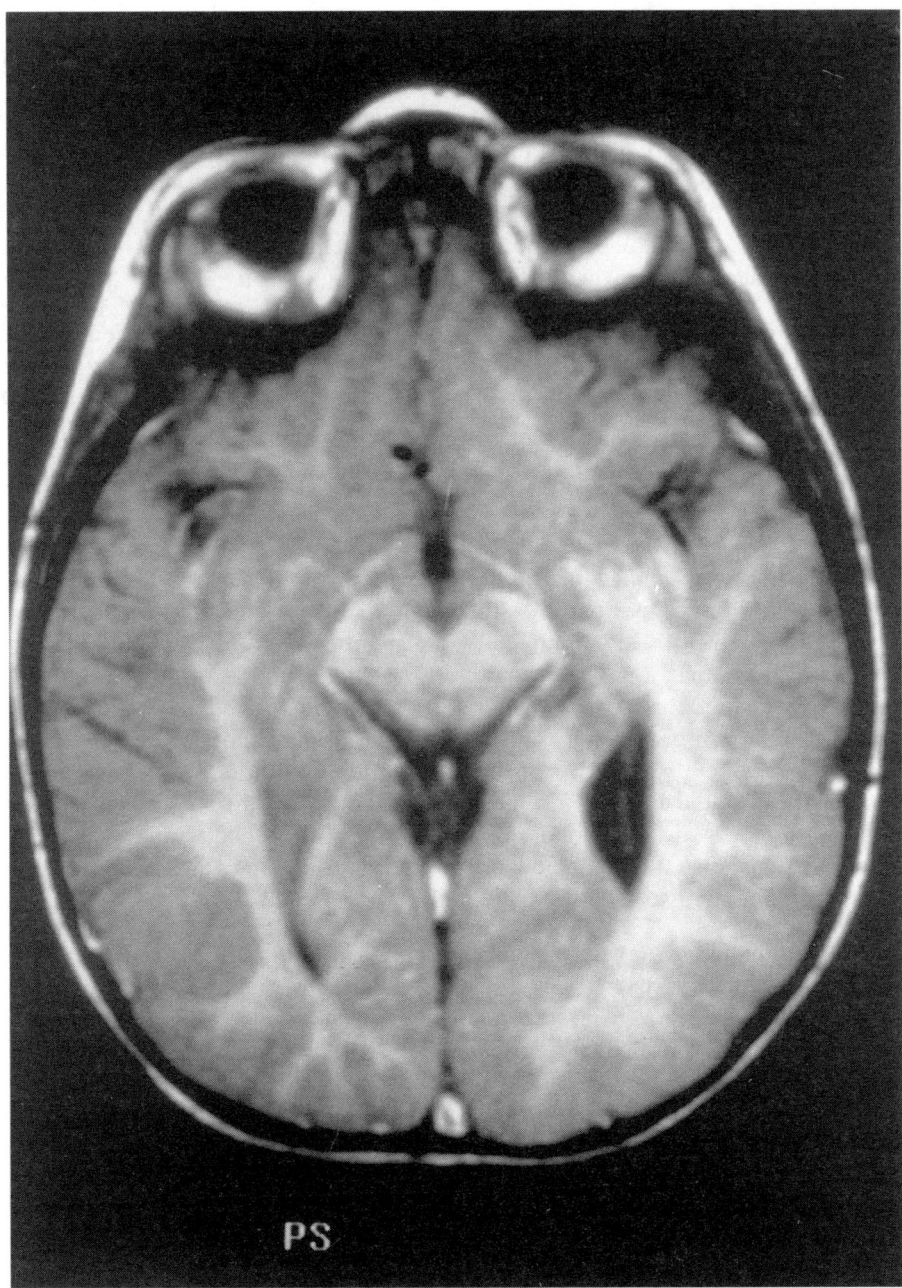

Figure 3. T1 weighted axial MR image in a 2 year old girl with medically resistant partial seizures that began on the second day of life. There is loss of the expected arborization of the white matter in the right parietal : temporal and occipital regions with thickening of the overlying cortex. Video-EEG monitoring revealed near-continuous epileptiform discharges in the right posterior quadrant and posterior temporal regions. Pathologic analysis of the resected tissue revealed widespread dysplastic changes including bizare neuronal elements: neuronal cytomegaly and dyslamination.

Table I. Clinico-pathologic diagnoses and excisional procedures for epilepsy in children under age 3 years at Miami Children's Hospital (1985-1994) (n=26).

Diagnosis	Tumors	Ganglioglioma (2) Gangliocytoma (4) DNET (2)
	Atrophic/Sclerotic (4)	
	Neurocutaneous disorder	Sturge-Weber syndrome (3) Tuberous sclerosis (1)
	Cortical dysplasia (4)	
	Developmental	Neuronal heterotopia (2) Schizencephaly (1) Hemimegalencephaly (1) Pachygyria (1) Polymicrogyria (1)
Procedure	Hemispherectomy (10)	
	Multilobar (3)	
	Lobar	Frontal (7) Temporal (5) Parietal (1)

Not unexpectedly, large developmentally abnormal regions of cortex are also difficult to define electrophysiologically from scalp EEG information. High field strength MR imaging may assist localization if electrophysiological studies are indeterminate. Occult abnormalities including mild degrees of cortical dysplasia or neuronal heterotopias may be overlooked even on state-of-the-art images [37, 38]. PET and SPECT reveal abnormal regions of metabolism or perfusion [39-41], and have been used to select surgical candidates at some centers. However, these procedures should be considered supportive since epilepsy is primarily an electrophysiologic disturbance and must be understood in these terms. Patients who are not localized by non-invasive electrophysiologic studies should be considered for intracranial electrode implantation.

Issues relating to the evaluation and localization of developmental lesions are not limited to pediatrics. Adults with developmental lesions and/or widespread EEG abnormalities have a poor postoperative prognosis [42]. Whereas lesionectomy guided by scalp EEG and electrocorticography has been advocated at some centers [43], this procedure is less beneficial for developmental lesions with spatial dimensions that are non-convergent with ictal or interictal EEG data [44, 45]. Comparable studies of lesionectomy in childhood have not been performed. Our personal experience with lesionectomy [46] and that of others [47] suggests that except for selected tumors [48], this approach is rarely successful in the majority of developmentally based epilepsies of childhood onset.

Anterior temporal spikes occur in a high proportion of adults with TLE [49], being bilateral in approximately half [47]. They are less frequent in the pediatric population [50, 51] where normal interictal EEGs, and multifocal or generalized discharges are commonplace, especially in infants and toddlers [50, 51]. Recording with anterior temporal electrodes may help detect antero-mesial temporal spikes [52] and are better tolerated by children than sphenoidal electrodes. Closely-spaced electrodes may further refine the parameters for defining the epileptogenic zone [53] and may on occasion differentiate temporal from extratemporal foci [11]. Extensive neocortical involvement usually mandates more invasive investigations.

Developmental influences on the intracranial EEG evaluation

Surgical candidates with poorly localized EEGs usually require intracranial EEG monitoring to define the epileptogenic region. Subdural electrodes, configured as strips and grids, are particularly advantageous for this purpose in the child as they permit extensive coverage of basal and interhemispheric neocortex [54]. Subdural electrodes can be positioned under direct observation at craniotomy, and used to record the EEG extraoperatively. They are well tolerated by children, infants and toddlers [55], and their position can be confirmed by routine skull X-ray or CT scan. Though considerably more expensive, platinum and nicrome electrodes are MRI compatible. Electrode thickness must be kept to a minimum to reduce pressure effects.

Extreme seizure activity in developmentally abnormal neocortex has recently been investigated during intraoperative monitoring [45]. Intraoperative ECoG recordings of dysplastic cortex reveal intense and complicated patterns including frequent and rhythmic seizure discharges, repetitive bursting and continuous or near-continuous rhythmical spiking. By contrast, electrophysiological abnormalities are less common for seizures due to other causes. *In vitro* recording confirms that dysplastic but not normal or sclerotic cortex is prone to seizure-like discharges in response to application of the convulsant drug 4-aminopyridine [56].

Patients with developmental lesions and well localized ictal onset zones may exhibit independent electrographic seizures in adjacent or remote cortical regions, a phenomenon termed "intraictal activation" [57]. Cortex that is intraictally activated during an electroclinical seizure may go on to exhibit independent epileptogenesis once the primary focus has ceased firing, and may even activate on the postexcision ECoG. Intraictally activated neocortex differs from mirror or homologous contralateral foci by virtue of its proximity to the primary focus and lack of spontaneous interictal firing. Intraictal foci are especially common in patients with developmentally based epilepsy, constituting an important potential reason for surgical failure. Removing the entire epileptogenic region including any structural lesion and the entire area of epileptogenic cortex is thus critical to outcome [45].

Compared to adults, children with medically resistant temporal lobe epilepsy especially benefit from intracranial EEG monitoring since acquired lesions such as HS are rarely the sole cause of their seizures. Temporal lobe seizures which begin early in life are typically neocortical in origin and posterior in location [12]. Posterior temporal seizures present as stereotyped episodes of behavioral arrest and motor symptomatology, with automatisms being either absent or late in the ictal sequence [12]. Subdural recording reveals electrographic seizure origin in basal neocortex, a region difficult to analyze by depth electrodes and well behind the surgical plane for standard temporal lobectomy. Temporal corticectomies tailored by subdural EEG data are successful in a high proportion of cases [12].

Functional cortical stimulation

The high incidence of extratemporal and multilobar epilepsy in children requires clarification of cortical function in many surgical candidates. Mapping eloquent cortical regions using electrical stimulation according to standard adult paradigms is of limited value in pediatrics [58]. In the adult paradigm, a baseline stimulus is increased in 0.5 to 1.0 mA steps until an afterdischarge, functional response or 15 mA ceiling is obtained. In adults, this procedure generates reliable responses at low levels of stimulation [59], but in patients younger than 4 years, sensorimotor responses are difficult to obtain, and are absent in infants below 2 years [58]. Electrical responsiveness increases in direct proportion to age while threshold for functional responsiveness decreases with age until adolescence [59].

Cortical responses are reliably elicited in childhood if stimulus intensity and duration are both increased in a stepwise fashion [59]. Increases in both domains rather than intensity alone cause the stimulus to converge towards the chronaxie on the strength-duration curve. Responses obtained at the chronaxie are elicited at the lowest expenditure of energy, a definite advantage when working in immature cortex. In comparison to the adult paradigm, only dual stimulation successfully evokes both afterdischarges and functional responses in patients 4 years and younger [59].

Sensorimotor mapping

Dual stimulation mapping of sensorimotor responses in pediatric epilepsy surgery candidates reveals an anatomic representation of cortical function that is similar to the adult schema. However, despite the similarities in organization, elicited responses display several important age related differences [9]. Children under age 4 show predominantly tonic rather than clonic movements, and movement of the tongue is unusual. Below age 6 years, hand but not individual finger movements can be elicited. As a rule, tonic finger movements appear earlier than clonic finger movements, a developmental sequence that mirrors the ontogenetic expression of motor seizure patterns in childhood [60, 61].

Below age 2 years, we have observed facial motor responses to more often be bilateral than unilateral [9], resembling a grimace lasting several seconds in duration. We have not seen bilateral facial movement in older children, leading us to speculate that bilateral facial movement is a transient postnatal response predating axonal and/or synaptic elimination [62, 63]. With maturation, ipsilateral lower facial innervation is gradually lost. The observed bilateral facial movement is also consistent with the facial sparing in congenital but not acquired hemiplegia [64].

Cortical mapping in patients with developmental pathology also reveals some interesting anomalies of the motor homunculus [9]. One patient exhibited a hand region superior to the primary shoulder region; another had a double shoulder region above and below hand and finger cortex. Aberrant patterns of cortical motor organization are probably more common in patients with dysplastic lesions, an observation recently confirmed by others [65]. Experimental studies in the primate brain indicate that prenatal lesions are capable of inducing anomalous cortical sulci and functional reorganization at remote cortical sites in both cerebral hemispheres [66, 67].

Language mapping

Much of our knowledge regarding the organization of primary language cortex in the child comes from studies of recovery from childhood aphasia [68]. It is generally acknowledged that complete or near-complete recovery is possible depending upon the age when the lesion was sustained as well as the size and location of the damage [69], and that recovery involves interhemispheric reorganization associated with a switch to right hemisphere dominance. While language recovery after early postnatal lesions is often impressive, deficits in non-language areas suggest that patterns of recovery are rarely complete or predictable [70].

While postnatally acquired lesions of the dominant cerebral hemisphere in early childhood cause significant reorganization of language cortex, there is relatively little information about language function and the cortical representation of language in children with partial seizures and developmental lesions. An understanding of this relationship has practical implications for the evaluation of children with seizures originating within or adjacent to language cortex [71].

We have recently investigated the effects of electrically stimulating language cortex in 34 patients with implanted subdural grid electrodes, 28 of whom had magnetic resonance imaging or histologic evidence of developmental tumors or cortical dysplasia [72]. In all instances, patients with developmental lesions had language in frontal and temporal cortex at sites anatomically similar to the adult. An "adult" representation has been documented in an epilepsy patient as young as 4 years, and has been encountered in a 2 year old being mapped prior to tumoral surgery. The actual amount of square surface area of cortex devoted to language (based on the number of subdural electrodes showing language representation) is also similar to the adult [73, 74] suggesting that language sites are designated in early life and conserved anatomically over the lifespan.

The increasing language competence of the child therefore cannot be attributed to increases in cortical surface area.

The permanence of language cortex in children with developmental lesions contrasts sharply with the relocation of language following early peri- and postnatally acquired lesions [75]. We have recorded relocation of language sites in 3 children with epilepsy whose language cortex was damaged before age 5 years. By contrast, developmental lesions which do not ablate language cortex do not cause its relocation to contralateral cortical regions. Furthermore, epileptic bombardment of language cortex is also incapable of displacing language cortex from predetermined sites.

Conclusions

There is much to be gained from the electrophysiologic evaluation of developmental lesions. Developmental issues remain at the core of the surgical treatment of pediatric epilepsy, but have important implications for adult surgery candidates, and indeed for all patients with or without epilepsy who are born with developmental brain anomalies. Since many patients with developmental pathology also manifest developmental disorders of intellect and behavior, a greater understanding of the electroclinical semiology of developmental pathology may provide important insights into mechanisms of brain development and organization.

References

1. Duchowny MS. Surgical outcome in children. In : Luders H, ed. *Epilepsy surgery*. New York : Raven Press, 1991 : 669-76.
2. Duchowny M. Epilepsy surgery in children. *Curr Op Neurol* 1995 ; 8 : 112-6.
3. Holmes GL. Surgery for intractable seizures in infancy and early childhood. *Neurology* 1993 ; 43 (suppl 5) : S28-37.
4. Luders HO. *Epilepsy surgery*. New York : Raven Press, 1992.
5. Engel J. Update on surgical treatment of the epilepsies. *Neurology* 1993 43 : 1612-7.
6. Lesser R, Fisher RS, Kaplan P. The evaluation of patients with intractable complex partial seizures. *Electroenceph Clin Neurophysiol* 1989 ; 73 : 381-8.
7. Duchowny M. Non-invasive evaluation of intractable seizures. *Int Pediatr* 1986 ; 1 : 74-7.
8. Duchowny M. The role of surgery in childhood epilepsy. *Int Pediatr* 1987 ; 2 : 205-11.
9. Duchowny M, Jayakar P. Functional cortical mapping in children. In : Devinsky O, Beric A, Dogali M, eds. *Electrical and magnetic stimulation of the brain and spinal cord*. New York : Raven Press, 1993 : 149-54.
10. Resnick T, Duchowny M, Jayakar P. Early surgery for epilepsy-redefining candidacy. *J Child Neurol* 1994 ; 9 : 2S36-41.
11. Duchowny MS, Shewrnon DA, Wyllie E, Andermann F, Mizrahi EM. Special considerations for preoperative evaluation in childhood. In : Engel J Jr ed. *Surgical treatment of the epilepsies*, 2nd edition. New York : Raven Press, 1993 : 415-27.

12. Duchowny M, Jayakar P, Resnick T, Levin B, Alvarez L. Posterior temporal epilepsy: electroclinical features. *Ann Neurol* 1994 ; 35 : 427-31.
13. Morrison G, Duchowny M, Resnick T, Alvarez L, Jayakar P, Prats AR, Dean P, Penate M. Epilepsy surgery in childhood: a report of 79 patients. *Pediatr Neurosurg* 1992 ; 18 : 291-7.
14. Shields WD, Duchowny M, Holmes GL. Surgically remedial syndromes of infancy and early childhood. In : Engel J Jr, ed. *Surgical treatment of the epilepsies,* 2nd edition. New York : Raven Press, 1993 : 35-48.
15. Eeg-Olofsson O, Petersen I, Sellden U. The development of the electroencephalogram in normal children from the age of 1 through 15 years. *Neuropediatrie* 1971 ; 2 : 375-404.
16. Cavazzuti GB, Cappella L, Nalin A. Longitudinal study of epileptiform EEG patterns in normal children. *Epilepsia* 1980 ; 21 : 43-55.
17. Farrell MA, DeRosa MJ, Curran JG. Neuropathologic findings in cortical resections (including hemispherectomies) performed for the treatment of intractable childhood epilepsy. *Acta Neuropathol* 1992 ; 83 : 246-59.
18. Duchowny M. The syndrome of partial seizures in infancy. *J Child Neurol* 1992 ; 7 : 66-9.
19. Chugani HT, Shields WD, Shewmon DA. Infantile spasms: I. PET identifies focal cortical dysgenesis in cryptogenic cases for surgical treatment. *Ann Neurol* 1990 ; 27 : 406-13.
20. Gaily EK, Shewmon DA, Chugani H, Curran SG. Asymmetric and asynchronous infantile spasms. *Epilepsia* 1995 ; 36 : 873-82.
21. Altman KD, Shewmon AD. Local paroxysmal fast activity: significance interictally and in infantile spasms. *Epilepsia* 1990 ; 31(5) : 623.
22. Harvey S, Jayakar P, Resnick TJ, Duchowny MS, Alvarez LA. *Focal interminent fast activity: clinical correlates*. Chicago : American EEG society meeting, 1994.
23. Panayiotopoulos CP. Basilar migraine? Seizures and severe epileptic EEG abnormalities. *Neurology* 1980 ; 30 : 1122-5.
24. Williamson PD, Thadani VM, Darcey MF, Spencer DD, Spencer SS, Mattson RH. Occipital lobe epilepsy: clinical characteristics, seizure spread patterns and results of surgery. *Ann Neurol* 1992 ; 31 : 3-13.
25. So N, Olivier A, Andermann F, Gloor P, Quesney F. Results of surgical treatment in patients with bitemporal epileptiforrn abnormalities. *Ann Neurol* 1989 ; 25 : 432-9.
26. Babb TL, Brown WJ. Pathological findings in epilepsy. In : Engel J Jr, ed. *Surgical treatment of the epilepsies*. New York : Raven Press, 1987 : 511-40.
27. Plate KH, Wieser H-G, Yasargil MG, Wiestler OD. Neuropathological findings in 224 patients with temporal lobe epilepsy. *Acta Neuropathol* 1993 ; 86 : 433-8.
28. Harvey AS, Duchowny M, Goldstein R, Bruce J, Jayakar P, Resnick T, Alvarez L, Altman N. Neuropathology in children with intractable partial epilepsy. *Ann Neurol* 1994 ; 36 : 487.
29. Harvey AS, Duchowny M, Bruce J, Altman N, Bean J, Jayakar P, Resnick T, Alvarez L. A proposed classification of cortical dysplasia in epilepsy surgery specimens. *Epilepsia* 1995 ; 36 : 139.
30. Mischel PS, Nguyen LP, Vinters HV. Cerebral cortical dysplasia associated with pediatric epilepsy. Review of neuropathologic features and proposal for a grading system. *J Neuropathol Exp Neurol* 1995 ; 54 : 137-53.
31. Kazee AM, Lapham LW, Torres CF, Wang DD. Generalized cortical dysplasia. Clinical and pathological aspects. *Arch Neurol* 1991 ; 48 : 850-3.
32. Sebire G, Goutières F, Tardieu M, Landrieu P, Aicardi J. Extensive macrogyri or no visible gyri; distinct clinical, electroencephalographic and genetic features according to different imaging patterns. *Neurology* 1995 ; 24 : 1105-11.

33. Bruce J, Harvey AS, Duchowny M, Altman A, Jayakar P, Resnick T, Alvarez L. Hippocampal sclerosis and developmental neuropathology in children with intractable partial seizures. *Epilepsia* 1995 ; 36 : 30.
34. Cendes F, Cook MJ, Watson C, Andermann F, Fish DR, Shorvon SD, Bergin P, Free S, Dubeau F, Arnold DL. Frequency and characteristics of dual pathology in patients with lesional epilepsy. *Neurology* 1995 ; 45 : 2058-64.
35. Engel JE Jr. Surgical treatment of the epilepsies. NewYork : Raven Press, 1993 (1st edition 1987) : 553-71.
36. Wyllie E, Baumgartner C, Prayson R, Estes M, Comair Y, Kosalko J, Skibinski C. The clinical spectrum of focal cortical dysplasia and epilepsy. *J Epilepsy* 1994 ; 7 : 303-12.
37. Kuzniecky R, Garcia JH, Faught E, Morawetz RB. Cortical dysplasia in temporal lobe epilepsy magnetic resonance imaging correlates. *Ann Neurol* 1991 ; 29 : 293-8.
38. Watanabe K, Negoro T, Aso K, Maeda N, Ohki T, Hayakawa F, Ito K, Kato T. Clinical, EEG and positron emission tomography features of childhood-onset epilepsy with localized cortical dysplasia detected by magnetic resonance imaging. *J Epilepsy* 1994 ; 7 : 108-16.
39. Harvey AS, Hopkins IJ, Bowe JM. Frontal lobe epilepsy: clinical seizure characteristics and localization with ictal ^{99m}Tc-HMPAO SPECT. *Neurology* 1993 ; 43 : 1980-96.
40. Chugani H, Shewmon DA, Khanna S, Phelps ME. Interictal and postictal focal hypermetabolism on positron emission tomography. *Pediatr Neurol* 1993 ; 9 : 10-5.
41. Cross JH, Gordon I, Jackson GD, Boyd SG, Todd-Pokropek T, Anderson PJ, Neville BGR. Children with intractable focal epilepsy: ictal and interictal ^{99}Tc^{M} HMPAO single photon emission computed tomography. *Dev Med Child Neurol* 1995 ; 37 : 673-81.
42. Palmini A, Andermann F, Olivier A, Tampieri D, Robitaille Y. Focal neuronal migration disorders and intractable partial epilepsy: results of surgical treatment. *Ann Neurol* 1991 ; 30 : 750-7.
43. Cascino GD, Kelly PJ, Sharborough F. Long-term follow-up of stereotactic lesionectomy in partial epilepsy predictive factors and electroencephalographic results. *Epilepsia* 1992 ; 33 : 639-44.
44. Rossi GF, Colicchio G, Scerrati M. Resection surgery for partial epilepsy. Relation of surgical outcome with some aspects of the epileptogenic process and surgical approach. *Acta Neurochir (Wien)* 1994 ; 130 : 101-10.
45. Palmini A, Gambardella A, Andermann F, Dubeau F, Jaderson CdC, Olivier A, Tampieri D, Gloor P, Quesney F, Andermann E, Paglioli E, Paglioli-Neto E, Coutinho L, Leblanc R, Kim HI. Intrinsic epileptogenicity of the human dysplastic cortex as suggested by corticography and surgical results. *Ann Neurol* 1995 ; 37 : 476-87.
46. Jayakar P, Resnick TJ, Duchowny MS, Alvarez LA, Morrison G. Epilepsy surgery in children with lesions. New Orleans, American epilepsy society meeting. *Epilepsia* 1994 ; 35 (8) : 154.
47. Berger MS, Ghatan S, Geyer JR, Keles GE, Ojemann GA. Seizure outcome in children with hemispheric tumors and associated intractable epilepsy: the role of tumor removal combined with seizure foci resection. *Pediatr Neurosurg* 1991 ; 17 : 185-91.
48. Raymond AA, Halpin SFS, Alsanjari N, Cook MJ, Kitchen ND, Fish DR, Stevens JM, Harding BN, Scaravilli F, Kendall B, Shorvon SD, Neville BGR. Dysembryoplastic neuroepithelial tumour. Features in 16 patients. *Brain* 1994 ; 117 : 461-75.
49. Sammaritano M, Gigli GL, Gotman J. Interictal spiking during wakefillness and sleep and the localization of foci in temporal lobe epilepsy. *Neurology* 1991 ; 41 : 290-7.
50. Dinner DS, Luders H, Rothner AD, Erenberg G. Complex partial seizures of childhood onset: a clinical and electroencephalographic study. *Cleve Clin Q* 1984 ; 51 : 287-91.
51. Holmes GL. Partial seizures in children. *Pediatrics* 1986 ; 77 : 725-31.
52. Sperling MR, Mendius JR, Engel J. Mesial temporal spikes: a simultaneous comparison of sphenoidal, nasopharyngeal and ear electrodes. *Epilepsia* 1986 ; 27 : 81-6.

53. Chartrian GE, Lettich E, Nelson PL. Ten percent electrode system for topographic studies of spontaneous and evoked EEG activities. *Am J EEG Technol* 1985 ; 25 : 83-92.
54. Jayakar P, Duchowny M, Resnick T. Subdural monitoring in the evaluation of children for epilepsy surgery. *J Child Neurol* 1994 ; 9 : 2S61-6.
55. Dean P. Grids for kids: the pediatric patient undergoing invasive extraoperative EEG monitoring. *J Neurosci Nursing* 1994 ; 28 : 352-6.
56. Mattia D, Olivier A, Avoli M. Seizure-like discharges recorded in human dysplastic neocortex maintained *in vitro*. *Neurology* 1995 ; 45 : 1391-5.
57. Jayakar P, Duchowny M, Alvarez L, Resnick T. Intraictal activation in the neocortex: a marker of the epileptogenic region. *Epilepsia* 1994 ; 35 : 489-94.
58. Alvarez L, Jayakar PB. Cortical stimulation with subdural electrodes: special considerations in infancy and childhood. *J Epilepsy* 1990 ; 3 (Suppl 1) : 125-30.
59. Jayakar P, Resnick TJ, Duchowny MS, Alvarez LA. A safe and effective paradigm to functionally map the cortex in childhood. *J Clin Neurophysiol* 1992 ; 9 : 288-93.
60. Jayakar P, Duchowny M. Complex partial seizures of temporal lobe origin in early childhood. *J Epilepsy* 1990 ; 3 (suppl 1) : 41-5.
61. Brockhaus A, Elger C. Complex partial seizures of temporal lobe origin in children of different age groups. *Epilepsia* 1995 ; 36 : 1173-81.
62. Innocenti GM, Caminitti R. Postnatal shaping of callosal connections from sensory areas. *Brain Res* 1980 ; 38 : 381-94.
63. Rakic P, Bourgeois JP, Eckenhoff MF, Zecevic N, Goldman-Rakic PS. Concurrent overproduction of synapses in diverse regions of the primate cerebral cortex. *Science* 1986 ; 232 : 231 -2.
64. Lenn NJ, Freinkel AJ. Facial sparing as a feature of prenatal-onset hemiparesis. *Pediatr Neurol* 1989 ; 5 : 291-5.
65. Maegaki Y, Yamamoto T, Takeshita K. Plasticity of central motor and sensory pathways in a case of unilateral extensive cortical dysplasia: investigation of magnetic resonance imaging, transcranial magnetic stimulation, and short-latency somatosensory evoked potentials. *Neurology* 1995 ; 45 : 2255-61.
66. Goldman PS. Neuronal plasticity in primate telencephalon: anomalous projections induced by prenatal removal of frontal cortex. *Science* 1978 ; 202 : 767-8.
67. Goldman-Rakic PS, Galkin TW. Prenatal removal of frontal association cortex in the rhesus monkey: anatomical and functional consequences in prenatal life. *Brain Res* 1978 ; 52 : 451-85.
68. Rapin I. Acquired aphasia in children. *J Child Neurol* 1995 ; 10 : 267-70.
69. Woods BT, Carey S. Language deficits after apparent clinical recovery from childhood aphasia. *Ann Neurol* 1979 ; 6 : 405-49.
70. Alajouanine TH, Lhermitte F. Acquired aphasia in children. *Brain* 1965 ; 88 : 653-62.
71. Berger MS, Kincaid J, Ojemann GA, Lettich E. Brain mapping techniques to maximize resection, safety, and seizure control in children with brain tumors. *Neurosurgery* 1989 ; 25 : 786-92.
72. Duchowny M, Jayakar P, Harvey AS, Resnick T, Alvarez L, Dean P, Levin B. Language cortex representation: effects of developmental *versus* acquired pathology. *Ann Neurol* 1996 (in press).
73. Lesser R, Gordon B, Fisher R, Hart J, Uematsu S. Subdural grid electrodes in surgery of epilepsy. In : Luders H, ed. *Epilepsy surgery*. New York : Raven Press, 1991 : 399-408.
74. De Vos KJ, Wyllie E, Geckler C, Kotagel P, Comair Y. Language dominance in patients with early childhood tumors near left hemisphere language areas. *Neurology* 1995 ; 45 : 349-56.
75. Basser LS. Hemiplegia of early onset and the faculty of speech with special reference to the effects of hemispherectomy. *Brain* 1962 ; 85 : 427-60.

6

Hemifacial spasm or subcortical (infratentorial) epilepsy : a case report of a child with Goldenhar's syndrome and a pontomedullary junction lesion

A.A. ARZIMANOGLOU

Child Neurology Unit and Epilepsy Research Group, Hôpital Salpêtrière, Paris, France.

"ἡγήσεσθαι μὲν τὸν διδάξαντά με την τέχνην ταύτην ἴσα γενέτησιν εμοῖσι..." [*]

Repetitive, stereotypic movements of the face and head may occur in focal epilepsy or as manifestations of nonepileptic movement disorders. Simple partial seizures, due to discharges in the motor cortex, may present as clonic movements of the face, head and neck. Segmental myoclonus, and particularly palatal myoclonus, refers to regular or irregular repetitive contractions of muscles innervated by single or contiguous levels of the brainstem or spinal cord. Hemifacial spasm is characterized by clonic and tonic contractions of the muscles innervated by the facial nerve and mostly occurs in adults.

---

[*] "I will honour him who has taught me this Art even as one of my parents..." (Hippocrates oath).

We had the rare opportunity to study a child with Goldenhar's syndrome [1] (oculo-auriculo-vertebral dysplasia) and clonic movements of the left hemiface, who later also developped abnormal eye movements at a rhythm similar to what is observed in palatal myoclonus [1].

Case report

A boy, now aged 16 years old, was first hospitalized at the age of 3 months for suspicion of left-sided facial motor seizures. He was the second child of healthy, unrelated parents.

He presented with moderate dysmorphic features associating facial asymmetry and a rather small mandible. Ophthalmologic examination revealed an epibulbar dermoid cyst of the right corneal limb associated to a pretragus tag. Mild atrophy of the inferior part of the left iris was also noted and considered as the equivalent of a minor coloboma. Fundus was normal. Spine radiographies showed fusion of the pedicles of the second and third thoracic vertebrae. These abnormalities suggested Goldenhar's syndrome (oculo-auriculo-vertebral dysplasia). Mild axial hypotonia was noted, otherwise neurological examination was rather unremarkable.

At that age paroxysmal episodes consisted of a mostly tonic involuntary contraction of the left side of the face, with narrowing of the palpebral fissure and reddening of the face. Slight acceleration of the respiratory rythm could preceede. A mild clonic twitching was occasionally observed. Attacks could be repeated more than ten times a day and infrequently during sleep. Duration was variable (5 to 60 seconds) and no triggering factor could be suspected. After the age of two years, elevation of the left shoulder and contraction of the trapezius and sternomastoid muscles could be observed in a few attacks. In some episodes, there was diminished muscle tone in the neck with slight head nod. A grunting, cough-like, noise could inaugurate the attack. There was no apparent impairement of awareness and memory.

Interictal EEG tracings were normal. Ictal recordings were usually normal or could occasionally evidence a run of rythmical slow waves (2Hz) concerning the rolandic regions. We never recorded any spikes or flattening or a recruiting rythm. A first CTscan was considered normal. These episodes were considered as simple partial seizures and antiepileptics were prescribed, but despite several trials no effect could be obtained.

---

1. All those who have the chance to work with Jean Aicardi know the importance he attaches to careful clinical observation and analysis. For him "child neurology is, and probably will remain, a clinical discipline". The clinical presentation and evolution of symptomatology of the case reported here raise interesting issues regarding both the topography and the nature of the underlying dysfunction. It also illustrates the importance a clinician should attach in trying to establish the relationship between the clinical symptoms of his patient and the findings of a rapidly developing world of paraclinical examinations.

Global psychomotor development took place in a rather slow rythm but always remained within normal limits. He walked when 19 months old, he used single words by the age of 26 months and he could later follow a normal scholarship. He remained rather slow in manipulating objects. When four years old he experienced a generalized tonic-clonic seizure, in a febrile context. No focal signs could be evidenced, despite detailed questionning of the family, and this episode remained unique. A few months later, he was submitted to an internal urethrotomie for urethral narrowing and later to a left nephrectomy for a small non functional kidney.

Neuro-opthalmological examination at the age of six years revealed paresis of the left VI cranial nerve and a convergent strabismus that the boy compensated by a slight rotation of the head to the right. When the child was 10 years old, Magnetic Resonance Imaging revealed the presence of a mass lesion (Figure 1), hyposignal in T1 sequences and hypersignal in T2, developing in the left cerebellar peduncle at the level of the pontomedullary junction. The lesion, impinging on the 4th ventricle and with a clear mass effect on the brainstem structures, did not cross the midline. It was considered to

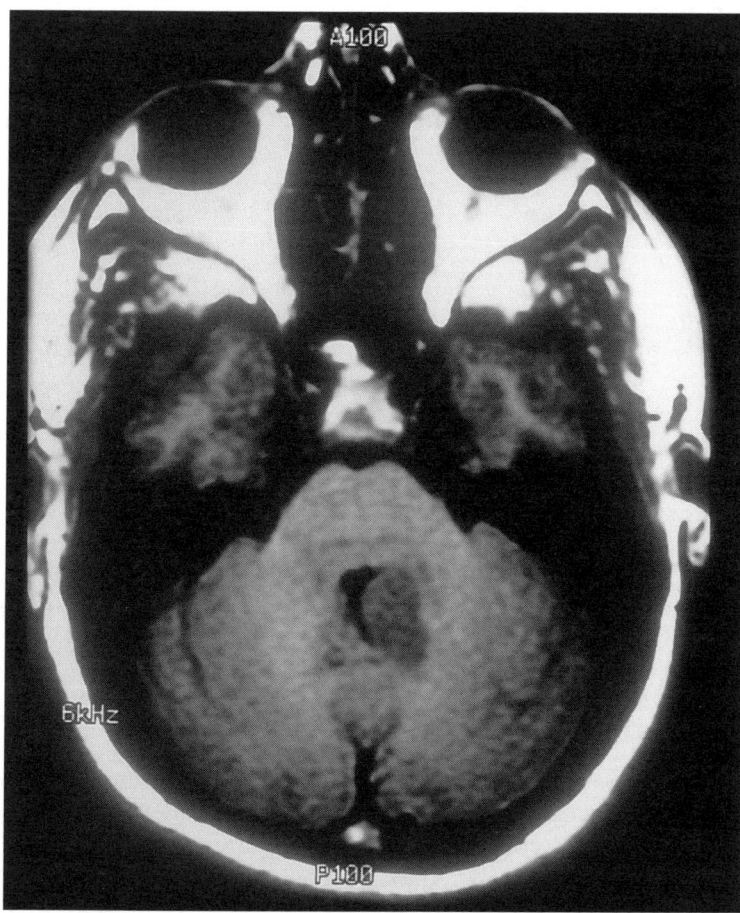

Figure 1. Mass lesion, returning a low signal in T1 sequences (high signal in T2), developing in the left pontomedullary junction impinging on the IV ventricle.

be a hamartoma. Repeated MRI examinations over the last 4 years did not show any change in shape, aspect, volume or mass effect.

At the age of 11 years, abnormal eye movements were noted for the first time. They had a rhythmical character and small amplitude, and were obliquely directed left and upwards with a clockwise rotatory component. They were synchronous with palpebral movements and contraction of chin muscles, identical to those in myorythmias but without involvement of the palate. They could persist during sleep. A concomitant mild contraction of the hemiface could be suspected.

Electrodiagnostic studies of facial muscles showed no clear signs of acute denervation. Minimal elements in favor of partial denervation were suspected. Voluntary activity of the orbicularis oculi was not strictly normal, but there was no significant difference between the involved and the uninvolved sides. Multiple discharges corresponding to rythmical movements could be registered. Brainstem auditory evoked potentials did not reveal any abnormality of the auditory pathways. The von Bekesy audiometer studies evidenced bilateral tone decay, with left predominance.

The patient is now a 16 year old young boy following normal school. Episodes of hemifacial twiching persist daily. Antiepileptic medication has been reduced to a minimal "security" dose. Surgical resection has been discussed but postponed, considering the infinitesimal interference of the attacks in the child's everyday life.

Discussion

Our patient presented with several dysmorphic features as observed in Goldenhar's syndrome [1]. For this syndrome the term of oculo-auriculo-vertebral spectrum is used by some authors [2] and it implies anomalies of the first and second branchial arches. While there is no agreement upon minimal diagnostic criteria, the facial phenotype is characteristic when enough manifestations are present. Involvement may not be limited to facial structures; cardiac, renal, skeletal, and other anomalies may also occur. In particular, the so-called "expanded Goldenhar complex" has demonstrated a wide spectrum of central nervous system malformations [3-8].

Daily episodes of hemifacial contraction rose several questions. Focal epilepsy originating in the facial area of the cortical motor strip seems highly improbable if we consider the character of the movement, the absence of any ictal EEG abnormality, the lack of response to numerous antiepileptic drugs, the topography of the jerks, and finally the presence of a bulbopontine mass lesion in contrast to the absence of any cortical lesion on several MRI examinations.

The tonic component of our patient's attacks, concerning mainly the lips, could evoke hemifacial spasm (HFS). This condition was described in 1888 by Gowers [9] and Cushing [10] referred to it as "tic convulsif" for cases occuring with trigeminal neuralgia. HFS is a disorder of adult life, characterized by rapid, irregular paroxysms of clonic twiching of one or more muscle groups innervated by the facial nerve. The twiches usually begin unilaterally about the eye and then spread to other facial muscles, but never beyond the domain of the facial nerve [11]. HFS is one of the few movement disorders that may persist during sleep.

The mechanism of HFS has been as elusive as the proposed locus of pathology, since even with pathologic data the exact location of lesion remains unknown. Digre and Corbett [12] recently discussed the different theories to explain HFS. In the early 1960s, Gardner and Sava [13] proposed that the facial nerve root exit zone at the pons was the most likely site of pathology and that irritation of the sensory portion of the VIIth cranial nerve may directly stimulate the motor segment. Auger [14], Janetta [15], and Nielsen [16] have adopted this theory and relabelled it "ephaptic transmission". Moller [17] proposed an alternative theory that he labeled "kindling" effect, according to which the root entry zone or "damaged" area becomes a trigger where impulses are generated and transmitted orthodromically as well as antidromically. The antidromic impulses activate facial nuclei motoneurons which cells in turn send impulses down the seventh cranial nerve and cause hemifacial spasm. For Digre and Corbett [12] both theories — the "ephaptic" and the "kindling" — are attractive but at this time there is no consensus regarding interpretation of the neurophysiologic data. In several reports the majority of patients with HFS have mechanical compression of the facial nerve at the root exit zone by an arterial loop or a compressive mass. Complete relief is usually obtained by surgery that supresses mechanical compression [15]. The "kindling" hypothesis seems difficult to accept, for cases that show immediate improvement following decompresive surgery.

To note that our patient presented with a mass lesion at the level of the pontomedullary junction. The initial symptomatology (repetitive left facial tonic contractions lasting 5 to 60 seconds) could be due to direct irritation of the VIIth nerve nucleus or of the depending fibers. However, hemifacial spasm is almost exclusively observed in adults or older children and association to a tumor is exceptionnal. Furthermore, our patient presented propagation of the discharge to bulbar centers (expressed by a grunting noise) and upper spinal cord (shoulder contraction and elevation). These elements reinforce the intial hypothesis of simple partial seizures.

We are aware of a case with similar symptomatology [18] where excision of a hamartomatous lesion permitted complete control of the twitching of the eyelid and the hemifacial jerks in a 3 year old child. Al-Shahwan et al. [19] recently reported two cases with what they consider to be "hemisomatic" spasms caused by a ganglioglioma in the region of the ipsilateral cerebellopontine angle. To our opinion, absence of paroxysmal activity on scalp EEG during the episodes does not necessarily exclude the hypothesis of seizures.

Later in life, the child presented with abnormal eye movements of a rhythmical character and small amplitude that could persist during sleep. They were identical to those seen in myorythmias, but without involvement of the palate. Rhythmic palatal myoclonus is a rare movement disorder characterized by rhythmic jerky movements of the soft palate and sometimes other brainstem-innervated muscles. Most of the cases reported in the literature are considered as symptomatic, secondary to brainstem or cerebellar disease. Some patients, however, fail to show evidence of a structural lesion [20]. The movements are usually bilateral and symmetric, occuring between 100 to 150 times per minute, and persist during sleep.

Compared with other movement disorders the pathology of this hyperkinesia is rather well established due to the pioneering work of Klien [21], Guillain and Mollaret [22], Lapresle and Ben Hamida [23, 24]. Palatal myoclonus, also referred to as palatal tremor or brainstem myorhythmia, is nowadays regarded as the prototype of a hyperkinetic movement disorder depending on a central pacemaker [25] chiefly because the rhythmic jerks are time-locked in different muscles [20]. The inferior olive is considered to be the pacemaker [26]. Furthermore, there is much evidence that "hypertrophic degeneration" of the inferior olive develops secondary to a lesion within a pathway from the contralateral dentate nucleus *via* the brachium conjonctivum and the ipsilateral central tegmental tract to the inferior olive [23, 24], originally referred to as the Guillain-Mollaret triangle.

Involvement of additional muscles or muscle groups in the rhytmic palatal myoclonic activity is a known phenomenon [20]. The general criterion for the involvement of a muscle in the hyperkinesia is that it shows jerks synchronous with those in the soft palate. The muscle groups concerned may be those of the eyes, the face, the tongue and larynx, and even the head, trunk, intercostal muscles and diaphragm. In patients with symptomatic rhythmic palatal myoclonus the pharynx is often also visibly involved in the hyperkinesia and the next more frequent manifestation is involvement of lower facial muscles, usually of the chin or periorally [20].

Focal rhythmic movements of the muscles innervated by the branchial arches can occur without palatal myoclonus [27]. Denny-Brown [28] referred to this as bulbar myoclonus. Branchial myoclonus may involve the lips, face, and platysma, the platysma only, or the neck and larynx. In general, the frequency of the movements and the clinical characteristics of the disorder are similar to those of palatal myoclonus, as are the etiologies [27]. Lapresle [29] also notes that these movements may be observed occasionally in skeletal muscles, that they may be associated and synchronous with palatal myoclonus or isolated, but that they always are rythmic and prolonged.

In our patient, ocular and skelettal myorhythmias suggest involvement of the Guillain-Mollaret triangle. In their original report Guillain and Mollaret discuss the possibilty of partial facial myoclonus without palatal involvement. They accept that absence of palatal myoclonus does not necessarily exclude a similar origin for the isolated myoclonic jerks, although they feel obliged to stress the characteristically rythmical aspect of the movement disorder. Furthermore, they point out the fact that in all known clinical observations in which symptomatology changed with time the only component that never regressed was myoclonus.

The variable involvement of additional muscles or muscle groups in the rhythmic palatal myoclonus may be the result of the somatotopic organization of the inferior olive

[30]. Only part of it could undergo hypertrophic degeneration [24, 31] and thereby somatotopic connections could determine the extent of muscles involved in the rhythmic movements. Future investigations will have to explain which principles govern the involvement of different muscles [20] and how myoclonus of the palate may be absent.

The mechanisms involved in our patient's symptomatology are rather difficult to elucidate. The aspect of the bulbopontine lesion and the absence of any sign of evolution on 4 repeated MRI's during a sixteen years follow-up highly suggests a lesion of dysplastic nature. The episodes of hemifacial tonic contraction were stereotyped and of a paroxysmal nature, thus being highly suggestive of an epileptic activity. Several recent reports [32-34] prove that lesions of this type may participate at the genesis of seizures. This hypothesis was confirmed by depth electrodes in patients with an hypothalamic hamartoma and gelastic seizures.

Harvey *et al.* (unpublished data) obtained ictal EEG recordings with posterior cranial fossa electrodes in an infant presenting with daily episodes of left hemifacial contraction and head and eye deviation. MRI revealed a mass in the left cerebellar hemisphere and peduncle. They demonstrated focal seizure activity in the region of the mass. Resection of the mass, which proved to be a ganglioglioma, resulted in remission of seizures.

We suggest that in our patient, the association of anomalies of the brachial arches to a pontine lesion, were responsible for paroxysmal attacks, that could represent epileptic activity due to the congenital lesion. Symptomatology progressively evolved to a more complex clinical syndrome involving the dentato-olivary pathway. Existing anomalies of the brachial arches and the presence of a compressive effect could be at the origin of a secondary "hypertrophic degeneration" of a part of the inferior olive, responsible for the appearance of focal rhythmic movements of muscles innervated by the brachial arches, but without involvement of the palate.

References

1. Goldenhar M. Associations malformatives de l'œil et de l'oreille, en particulier le syndrome dermoïde epibulbaire-appendices auriculaires-fistula auris congenita et ses relations avec la dysostose mandibulo-faciale. *J Genet Hum* 1952 ; 1 : 243-82.
2. Gorlin RJ, Cohen MM Jr, Levin LS. Branchial arch and oro-acral disorders. In : *Syndromes of the head and neck*. Oxford Monographs on Medical Genetics n° 19. Oxford University Press, 1990 : 641-91.
3. Aleksic S, *et al.* Unilateral arhinencephaly in Goldenhar-Gorlin syndrome. *Dev Med Child Neurol* 1975 ; 17 : 498-504.
4. Aleksic S, *et al.* Congenital ophthalmoplegia in oculoauriculovertebral dysplasia in hemifacial microsomia (Goldenhar-Gorlin syndrome). *Neurology* 1976 ; 26 : 638-44.
5. Aleksic S, *et al.* Encephalocele (cerebellocele) in the Goldenhar-Gorlin syndrome. *Eur J Pediatr* 1983 ; 140 : 137-8.

6. Aleksic S, et al. Intracranial lipomas, hydrocephalus and other CNS anomalies in oculoauriculo-vertebral dysplasia (Goldenhar-Gorlin syndrome). *Child's Brain* 1984 ; 11 : 285-97.
7. Pauli R, et al. Goldenhar association and cranial defects. *Am J Med Genet* 1983 ; 15 : 177-9.
8. Wilson GN. Cranial defects in Goldenhar's syndrome. *Am J Med Genet* 1983 ; 14 : 435-43.
9. Gowers WR. *A manual of diseases of the nervous system.* Philadelphia : P Blakinston and Company, 1888 : 660-9.
10. Cushing H. The major trigeminal neuralgias and their surgical treatment based on experience with 332 gasserian operations. *Am J Med Sci* 1920 ; 160 : 157-84.
11. Hanson MR, Sweeney PJ. Lower cranial neuropathies. In : Bradley WG, Daroff RB, Fenichel GM, Marsden CD, eds. *Neurology in clinical practice* Butterworth-Heinemann, 1991 : 217-30.
12. Digre K, Corbett JJ. Hemifacial spasm : differential diagnosis, mechanism and treatmen. In : Jankovik J, Tolosa E. eds. *Advances in neurology, vol. 49 : Facial dyskinesias.* New York : Raven Press 1988 : 151-76.
13. Gardner WJ, Sava G. Hemifacial spasm - a reversible pathophysiologic state. *J Neurosurg* 1962 ; 19 : 240-7.
14. Auger RG. Hemifacial spasm: clinical and electrophysiologic observations *Neurology* 1979 ; 29 : 1261-72.
15. Janetta PJ, Abbasy M, Maroon JC, et al. Etiology and definitive microsurgical treatment of hemifacial spasm: operative techniques and results in 47 patients. *J Neurosurg* 1977 ; 47 : 321-8.
16. Nielsen VK. Electrophysiology of the facial nerve in hemifacial spasm: ectopic/ephaptic excitation. *Muscle Nerve* 1985 ; 8 : 545-55.
17. Moller AR, Janetta PJ. On the origin of synkinesis in hemifacial spasm: results of intracranial recording. *J Neurosurg* 1984 ; 61 : 569-76.
18. Rodriguez D, Delalande O, Jedynak J, Ponsot G. Hamartome du plancher du IV ventricule responsable d'hemispasmes faciaux à début néonatal. 3rd Congress of the French Child Neurologie Society, Lille, January 1993 (personal communication).
19. Al-Shahwan SA, Singh B, Riela A, Roach ES. Hemisomatic spasms in children. *Neurology* 1994 ; 44 : 1332-3.
20. Deuschl G, Mischke G, Schenck E, et al. Symptomatic and essential rhythmic palatal myoclonus. *Brain* 1990 ; 113 : 1645-72.
21. Klien H. Zur pathologie der kontinuierlichen rhythmischen Krämpfe der Schlingmuskulatur (2 Fälle von Erweichungsherden im Kleinhirn). *Neurologisches Centralblatt* 1907 ; 26 : 245-54.
22. Guillain G, Mollaret P. Deux cas de myoclonies synchrones et rythmées vélo-pharyngo-laryngo-oculo-diaphragmatiques. Le problème anatomique et physio-pathologique de ce syndrome. *Rev Neurol* 1931 ; 2 : 545-66.
23. Lapresle J, Ben Hamida M. Correspondance somatotopique, secteur par secteur, des dégénérescences de l'olive bulbaire consécutives à des lésions limitées du noyau dentelé contro-latéral : étude de 4 observations anatomiques. *Rev Neurol* 1965 ; 113 : 439-48.
24. Lapresle J, Ben Hamida M. Contribution à la connaissance de la voie dento-olivaire : étude anatomique de deux cas de dégénérescence hypertrophique de l'olive bulbaire secondaire à un ramollissement limité de la calotte mésencéphalique. *Presse Med* 1968 ; 76 : 1226-30.
25. Llinas RR. Rebound excitation as the physiological basis for tremor: a biophysical study of the oscillatory properties of mammalian central neurones *in vitro*. In : Findley LJ, Capildeo R, eds. *Movement disorders: tremor.* London : Macmillan, 1984 : 165-82.
26. Trelles JO. Les myoclonies vélo-palatines. Considérations anatomiques et physiopathologiques. *Rev Neurol* 1968 ; 119 : 165-71.
27. Dubinsky RM, Hallett M. Palatal myoclonus and facial involvement in other types of myoclonus. In : Jankovik J, Tolosa E, eds *Advances in neurology, vol. 49 : Facial dyskinesias.* New York : Raven Press, 1988 : 263-78.

28. Denny-Brown D. Discussion. *Trans Am Neurol Assoc* 1956 ; 8 : 62-3.
29. Lapresle J. Rhythmic palatal myoclonus and the dentato-olivary pathway. *J Neurol* 1979 ; 220 : 223-30.
30. Beitz AJ. The topographical organization of the olivo-dentate and dentato-olivary pathways in the cat. *Brain Res* 1976 ; 115 : 311-7.
31. Gautier JC, Blackwood W. Enlargement of the inferior olive nucleus in association with lesions of the central tegmental tract or dentate nucleus. *Brain* 1961 ; 84 : 341-61.
32. Kahane P, Tassi L, Hoffmann D, *et al.* Crises dacrystiques et hamartome hypothalamique. A propos d'une observation Vidéo-SEEG. *Epilepsies* 1994 ; 6 : 259-79.
33. Munari C, Kahane P, Francione S, *et al.* Role of the hypothalamic hamartoma in the genesis of gelastic fits (Video-SEEG study). *Electroenceph Clin Neurophysiol* 1995 ; 95 : 154-60.
34. Francione S, Kahane P, Tassi L, *et al.* Stereo-EEG of interictal and ictal electrical activity of a histologically proved heterotopic grey matter associated with partial epilepsy. *Electroenceph Clin Neurophysiol* 1994 ; 90 : 284-90.

7

Epilepsy, autistic regression and disintegrative disorder

I. RAPIN

Saul R. Korey Department of Neurology, Department of Pediatrics, and Rose F. Kennedy Center for Research in Mental Retardation and Human Development, Albert Einstein College of Medicine, Bronx, NY, USA.

Disorders on the autistic spectrum: definitions

Autism is a behaviorally defined disorder of the immature brain for which there is no biologic test. It is defined on the basis of a series of aberrant behaviors involving interpersonal interaction (sociability and affect), verbal and nonverbal communication, symbolic play, range of interests and activities, and perseveration. As pointed out by Lorna Wing [1], autism has a wide range of severity so that it is helpful to think of the autistic spectrum rather than of autism as a disorder with a narrow symptomatology. At the biologic level, autism has many etiologies, some genetic, others acquired, and in some cases it may arise as a consequence of the interaction of a genetic vulnerability with some deleterious environmental circumstance. At the central nervous system level, the meager anatomic evidence uncovered by Bauman and Kemper [2] points to cellular maldevelopment in the hippocampus, amygdala, other limbic areas, and neocerebellum dating to early gestation. There is also suggestive evidence for distinctive cellular findings in children and adult autistic individuals, but the evidence is so sparse that further well studied cases are needed for secure interpretation.

In the 1994 Diagnostic and Statistical Manual of the American Psychiatric Association (DSM IV) [3] the term pervasive developmental disorder (PDD), and in the 1993 10th edition of the International Classification of Diseases (ICD-10) [4], the term autism are the umbrella categories for a group of disorders with this common core of behavioral symptoms. Autistic disorder (AD) (DSM IV) or childhood autism (ICD-10) are the categories for the full classic syndrome, manifest before age 3 years, whereas disintegrative disorder (DD) denotes regression of language, sociability and cognition after fully normal early development in a child of at least 2 years who was speaking in sentences. Asperger syndrome is to be used for a child with autistic symptomatology who did not speak late, is not mentally deficient but may be clumsy, and, unlike the majority of children on the autistic spectrum, may have a higher verbal than performance IQ. Pervasive developmental disorder-not otherwise specified (PDD-NOS) (DSM IV) or atypical autism (ICD-10) for children who do not fit these categories nor that of Rett syndrome, a biologically-defined syndrome of girls described by Hagberg, Aicardi, Dias, and Ramos [5].

Cognitive level is not a defining feature of AD or PDD-NOS, although the literature states that a majority, some 70% of autistic individuals, are mentally deficient. A most important point for pediatricians and child neurologists: one cannot predict cognitive outcome reliably in preschool children on the autistic spectrum; the ability to speak at that age, although of course encouraging, is not necessarily the harbinger of normal or near normal intelligence, nor is lack of speech beyond the age of 5 years a completely reliable sign of poor outcome. Neither are exceptional but isolated nonverbal skills encountered in a number of mentally deficient autistic persons.

Language regression with/without behavioral regression

Some 30% of parents of autistic children report that their child, who may or may not have been entirely normal until then, underwent an usually insidious, rarely abrupt, loss of the words he or she had acquired. This loss is associated with regression in social skills and play and usually takes place between 18 and 30 months, but may occur as early as one year and as late as 3 years [6]. Disintegrative disorder (DD) refers to regression in a child of at least 2 years, or at any age thereafter, who was speaking and behaving entirely normally up to then. The regression in DD impairs cognition as well as sociability, language, and range of interests and activities, and thus has essentially the same characteristics as autistic regression. The term disintegrative disorder is preferable to disintegrative psychosis; although children with DD may have very deviant behaviors such as smearing feces, destructiveness, or self-injury, these same aberrant behaviors may occur in severely affected autistic children without regression, and it is doubtful that children with DD hallucinate or have a primary thought disorder. Furthermore the demarcation between autistic regression and DD is not sharp, especially in children who regress between ages 2 and 3 years [7]. Prognosis for significant improvement of language and behavior is generally better in autistic regression than in DD which tends to have a dismal prognosis [8], but, again, prognosis is unpredictable early on.

When language loss occurs without significant behavioral or cognitive regression in the context of either clinical seizures or a paroxysmal EEG, the disorder is called acquired epileptic aphasia or Landau-Kleffner syndrome (LKS) [9]. Confusion arises because LKS overlaps with autistic regression and disintegrative disorder in those children in whom global behavioral regression is associated with seizures or a paroxysmal EEG. The term LKS, which implies acquired epileptic aphasia, is clearly inappropriate for children with regression who have neither clinical seizures nor a paroxysmal EEG.

By far the most prevalent language disorder in children with classic LKS is a severe receptive language deficit of the verbal auditory agnosia (VAA) type. VAA also occurs in children with developmental language disorders (DLD), but it is particularly prevalent in autistic children with or without regression [10]. Recent evidence points to an auditory perceptual deficit with secondary inability to decode phonology so that, strictly speaking, the terms VAA or word deafness may not be exactly correct, although auditory perceptual deficit results in a profound impairment in consonant discrimination and thus in the language deficit [11]. Because young children are in the process of acquiring language, a mixed receptive/expressive disorder is the inevitable consequence of inadequate reception. If children with VAA speak at all their phonology is very distorted. In a few children with VAA, Lou [12] and others have shown hypoperfusion of the temporal region. The EEG in LKS is similar to that of Rolandic epilepsy.

In a minority of children with LKS it is expression that is affected, with spared reception [*e.g.*, 13]. In such cases, the language disorder may have the characteristics of verbal dyspraxia, with or without oromotor dyspraxia, and resemble the anterior opercular syndrome of Foix-Chavany-Marie. Children with anterior foci may be less likely to have associated autistic features than those with posterior foci and comprehension deficits. However, Roulet-Perez *et al.* [14] point out that frontal epileptic foci may be responsible for some cases of severe but reversible language and behavioral regression associated with electrical status epilepticus in slow wave sleep (ESES) [15].

Epilepsy, autism, and the Landau-Kleffner syndrome

It is well established that epilepsy is considerably more prevalent in autism than in the general population; in fact this observation was one of the first irrefutable arguments against its psychogenic cause. According to a number of studies, including those performed by Tuchman *et al.* [16] and Ballaban-Gil *et al.* [17], in my patients, the cumulative probability of epilepsy increases across childhood to reach some 30%, with a second peak in adolescence. All seizure types occur in children with DLD and AD. Tuchman [16] showed that the probability of seizures among autistic children is correlated with motor deficit and mental deficiency and therefore with the severity of the underlying brain dysfunction. In contrast, although the prevalence of epilepsy is somewhat higher in early childhood in autistic children with normal or near normal intelligence than in controls, there is no increase in the prevalence of epilepsy with age. Tuchman [16] found a link between the VAA type of language disorder and the prevalence of epilepsy in both DLD and AD, presumably because VAA denotes temporal dysfunction and the temporal lobe has the lowest seizure threshold.

An unresolved question is whether epilepsy is the cause of LKS (and perhaps of some cases of autistic regression and DD), as argued persuasively by Deonna [18, 19] and others, or whether both the epilepsy and language loss are the common manifestations of some as yet undefined underlying brain dysfunction. In the majority of cases of LKS the seizures and EEG abnormality have a much more benign course and are more amenable to medical treatment than the language disorder which tends to persist for many weeks, months, or even years. On the other hand, there are well documented case reports of LKS in which antiepileptic treatment resulted in prompt and convincing improvement in both language and behavior. Unfortunately the efficacy of anticonvulsant medications or ACTH/steroids is unpredictable because they are often ineffective, whether because the wrong drug was used, the dose was inadequate, the treatment was not started early enough, or because epilepsy was not the responsible pathogenetic agent in these cases remains undetermined.

There are no reliable figures on the prevalence of epilepsy or paroxysmal EEGs in autistic regression and DD because few systematic studies have been performed in either disorder. Among 239 children I saw in consultation prior to 1988, 104 (39%) were reported to have undergone a regression, but only 20 (19%) of them had epilepsy. This figure may be an underestimate because many of the children were still preschoolers when seen and there was no systematic sleep EEG recording or follow-up. Kurita et al. [6] found that there was no difference in the prevalence of abnormal EEGs (28%) in 192 autistic children with and without a history of regression, whereas the prevalence was much higher (61%) in 18 children with DD, although even in these children the prevalence of clinical epilepsy was only 11%. Perhaps some of these children had undetected ESES. Some but not all children with ESES present the clinical picture of DD. Other children with DD have an EEG abnormality or seizures similar to those of children with LKS, and some children have neither seizures nor EEG abnormalities. Roulet-Perez et al. [14] described variable combinations of epilepsy, language and behavioral regression in ESES and suggested that such cases may be due to frontal epileptogenic foci that may improve with appropriate antiepileptic therapy.

Conclusion

Much remains to be done in sorting out the role of epilepsy in LKS, autistic regression, and DD. For the time being, it is unwarranted to substitute the diagnosis of LKS for that of autism or DD with epilepsy in a child who lost his language, has seizures or a paroxysmal EEG, and has clear autistic behaviors. Whereas, by definition, epilepsy or a paroxysmal EEG is required for a diagnosis of LKS, data available thus far indicate that only in a minority of cases are autistic regression and DD associated with epilepsy. It is of course extremely important to identify those children who have evidence of subclinical epilepsy because of the possibility that treatment of the epilepsy may, in some of them, have a favorable influence on both the epilepsy and the language and behavioral deficits. The question of whether epilepsy is the cause or simply a concomitant of the language and/or behavioral regression remains to be determined. Unfortunately, although the seizures may respond to steroids or anticonvulsants, there is no guarantee that either the language or the behavior will improve substantially, although they may. Therefore pessimism is unwarranted and a trial of therapy, making no promise of success, is justified if a prolonged sleep EEG uncovers paroxysmal activity. Answers to these puzzles await an understanding of the pathophysiology of LKS, autistic regression, and DD.

Acknowledgement

Supported in part by Program Project Grant NS 20489 from the National Institute of Neurological Disorders and Stroke, United States Public Health Service.

Abbreviations

AD: autistic disorder
DD: disintegrative disorder
DLD: developmental language disorder
LKS: Landau-Kleffner syndrome
PDD: pervasive developmental disorder
PDD-NOS: pervasive developmental disorder - not otherwise specified
VAA: verbal auditory agnosia

References

1. Wing L. The relationship between Asperger's syndrome and Kanner's autism. In : Frith U, ed. *Autism and Asperger syndrome*. Cambridge UK : Cambridge University Press, 1991 : 93-121.
2. Bauman ML, Kemper TL. Neuroanatomic observations of the brain in autism. In : Bauman ML, Kemper TL, eds. *The neurobiology of autism*. Baltimore MD : The Johns Hopkins University Press, 1994 : 119-45.
3. American Psychiatric Association. *Diagnostic and statistical manual of mental disorders* 4th ed. Washington DC : American Psychiatric Association, 1994.
4. World Health Organization. *Mental disorders: glossary and guide to their classification in accordance with the tenth revision of the international classification of diseases*. Geneva ; WHO, 1993.
5. Hagberg B, Aicardi J, Dias K, Ramos O. A progressive syndrome of autism, dementia, ataxia, and loss of purposeful hand use in girls: Rett's syndrome: report of 35 cases. *Ann Neurol* 1983 ; 14 : 471-9.

6. Kurita H, Kita M, Miyake Y. A comparative study of development and symptoms among disintegrative psychosis and infantile autism with and without speech loss. *J Aut Dev Disord* 1992 ; 22 : 175-88.
7. Rapin I. Autistic regression and disintegrative disorder: how important the role of epilepsy? *Semin Pediat Neurol* 1995 (in press).
8. Volkmar FR, Cohen DJ. Disintegrative disorder or "late-onset autism". *J Child Psychol Psychiatr* 1989 ; 30 : 717-24.
9. Dugas M, Gérard CL, Franc S, Sagar D. Natural history, course and prognosis of the Landau and Kleffner syndrome. In : Pavao Martins I, Castro-Caldas A, van Dongen HR, van Hout A, eds. *Acquired aphasia in children: acquisition and breakdown of language in the developing brain.* Dordrecht NL : Kluwer Academic Publishers, 1991 : 263-77.
10. Allen DA, Rapin I. Autistic children are also dysphasic. In : Naruse H, Ornitz EM, eds. *Neurobiology of infantile autism.* Amsterdam : Excerpta Medica, 1992 : 157-68.
11. Tallal P, Miller S, Fitch RH. Neurobiological basis of speech: a case for the preeminence of temporal processing. In : Tallal P, Galaburda AM, Llinas RR, von Euler C, eds. *Temporal information processing in the nervous system: special reference to dyslexia and dysphasia.* New York : New York Academy of Sciences, 1993 : 27-49.
12. Lou HC. Cerebral single photon emission tomography (SPECT) and positron emission tomography (PET) during development and in learning disorders. In : Rapin I, Segalowitz SJ, eds. *Child neuropsychology.* Amsterdam : Elsevier Science, 1992 : 331-8.
13. Deonna T, Roulet E, Fontan D, Marcoz J-P. Speech and oromotor deficits of epileptic origin in benign partial epilepsy of childhood with rolandic spikes (BPERS): relationship to the acquired aphasia-epilepsy syndrome. *Neuropediatrics* 1993 ; 2 : 83-7.
14. Roulet Perez E, Davidoff V, Despland P-A, Deonna T. Mental and behavioural deterioration of children with epilepsy and CSWS: acquired epileptic frontal syndrome. *Dev Med Child Neurol* 1993 ; 35 : 661-74.
15. Jayakar PB, Seshia SS. Electrical status epilepticus during slow-wave sleep: a review. *J Clin Neurophysiol* 1991 ; 7 : 299-311.
16. Tuchman RF, Rapin I, Shinnar S. Autistic and dysphasic children. I: clinical characteristics. II: epilepsy. *Pediatrics* 1991 ; 6 : 1211-8, 1219-25.
17. Ballaban-Gil K, Rapin I, Tuchman RF, *et al.* Autism: longterm outcomes in adolescents and young adults. 1995 (submitted).
18. Deonna TW. Acquired epileptiform aphasia in children (Landau-Kleffner syndrome). *J Clin Neurophysiol* 1991 ; 3 : 288-98.
19. Deonna T, Ziegler A-L, Mourra-Serra J, Innocenti G. Autistic regression in relation to limbic pathology and epilepsy: report of two cases. *Dev Med Child Neurol* 1993 ; 35 : 186-96.

8

Cognitive disorders in childhood epilepsy

O. DULAC

Neuropediatrics Department, Hôpital Saint-Vincent-de-Paul, Paris, France.

The occurrence of cognitive disorders is a major issue of epilepsy in childhood. It is correlated with duration of epilepsy, but may occur in patients who exhibit very few or even no seizures at all. Therefore, the mechanisms involved are various. The etiology of the disease and the type of epilepsy play a major role in determining the type of cognitive disorder.

In progressive diseases due to inborn errors of metabolism in which brain atrophy progresses over a period of several months or years, cognitive deterioration occurs even if seizures are properly controlled. In this setting, neuronal damage by endogenous toxicity is of course the major cause of cognitive deterioration.

In partial epilepsy, patients exhibit selective cognitive troubles corresponding to the epileptogenic zone. There may be speech trouble in left temporal epilepsy, memory disorders in mesial temporal epilepsy, or change in laterality in left parietal epilepsy. The defect is often correlated with hypoperfusion or hypometabolism on functional imaging. The cause of cognitive disorder may be partly due to a focal lesion, but partly to the seizures themselves, and improve therefore after the control of seizures is obtained. Thus the mechanism is similar to troubles observed in adults with partial epilepsy. There is therefore a combination of functional and lesional phenomena.

In generalized epilepsy with convulsive seizures, seizures play an important role. However, even after full-control of seizures, it is relatively common to observe behaviour difficulties with hyperkinesia, and visual memory disorders [1]. The occurrence of convulsive status epilepticus in the first year of life is a frequent characteristic of intractable epilepsy with convulsive seizures in the first year of life, called either severe myoclonic epilepsy of infancy [2] or polymorphous epilepsy of infancy [3]. It is often followed by the development of autistic-like behaviour. It is likely that lesions produced in areas experiencing rapid development at this age, *i.e.* gnosic functions, account for such cognitive and behavioural troubles.

The most difficult situation involves epileptogenic encephalopathies, West syndrome (WS), Lennox-Gastaut syndrome (LGS) and the syndrome of Continuous Spike Waves during Slow Sleep (CSWS). These conditions seem to be intermediate disorders between epilepsy (*e.g.* recurrent seizures separated by interictal periods) and status epilepticus (*e.g.* a prolonged epileptic condition). Indeed, in epileptogenic encephalopathies, seizures are separated by periods that are not properly interictal since there are permanent neurological manifestations consisting of cognitive or motor defects. Some patients exhibit rare or even no seizures throughout the disorder, and there is no correlation of the type of defect with the type of seizures. A patient may exhibit speech troubles with spasms or with massive myoclonus, two seizure types that do not involve the temporal lobe. On the other hand, selective cognitive or motor trouble correlate well with the topography of so-called interictal spike activity, and the function involved is usually the most recently acquired as if areas in development were particularly prone to experience such a phenomenon during the period of development, of the given function [4, 5]. When the spike activity disappears with acute administration of antiepileptic medication, cognitive functions do not improve immediately. It is only within several weeks or months that progressive recovery may be obtained if paroxysmal EEG activity is controlled, as if the patient had recovered the ability to develop the cognitive function, not the cognitive function itself.

The age of occurrence of these encephalopathies involves 2 major periods: between 3 and 12 months, and between 2 and 8 years. The first period corresponds to the development of visual and auditive gnosis functions. The second one to more elaborated functions such as speech and functions of the frontal lobe that can only develop after the gnosis functions have been acquired. It is interesting to notice that the functions that are the most affected in West syndrome are gnosic functions, particularly visual agnosia [4]. In CSWS syndrome, the cognitive troubles consist mainly of speech deterioration or frontal lobe syndrome [5]; the latter is also the most affected in Lennox-Gastaut syndrome. Therefore, the most affected cognitive functions are those that are presently developing when the epileptogenic encephalopathy develops. The period during which the syndrome may develop is limited, with either spontaneous recovery or conversion to another type of epilepsy with aging. Spasms and hypsarrhythmia usually disappear in early childhood; CSWS disappear before puberty. Although tonic seizures of LGS persist into adulthood, atypical absence seizures and slow spike waves also tend to diminish in the second decade. The risk period for syndrome onset corresponds, therefore, to what may be considered as a "critical developmental period" for the specific affected cognitive function. Similarly, the usual remission age of the complete pattern of these syndromes also corresponds to the end of this "critical period". If the epilepsy has persisted during this time, spontaneous recovery occurs at the cost of loss of the ability to recover the corresponding function, *i.e.* agnosia, language, and judgment. In addition, abnormal development of the elementary functions may result in abnormal development of the more elaborate functions, *i.e.* auditory agnosia precludes the later language development.

In the first years of life, the brain undergoes rapid maturation; it is not a miniature adult brain. This early postnatal period is indeed a critical period for epilepsy. During the early postnatal period in animals, which could correspond to the first or the second year of life in humans, the cortex is more excitable than it is in later life, and a focal discharge is more likely to become generalized, asynchronously, to the entire cortex. Indeed, N-methyl-D-asparate (NMDA) receptors are in excess, in relation to the development of the neuronal network, as shown in animal visual pathways during the critical developmental period. Axonal collaterals are redundant and subcortical structures that contribute to prevent generalization in later life, such as the substantia nigra, are ineffective. Myelination of the hemispheric white matter is immature during the first 2 years of life (for review [6]).

Similar neuronal networks are involved by cognitive functions and by epilepsy; therefore both are likely to compete. Any potentially epileptogenic area, *i.e.* brain dysplasia, is likely to initiate epileptic phenomena when the surrounding cortex undergoes rapid maturation, and therefore experiences an increase in excitatory pathway activity, during this entire critical period. The occurrence of epilepsy within this developing network is likely to produce much greater disorganization than epilepsy involving a previously structured network, *i.e.* that of an adult brain or of the childhood motor pathway.

However, not all functions presently developing are involved: in a given age range it may consist either in visual or auditive agnosia for infantile epilepsy, either in speech trouble or frontal lobe syndrome for childhood epilepsy, and each one is correlated with the topography of predominant spike and that of an eventual brain lesion demonstrated by MRI.

There seems to be a predominant role of so-called "interictal" spike activity as a causal factor of cognitive disorders. Indeed, the latter are correlated with the topography of spike focus, not the type of seizure. The role of the slow wave activity appears clearly in cases with rolandic focus in which negative myoclonus is time-locked to the slow wave of the spike wave complex, thus expressing the inhibitory role of the neurophysiological event expressed by the slow wave [7]. One can easily imagine what happens in areas corresponding to cognitive functions when a nearly continuous inhibitory activity takes place for months, either during waking or sleep, and on both hemispheres. Not only does it prevent the development of the function in the area devoted to it, but it also prevents the contralateral hemisphere from taking over.

Therefore, cessation of WS, LGS, or CSWS is not sufficient for cognitive functions to recover, although it is a prerequisit. Cessation of spike and slow wave activity permits learning abilities to recover; from then on, the corresponding cognitive function may resume development.

In conclusion, early identification and understanding, rehabilitation and appropriate choice of anti-epileptic treatment of the cognitive, including behaviour troubles, are major and complementary features of prognosis in early childhood epilepsy. Neuropsychological work-up is a major component of investigation, follow-up and rehabilitation of infants and children with epilepsy. In epileptogenic encephalopathy, there is a clear correlation between the type of syndrome, the topography of predominant interictal spike activity and the eventual brain lesion, and the cognitive pattern.

References

1. Jambaque I, Dellatolas G, Dulac O, Ponsot G, Signoret JL. Verbal and visuel memory impairment in children with epilepsy. *Neuropsychologia* 1993 ; 31 : 1321-37.
2. Dravet C, Bureau M, Guerrini R, Giraud N, Roger J. Severe myoclonic epilepsy in infants. In : Roger J, Bureau M, Dravet C, Dreifuss FE, Perret A, Wolf P, eds. *Epileptic syndromes in infancy, childhood and adolescence* (2nd edition). London : John Libbey and Company Ltd, 1992 : 75-88.
3. Aicardi J. *Epilepsy in children, international review of child neurology series.* New York : Raven Press, 1986 : 413.
4. Jambaque I, Chiron C, Dulac O, *et al.* Visual inattention in West syndrome: a neuropsychological and neurofunctional imaging study. *Epilepsia* 1993 ; 34 : 692-700.
5. Roulet-Perez E, Davidoff V, Despland PA, Deonna T. Mental and behavioural deterioration of children with epilepsy and CSWS: acquired epileptic frontal syndrome. *Dev Med Child Neurol* 1993 ; 35 : 661-74.
6. Dulac O, Chiron C, Robain O, Plouin P, Jambaque I, Pinard JM. Infantile spasms: a pathophysiological hypothesis. *Sem Pediatr Neurol* 1994 ; 1 : 83-9.
7. Guerrini R, Dravet C, Genton P, *et al.* Epileptic negative myoclonus. *Neurology* 1993 ; 43 : 1078- 83.

9

Comments about the assessment and treatment of some dysphasic children

D. TRUSCELLI

Service de Rééducation Neurologique, Centre Hospitalier de Bicêtre, Le Kremlin-Bicêttre, France.

In order to comment on the assessment, treatment and prognosis of children with specific difficulties in language development, we particularly studied 9 children followed and treated in our Reabilitation Unit. All children were referred to us by J. Aicardi and his colleagues. Some aspects of their personal history were rather common: a neuropediatrician's advice was seeked only after some years of evolution which led to a rather late diagnosis of their pathology; at least one member of their close family suffered from some kind of speech and language disorder responsible for many difficulties at school; all of them had to repeat the programme of one or more school years during primary education and were finally excluded from mainstream school; they have all attended speech therapy sessions, sometimes in conjunction with some form of psychotherapy; all, except one, were right handed. Three out of nine had or have experienced seizures; a 24 hours EEG recording was normal in all the others and no patient presented with continuous spike-waves during slow sleep. MRI was normal in all but one. This girl presented some abnormal high signals mainly concerning the temporo-parietal regions, in relation with complications during pregnancy. Neurological examination was normal in all nine children. They all used some words, mimics, gestures or cartoons in their effort to communicate.

They were all young patients, 7 boys and 2 girls, born between 1979 and 1985, suffering from a severe phonologico-syntactic form of developmental dysphasia - a specific trouble of language development. They were all tested by the Chevrie-Muller neuropsychologic battery and other syntactic tasks. One out of 9 had an articulation disorder related to bucco-facial dyspraxia associated with a mild degree of drooling.

It is of interest to emphasize the fact that 8-year-old children, even after many years of reeducation, fail completely the phonological and vocabulary tests observed in naming pictures, being situated out of the three standard deviation limits. There is a discrepancy with a standard comprehensive skill measured on the capacity to extract the main idea contained in a short story read to the child by an adult. It is necessary to move beyond the appraisal of the child's level of language towards a qualitative analysis of the pattern; it would be invaluable to know the meaning of the bad performances in syntax or vocabulary. For example, if the correct word cannot be found, a semantic paraphasia or a generic term is often used by the subject: tool instead of scissors or gadjet for any kind of tool. The delineation of such patterns is important for the remediation programme.

All these children are considered as of normal intelligence because of the results obtained at the WISC-Performance. In our group IQ was evaluated within the range of 113 to 67. But a great heterogeneity is usually observed in the subtest scores. The digit symbol scores are very low; the same applies to picture arrangement, thus also focussing on the difficulty for temporal organisation. Extremely low scores are obtained at the verbal tests, especially those implicating digit memory, and should be interpreted as a prognosis indicator of severe trouble. The K-ABC evidences, as it could be foreseen, failure in the sequential subtest and the sub-normality of the ability for the so-called simultaneous activity. Analysis of the results may provide us with some indications for the remediation programme, but we are far from a "true picture" of the patient even if we are used to work with the idea of the independance of upper functions. However, examples of a different orientation in diagnosis, resting on a similar evaluation, are relatively frequent. This phenomenon can be understood in the light of the close connection between language and emotional domains. We need, once more, to deal with process-oriented tasks. We have chosen for this aim to test the child with the EDEI (*Échelles Différentielles d'Efficiences Intellectuelles*) (Perron-Borelli, 1978), to evaluate his capacity in categorial activities, in classification and categorial analysis. These non-verbal standardized tests are prepared to be used in groups of children aged 3 to 11 years. The basic principle in classification consists in finding the logical assembling or representative objects. The second test of categorial analysis is based on the same logical approach and it requires to group together tokens of various color, size and shape (Barbot, 1993). Good results in these tests enable us to pick out some talented patients who had done poorly on WISC-Performance (Table I). Another observation is the discrepancy between the classification (more heavily weighted in verbal factor) and categorial analysis; the third observation concerns the intrinsic quality of the patient's response which may not refer to logical classes but to natural ones. Following this reference to cognitive assessment, we shall not dwell here on the psychological approach, on the importance to understand how the interrelations with the environment have been built, especially with the mother.

Reeducation procedures should invite collaboration between speech therapists and teachers; they have to be attractive to the child. One of the well-known techniques consists of staging a story which has been read by an adult or invented by the child. The

TREATMENT OF SOME DYSPHASIC CHILDREN

Table I.

	WISC-R	EDEI	Class	An cat.	WISC-R	EDEI	Class	An cat.	SCHOOL LEVEL
MTM March 1979	1989 V (MC 0) 1989 P 86	1988	60	64	1992 V (MC 0) 1992 P 80 (code 4, AI 12)	1988	66	90	reads, does not understand oriented : IME
FEL De Oct 1980	1990 V (MC 2) 1990 P 84 (code 4, AI 8)	1990	77	78	1992 V (MC 2) 1992 P 84				CE2 in 1994 EREA
RAM Se March 1982	1991 V - ? (MC 3) 1991 P 110 (code 10, AI 12)	1991	58	90	1993 V ? (MC 3) 1993 P 102	1991	100	100	level CP oriented : IME
PIC-CL Fr July 1982	1993 V 1993 p 80 (code 2, AI 7)	1993	50	60	1994 V 56 (MC 3) 1994 P 80	1994	70	70	reads only 2 syllabes oriented : IME
DEM Se Sept 1983	1992 1992 P 77 (code 7, AI 4)	1993	89	60	1995 V 60 (MC 6) 1995 P 59	1995			reads, does not understand oriented : IME
ROD Emm March 1984	1991 V 1991 P 68 (code 4, AI 7)	1991	78	49	1994 V 58 (MC 2) 1994 P 73	1991	70	50	reads syllabes, can copy oriented : IME
SIM al Oct 1984	1993 V 1993 P 85 (code 5, AI 10)	1991	83	83	1994 v 57 (MC 7) 1994 P 92	1994	76	100	reads, understand easy texts oriented
AM Abd Nov 1985	1991 V 54 1991 P 67 (code 1, AI 7)	1992	80	80	1995 V 73 (MC 5) 1995 P 89 (code 6, AI 12)	1995	81	80	does not read, can copy LO simple, CP
MES Ca June1986	1992 V 1992 P 58	1990	75	79	1994 V 64 (MC 2) 1994 P 79 (code 8, AI 4)	1994	87	100	reads syllabes, can copy LO telegraph, CP

MC = digit memory
Code = digit symbol
AI = picture arrangement

LO = oral language
IME = institut médico-éducatif
CP = classe primaire préparatoire

use of comic strips enables us to work on the notion of time and, whenever this is possible, on the adequacy with written dialogue. Such a procedure aims to provide the child with a visual representation of words in their context, treated at different levels. Beyond the ability of reading which particularly improves the phonological deficits, one should emphasize the need for the child to understand the text he is reading. Many of them do not succeed; they can only acquire the reading techniques. Moreover, the communication by written language is not as useful as expected; few of these patients are able to write short messages which may be quite informative. But even if they do, they are unable to respect syntax or grammar. Many authors (Haynes, 1994; Rutter, 1987) insist on these learning difficulties and limits. The use of the sign language is of no help and in any case difficult to learn. Its grammar rules overpass the capacities of these children.

For all these reasons we should try to provide them with Alternative and Augmentative means of Communication (AAC) such as boards filled with pictures or Bliss symbols: speaking becomes pointing the finger at a succession of cartoons. But the patients and their families do not cope with it even when the speech is far from clear. It remains a good professional support to teach the written language and illustrate the grammatical groups. The microtechnology can be seen as a complement and as a new approach for reciprocal communication. Speech synthesiser may work with non-verbal inputs such as symbolic ones and can provide a clear speaking voice with syntactically correct sentences. However, these techniques seem to be too far from the expectations of all the partners....

Prognosis is very difficult to define. A positive evolution is not always predictable, even when the child succeeds in WISC-Performance tests (Billard, 1992) or demonstrates even during the first tests a certain superiority in some comprehensive verbal capacities as compared to the expressive ones. A general improvement is possible with time, but in the severe forms of language deficiency the child is very handicapped in his relations with the environment. There is a poor spontaneous linguistic capacity and the reactive capacities when the child is helped by a speech therapist or a teacher he trusts.

In conclusion, we suggest that these patients must be evaluated early and receive specific help. Progression is possible, although it takes place slowly and is time consuming. Reeducation has to prevent the patients tendency to withdraw when reaching adulthood and to avoid emotional complications. Recently, the ways of communication adopted by the mothers of these children have been studied; it sems obvious that they are used to speaking sentences without the ability to know how to link one with another, as if they lack the sense of continuity of speech.

Language reeducation has to be inserted in a larger programme of cognitive development. To our experience, with this small group of patients, working on mental process may improve the results when the evaluation of the construction of the process of the thinking is done. To note that when the IQ is measured for a second time the results are similar to those calculated when using classic level tests. Following this observation we are led to suppose that it is important to modify the learning schedule and to introduce a global programme based not only on language reeducation but also on developing the child's ability to express self-criticism based on common sense. The remediation work must take into account the emotional content and context of the communication.

Bibliography

1. Ajuriaguerra J, *et al.* Organisation psychologique et troubles du langage. In : *Problèmes de psycholinguistique*. Paris : PUF, 1963.
2. de Barbot F. Étude de l'activité catégorielle chez les enfants dysphasiques. Actes du Colloque sur les dysphasies. Dijon, Université de Bourgogne, 1992.
3. Billard C, Loisel Dufour ML, *et al.* Évolution du langage oral et du langage écrit dans une population dysphasique de développement de forme expressive. *ANAE* 1989 ; 1 : 16-20.
4. Chevrie-Muller C. Évaluation neuropsycholinguistique chez l'enfant. *Glossa, les cahiers de l'Unadrio*, 1991 ; 25 : 8-13.
5. Gérard C. Troubles du langage oral et troubles de la lecture. In : Van Hout A, Estienne F, éds. *Les dyslexies*. Paris : Masson, 1994 : 158-65.
6. Haynes C, Naidoo S. *Children with speech and language impairment*. London : Mc Keith Press, 1991 : 206-25.
7. Klees M, Szliwowski H. Les dysphasies sévères chez l'enfant. *Rev Intern Ped* 1993 ; 232 : 34-7.
8. Perron-Borelli M. *Les échelles différentielles d'efficiences intellectuelles*. Issy les Moulineaux : EAP, 1978.
9. Rice ML, Sell MA, Hadley PA. Social interactions of speech and language impaired children. *J Speech Hearing Res* 1991 ; 34 : 1299-307.
10. Tallal P, *et al.* A reexamination of some non verbal perceptual abilities of language impaired and normal children as a function of age and sensory modality. *J Speech Hearing Res* 1981 ; 24 : 351-7.
11. Van Hout A. Aspect du diagnostic des dysphasies. *ANAE* 1989 ; 1 : 11-5.

10

Developmental defects of the corpus callosum

G. LYON

50, rue d'Assas, Paris, France.

Congenital abnormalities of the corpus callosum are among the most frequent developmental defects of the brain. Curiously, their morphologic features are poorly described in most reports, and little is known of their pathophysiology. Total or partial aberrations of this commissure come as one element of a complex developmental syndrome, or as an apparently isolated abnormality. In the latter case, cognitive impairment and minor dysmorphic signs are frequent. Isolated callosal defects are usually sporadic, but the accompanying mental deficiency may be familial.

Abnormalities of the corpus callosum apparently play no role, or a very limited role, in the genesis of associated neurologic signs. They constitute, in this case, clinically mute stigmata of a more diffuse developmental encephalopathy.

Development and function of the corpus callosum

A brief reminder of the principal data concerning the development and function of the corpus callosum is useful at this point. Callosal fibers cross the midline in the commisural plate at 12 weeks gestation (after the anterior commissure). Formation of the commissure proceeds antero-posteriorly (partial agenesis usually involves the splenium). The primitive corpus callosum is completed at 16 weeks.

Callosal neurons are essentially situated in layers II and III of the cortex, in the rat, the cat and primates. Their axons cross the midline and terminate in homologous areas of the controlateral hemisphere. There are regional differences in the density of the projections: they are numerous in the association areas and minimal in cortical areas representing the hands and feet.

During late intra-uterine and early post-natal development, numerous callosal fibers (axonal collaterals) are normally eliminated [1]. Up to 70% of callosal collaterals disappear in the cat, with preservation of their neurones of origin in the cortex (an abnormality of developmental axonal restriction may play a role in some human defects of the corpus callosum; see below). Myelination starts after birth at approximately 3 months in humans, is well advanced at 6 months, and continues slowly until the age of 6 years, with a dorsofrontal progression. Many callosal fibers are unmyelinated. Individual variations in the profile of this commissure are marked.

The functions of the corpus callosum are not entirely understood. This large transverse commissure certainly plays a role in the transfer of information between two differently specialized hemispheres, allowing them to cooperate. However, when the hemispheres are disconnected by sectionning of the corpus callosum, the "disconnection syndrome", revealed by specialized tests, is transitory and of no real inconvenience for the individual. A developmental role of the corpus callosum in establishing the lateralization of cortical fonctions has been postulated.

Morphology and pathophysiology of development defects of the corpus callosum

Very little is known of the sequence of events leading to developmental defects of the corpus callosum. Deviation from the normal path of axonal growth or a disorder of the mechanisms of axonal stabilisation during development, not an abnormality of neurons, are among possible causes. There are different structural types. The defect may be total or partial. In the latter case, it usually affects the posterior part of the commissure. We believe the following morphologic forms should be distinguished, at least provisionally.

The most frequent form is the classic agenesis of the corpus callosum with absence of transverse fibers and presence of longitudinal "Probst bundles"

Callosal fibers do not cross the midline (absence of "commissuration") [2]; a normal or reduced amount of fibers are condensed in bilateral longitudinal bundles running in a fronto-caudal direction (Probst bundles) (in some cases a few transverse fibers may be seen) (Figure 1). Other characteristics are a bilateral dilatation of the posterior segment of the lateral ventricles and a verticalization of the sulci of the medial, supra callosal, surface of the cortex. This latter abnormality which can be detected before or at birth serves to differentiate an agenesis of the corpus callosum from an incipient hydrocephalus. In some instances, the anterior commissure is missing.

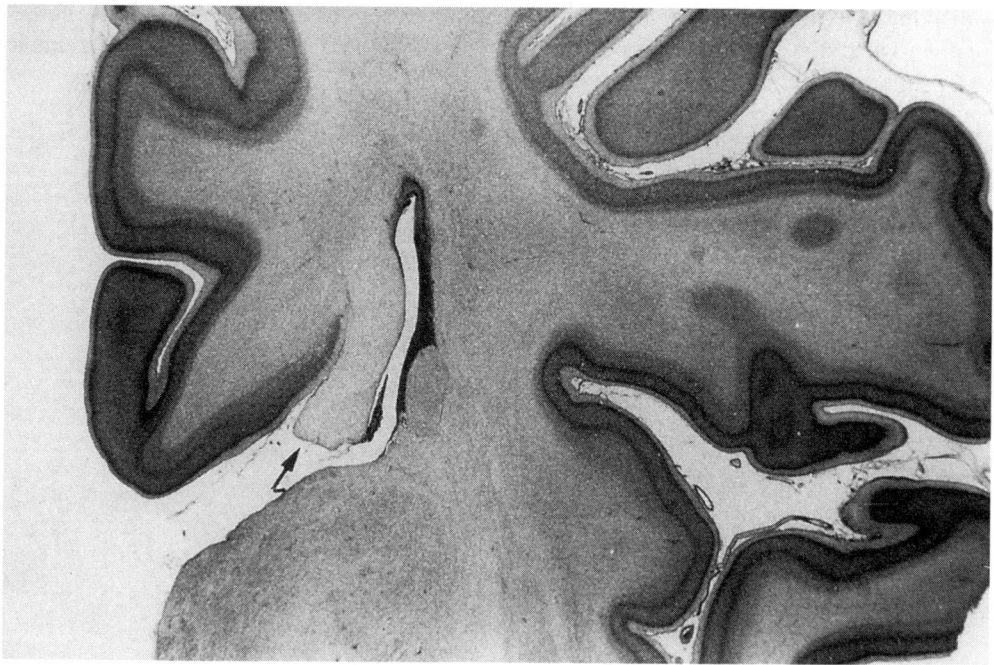

Figure 1. Frontal section of hemisphere. Agenesis of the corpus callosum with longitudinal Probst bundle (arrow).

Acallosal mice related to different mutations (BALB/C and ddN strains) reproduce the picture of classical agenesis in humans [3, 4]. Their study has confirmed that, normally, callosal axons when reaching the midline penetrate into a median extension of the subventricular cellular tissue, referred to as the "sling". Possibly, a defect of this substrate for axonal guidance plays a role in the absence of commissuration. No evident behavioral changes have been observed in acallosal mice, but further studies are needed into this field. No primate models of agenesis of the corpus callosum are known. Classic agenesis of the corpus callosum is usually sporadic (see below).

Extreme thinness of the corpus callosum due to a disorder of axonal stabilisation

In this type of autosomal recessive hereditary condition (Figure 2), a marked atrophy or hypolasia of the corpus callosum is associated with a volumetric reduction of the central white matter, and an absence of the bulbar pyramids. The cortex and the hypoplastic white matter are normal. This disorder has previously been reported as "familial hypoplasia of the central white matter" and considered to be the consequence of hypomyelination [5-7]. In our view, this opinion is not tenable: the absence of bulbar pyramids and the marked thinness of the corpus callosum can in no way be explained by an absence of myelination; they are the expression of an axonal disorder. Lyon et al. [8] reported 3 patients with this condition, two of them in the same sibship. There was indisputable evidence of axonal lesions. The authors suggested that this anomaly could be due to an extension of the normal phenomenon of axonal restriction, possibly related to a primary defect of the axonal cytoskeleton.

Developmental hypophasia must be distinguished from acquired atrophy of the corpus callosum secondary to diffuse cortical or white matter lesions.

Other callosal defects

They include:
- complete absence of the corpus callosum. This form has been poorly studied and its possible relationship with (1) or (2) is uncertain;
- absence of the corpus callosum in holoprosencephaly;

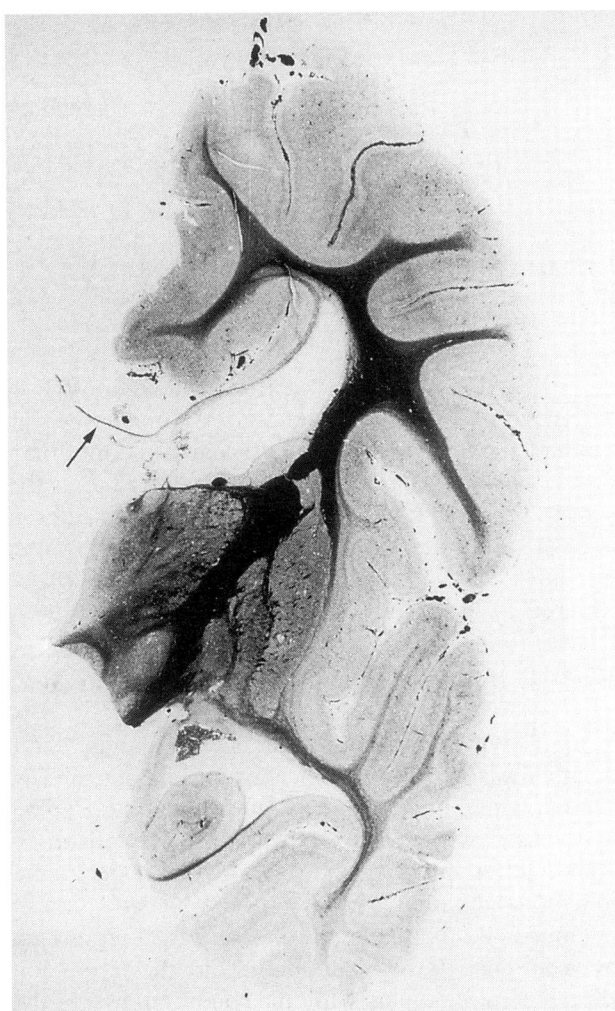

Figure 2. Extreme atrophy of the corpus callosum (arrow) due to a disorder of axonal development. Poor development of central white matter. There was an absence of pyramids.

- a poorly developed corpus callosum with a fused interhemispheric fissure is very characteristic of Walkers (Type II) lissencephaly [9];
- defects of the corpus callosum can be associated with median lipomas and cysts;
- hypertrophy of the corpus callosum is a frequent feature of lissencephaly type I (Miller-Dieker syndrome), according to our experience. Of six cases with this condition the corpus callosum was large in five and normal in one. Absence of the corpus callosum may occur but is not frequent in lissencephaly type I.

Etiology and developmental context of defects of the corpus callosum

A) A developmental abnormality of the corpus callosum is a usual or constant feature of a few specific malformative syndromes, the most important of which is Aicardi syndrome (Figure 3). This sporadic condition occurring only in girls and probably due to an X-linked dominant mutation is characterized by infantile spasms, severe mental deficiency, typical retinal lesions, vertebro-costal defects, asynchronous independent EEG abnormalities of both hemispheres, total or partial absence of the corpus callosum (inconstant), cortical dysplasias, subventricular heterotopias and posterior-fossa

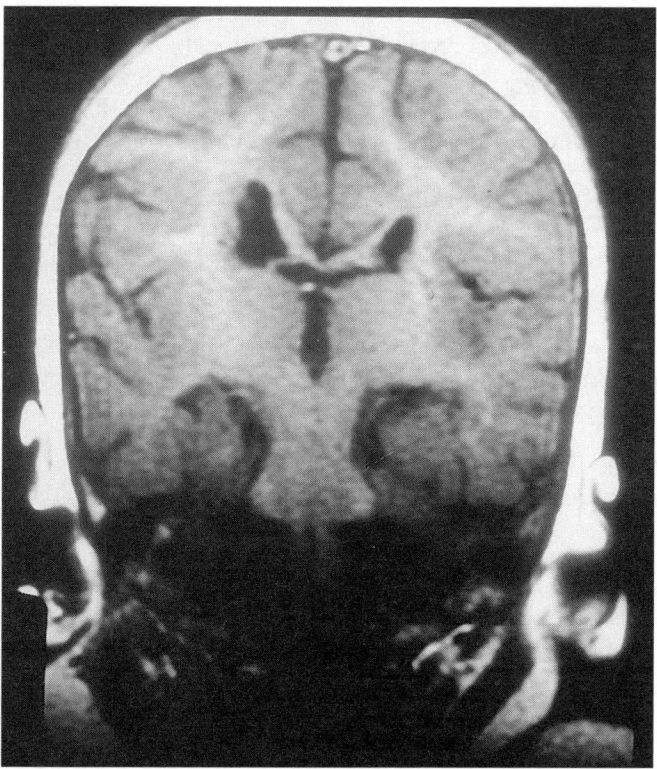

Figure 3. Aicardi syndrome with persistence of an hypoplastic corpus callosum. Typical subependymal cortical heterotopias protrude into the slightly dilated ventricle on the left side of the figure (courtesy of Dr Darryl De Vivo).

malformations. The callosal defect plays no, or a minimal, role in the symptomatology of Aicardi syndrome (see below).

Other developmental syndromes with usual callosal defects include: Andermann syndrome, Shapiro syndrome, acrocallosal syndrome, trisomy 18, Apert syndrome, orofacio-digital syndrome. Also, agenesis of the corpus callosum may be observed occasionally in practically every type of developmental defect of the brain.

B) Interestingly, prenatal defects of the corpus callosum occur in a number of hereditary metabolic disorders [10], essentially pyruvate dehydrogenase (PDH) E1α deficiency and non-ketotic hyperglycinemia. In PDH deficiency the abnormality of the corpus callosum is associated with other lesions, such as widespread necrosis of the white matter and cortex, absence of pyramidal tracts and heterotopias of inferior olives. From three personal cases and a review of the literature, it appears that the callosal defect does not correspond to classical agenesis. There is thinning or partial absence of the commissure which is most probably the result of severe hemispheric necrosis or direct destruction of the commissure. This prenatal X-linked encephalopathy is seen both in boys and in heterozygous females, and has been related to different types of mutations in the PDH E1α gene. There is only scant information concerning the type of callosal defect in non-ketotic hyperglycinemia.

C) Apparently isolated defects of the corpus callosum with no known cause. The exact frequency of "isolated" cryptogenetic agenesis of the corpus callosum is unknown, but this morphologic abnormality is certainly not exceptional. Most cases are sporadic, although a few familial cases have been reported. Associated clinical signs are usual but probably not constant. They include mental deficiency, learning disorders, occasionally seizures, hypertelorism, macrocephaly, or more rarely microcephaly.

Heredity: reports of familial cases are remarkably rare. They are usually inherited as an autosomal recessive trait, rarely as dominant or X-linked disorders. However, cognitive impairment with a normal commissure is not infrequently found in sibling or other members of the family.

These then are cases of a familial encephalopathy with cognitive impairment in which the incidental presence of an agenesis of the corpus callosum in one sibling merely points out to the developmental nature of the disorder.

Clinical significance: two questions may be raised: does the absence of corpus callosum have an incidence on the determinism and type of cognitive impairment and on seizures? Is there a "disconnection syndrome" in agenesis of the corpus callosum?

Available clinical data - particularly the existence of families with two mentally retarded siblings, one of which has agenesis of the corpus callosum - are not in favor of a significant role of the corpus callosum in the genesis of cognitive deficits. Associated cortical developmental abnormalities probably underly the intellectual impairment. However, a limited role of the callosal defect cannot be totally excluded: callosal projections are more numerous in frontal associative areas; also, the corpus callosum might possibly contribute to cortical development and specialization.

A "developmental disconnection syndrome" has been described by Ramackers and Njiukiktjien in their comprehensive work on the corpus callosum [11]. However the changes (in mentally subnormal children) were subtle and probably clinically negligible.

The absence of the corpus callosum appears to have little or no effect on the EEG and on the pattern of seizures. Alpha-rythms are generally symmetrical. Asymmetry of sleep spindles has been reported. In Aicardi syndrome, the so-called "split-brain EEG" and the seizure pattern are not related to the callosal defect: these abnormalities are also observed when the commisure is totaly or partially preserved, as may happen in this syndrome.

It can be concluded that prenatal defects of the corpus callosum are clinically mute stigmata of a more diffuse developmental encephalopathy which underlies the clinical manifestations.

Medical counselling of families having a child with "isolated" cryptogenetic "agenesis" of the corpus callosum

When an isolated defect of the corpus callosum is discovered before birth, or is revealed in a young infant, counselling is very difficult. Chances of future cognitive impairment are high, although its incidence is unknown, and the degree of mental deficit may be modest. In a recent series of twelve children with a callosal defect detected before birth, which were followed during 2 to 8 years, six were said to have a normal development [12]. Further prospective studies are needed.

Counselling should be made on an individual basis; on the whole an isolated agenesis of the corpus callosum is certainly not a strong indication for terminating pregnancy.

The chances for another sibling to have a callosal defect are probably low, but the occurrence of mental deficiency without callosal changes in a future child constitutes a real possibility, although no statistical data are available.

References

1. Innocenti GM. Growth and reshaping of axons in the establishment of visual callosal projections. *Science* 1981 ; 212 : 824-6.
2. Rakic P, Yakovlev PI. Development of the corpus callosum and cavum septi in man. *J Comp Neurol* 1968 132 : 45-72.
3. Wahlsten D. Deficiency of corpus callosum varies with strain and supplier of mice. *Brain Res* 1982 ; 239 : 329-47.

4. Ozaki HS, Murakami TH, Toyoshima T, *et al.* The fibers which leave the Probst longitudinal bundle seen in the brain of an acallosol mouse: a study with the horseradish peroxidase technique. *Brain Res* 1987 ; 400 : 239-46.
5. Chattha AS, Richardson EP. Cerebral white-matter hypoplasia. *Arch Neurol* 1977 ; 34 : 137-41.
6. Guazzi GC, Stoppoloni G, Ventruto V, *et al.* Immaturité neuronale corticale avec agénésie des grandes commissures interhémisphériques et hypoplasie des voies optico-pyramidales chez trois enfants issus d'une même famille. *Acta Neurol (Napoli)* 1974 ; 39 : 659-74.
7. Volpe JJ. *Neurology of the new-born,* 3rd ed. Philadelphia : Saunders, 1995.
8. Lyon G, Arita F, Le Galloudec E, *et al.* A disorder of axonal development, necrotizing myopathy, cardiomyopathy and cataracts: a new familial disease. *Ann Neurol* 1990 ; 27 : 193-9.
9. Lyon G. Congenital malformations of the brain. In : Levene MI, Lilford RJ, Bennett MJ, Punt J, eds. *Fetal and neonatal neurology and neurosurgery*. Edinburgh : Churchill Livingstone, 1995 : 193-214.
10. Kolodny EH. Agenesis of the corpus callosum: a marker for inherited disease? *Neurology* 1989 ; 39 : 847-8.
11. Ramakaers G, Njiokiktjien. *The child's corpus callosum*. Amsterdam : Suji Publications, 1991.
12. Blum A, André M, Droullé D, Husson S, Leheut B. Prenatal echographic diagnosis of corpus callosum agenesis. The Nancy experience 1982-1989. *Genetic Counselling* 1990 ; 1 : 115-26.

11

Aicardi syndrome with normal developmental progress, remission of epilepsy and bilateral intraventricular tumours

I.J. HOPKINS

Royal Children's Hospital, Melbourne, Australia.

The condition which has become known as a Aicardi syndrome (AS) was first reported by Aicardi, Lefebre and Lerique-Koechlin in 1965 [1], followed by a second paper by Aicardi, Chevrie and Rousellie in 1969 [2] which delineated the clinical features in more detail. It has generally been accepted that the classical clinical findings are female sex, infantile spasms, intellectual disability, retinal lacunae, a characteristic EEG pattern, agenesis of the corpus callosum (ACC) and vertebral anomalies. However, patients with most but not all of these features have been included by some authors. Donnenfeld et al. [3] reported complete ACC in 72% of their cases, and partial agenesis in 28%. It is the present author's contention that there is a greater clinical heterogeneity in AS, than is usually accepted, and using a definition that includes all the classical features as being essential for diagnosis and case finding will exclude some milder and variant forms. A child illustrating this is the basis of this report.

Patient report

After a 38 week pregnancy, normal apart from mild gestational diabetes, a female infant was born without incident after a normal labour. Birth weight was 3560 g. She was slightly jittery in the neonatal period but required no special care. Early developmental progress was normal and at 4.5 months she was able to roll supine to prone, and reach to grasp objects. At 5 months she had the onset of infantile spasms and became less responsive. Physical examination revealed bilateral retinal lacunae (Figure 1) that were typical of AS, and mild hypoplasia of the right optic disc. Her EEG showed the pattern of typical hypsarrhythmia. MRI showed a normal corpus callosum, and no evidence of neuronal migration abnormalities. However, bilateral choroid plexus masses that enhanced brilliantly with gadolinium were present (Figure 2).

She was treated with prednisolone 2mg/kg/day for 6 weeks and clonazepam. Infantile spasms diminished in number and ceased completely by 8 months of age. Clonazepam was ceased at 1 year. She walked independently at 14 months. When seen at 20 months of age she was saying approximately 20 single words and followed simple instructions. At 2.5 years her developmental progress was within the range of normal and no further seizures have occurred.

Discussion

Diagnosis of AS in this patient is based on the presence of infantile spasms occurring in a female infant who has the typical retinal abnormalities of AS, with bilateral lacunae, and unilateral optic disc hypoplasia being present. Aicardi (personal

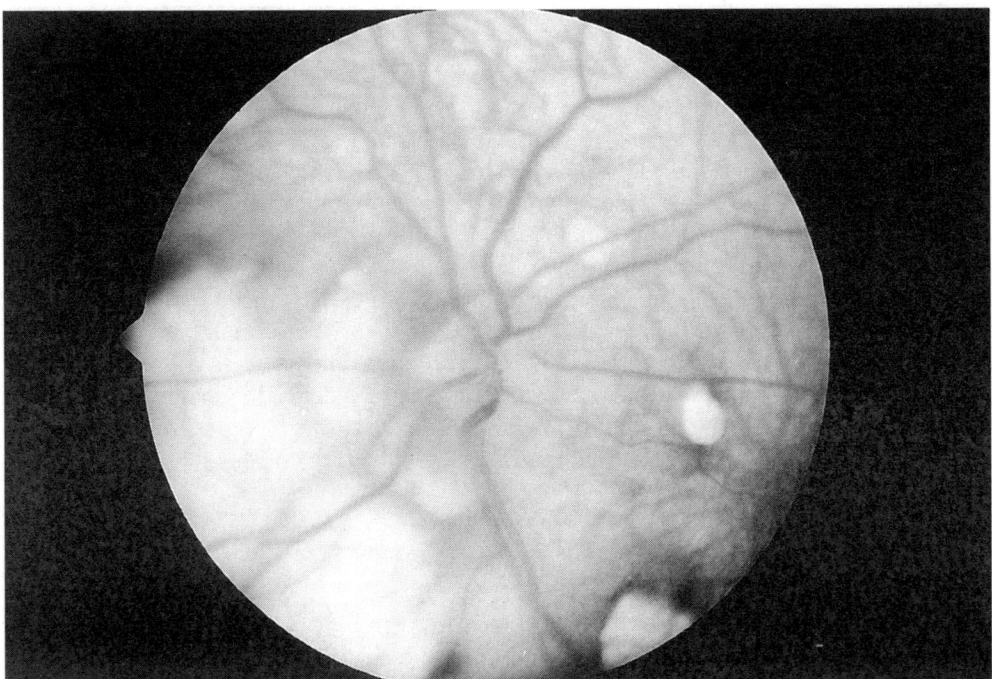

Figure 1. Fundal photograph showing the typical retinal lacunae of Aicardi syndrome.

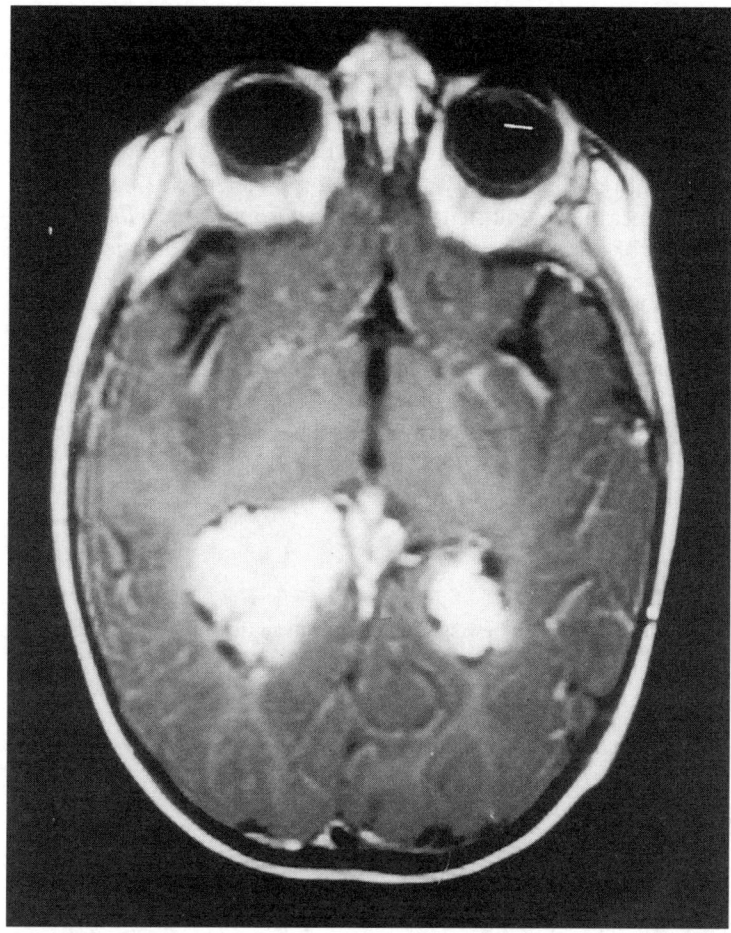

Figure 2. MRI scan showing bilateral choroid plexus masses enhancing with gadolinium. T1-weighted image.

communication) no longer considers that ACC is an essential feature of the syndrome that has his name. The presence of the choroid plexus tumours, which have only increased minimally in size in the past two years, and have not been associated with development of hydrocephalus, can in fact be regarded as a finding supporting the diagnosis of Aicardi syndrome, as the author is aware of seven cases of Aicardi syndrome with intraventricular tumours. Five of these have been reported [4-6]. In contrast to the more usual situation with choroid plexus tumours, *i.e.* those unassociated with AS, which are nearly always single, it is suggested that AS should always be considered in differential diagnosis if bilateral choroid plexus tumours of the lateral ventricles are present. The favourable course of the epilepsy, which is in complete remission, and the normal developmental progress are features of great interest in the patient reported above. It seems likely that the severity of intellectual disability, and perhaps also of epilepsy, would correlate with the severity of neuronal migration abnormalities. The extent of these in AS has only become apparent with more recent reports dealing with pathology and MRI findings.

There are no previous reports of normal developmental progress in Aicardi syndrome, although Abe *et al.* [7] have reported a single case and noted ten additional cases of mild mental retardation in a literature survey. Menezes *et al.* [8] found that none of 28 neurologic features were predictive of cognitive development. However, of their 11 patients with severe mental retardation nine had complete ACC whereas of three children with mild mental retardation only one had complete ACC. In a separate study Menezes [9] reported, in a paper entitled "*Aicardi syndrome - the elusive mild case*", a child with hypoplasia of the corpus callosum and mild intellectual disability.

Until a biological marker for AS is found it will be a matter of speculation as to the variability of the clinical features, and validity of diagnosis in mild or unusual cases. Hopefully further genetic studies of heterogeneity of the molecular lesion, as reported by Neidich *et al.* [10] using X-inactivation and other molecular biological techniques, will eventually shed light on this facet of Aicardi syndrome. Studies of this type are planned for the infant reported in this paper.

References

1. Aicardi J, Lefebre J, Levique-Kaechlin A. A new syndrome: spasms in flexion, callosal agenesis, and ocular abnormalities. *Electroencephalog Clin Neurophysiol* 1965 ; 19 : 609-10.
2. Aicardi J, Chevrie JJ, Rousselle F. Le syndrome spasmes en flexion, agénésie calleuse, anomalies chorio-rétiniennes. *Arch Fr Pediatr* 1969 ; 26 : 1103-20.
3. Donnenfeld AE, Graham JM Jr, Packer RJ, Aquino R, Berg SZ, Emanuel BS. Microphthalmia and chorioretinal lesions in a girl with an Xp22.2-pter deletion and partial 3p trisomy: clinical observations relevant to Aicardi syndrome gene localization. *Am J Med Gene* 1990 ; 37 : 182-6.
4. Font RL, Marines HM, Cartwright J Jr, Bauserman SC. Aicardi syndrome. A clinicopathologic case report including electron microscopic observations. *Ophthalmology* 1991 ; 98 : 1727-31.
5. Hamano K, Matsubara T, Shibata S, *et al.* Aicardi syndrome accompanied by auditory disturbance and multiple brain tumors. *Brain Dev* 1991 ; 13 : 438-41.
6. Robin WM, Johnson GF, Minilla PA. Aicardi syndrome, papilloma of the choroid plexus, cleft lip and cleft of the posterior palate. *J Paediatr* 1984 ; 104 : 404-5.
7. Abe K, Mitsudome A, Ogata H, Ohfu M, Takakusaki M. A case of Aicardi syndrome with moderate psychomotor retardation. *No To Hattastsu* 1990 ; 22 : 376-80.
8. Menezes AV, MacGregor DL, Buncic JR. Aicardi syndrome: natural history and possible predictors of severity. *Pediatr Neurol* 1994 ; 11 : 313-8.
9. Menezes AV, Enzenauer RW, Buncic JR. Aicardi syndrome - the elusive mild case. *Br J Ophthal* 1994 ; 78 : 494-6.
10. Neidich JA, Nussbaum RL, Packer RJ, Emanuel BS, Puck JM. Heterogeneity of clinical severity and molecular lesions in Aicardi syndrome. *J Pediatr* 1990 : 116 : 911-7.

12

Subcortical laminar heterotopia and other X-linked cerebral cortical dysgenesis

J.-M. PINARD

Service de Neuropédiatrie, Hôpital Raymond Poincaré, Garches, France.

Cerebral cortical dysgenesis (CD) is a heterogeneous group of disorders of cortical development and organization, and an important cause of mental retardation and epilepsy. The term neuronal migration disorder is often improperly used. Indeed, these malformations may result from failure of neuronal and glial proliferation, from defective neuroblast migration, or from defective maturation of cortical organization [1]. Generalized cerebral malformations with CD such as lissencephaly (or agyria-pachygyria complex) are frequently genetic. Miller-Dieker syndrome and a part of isolated lissencephalies are caused by deletions or microdeletions in the short arm of chromosome 17p13, involving the gene LIS 1 [2]. Several other CD such as Walker-Warburg syndrome or tuberous sclerosis have an autosomal recessive inheritance. Recently, two cerebral cortical dysgenesis can be readily diagnosed on routine MRI. The first one is subcortical laminar heterotopia (SCLH) observed as sporadic cases [3-5] or familial cases, associated with lissencephaly in some families [6-8]. The second one is bilateral subependymal nodular heterotopia (BSENH) [9]. There are some strong arguments for their linkage to X chromosome [6-10]. Several data support the hypothesis of a distinct genetic origin of these 2 X-linked cortical dysgenesis. In other respects, the place of familial lissencephaly described by some authors is not clear [11-13]. However, some of these previously described families with lissencephaly in males and SCLH could have a same genetic origin.

Subcortical laminar heterotopia

This cerebral malformation, also called "band heterotopia" or "double cortex", consists ususally of bilateral, more or less symmetrical extensive plates or bands of grey matter located between the cortex and the ventricle, well separated from both by white matter. The heterotopic grey matter structure can be circumferential or may have a regional, anterior or posterior, distribution. The inner margin of the heterotopic structure is usually smooth and the white matter in the frontal area often has, on axial CT or MRI scan, a butterfly wings shape. The outer margin may be smooth, and the overlying cortex seems to be normal. When the outer margin undulates with the cortical interdigitations, the underlying cortex appears to be pachygyric (Figure 1). Sometimes, the inner and the outer margins of the layer undulate. The thickness of the heterotopic structure is variable from a thick layer of heterotopia, to discontinuous islands of heterotopic grey matter arranged in series [1, 14]. Furthermore, various thickness of SCLH may be observed in a same family [6].

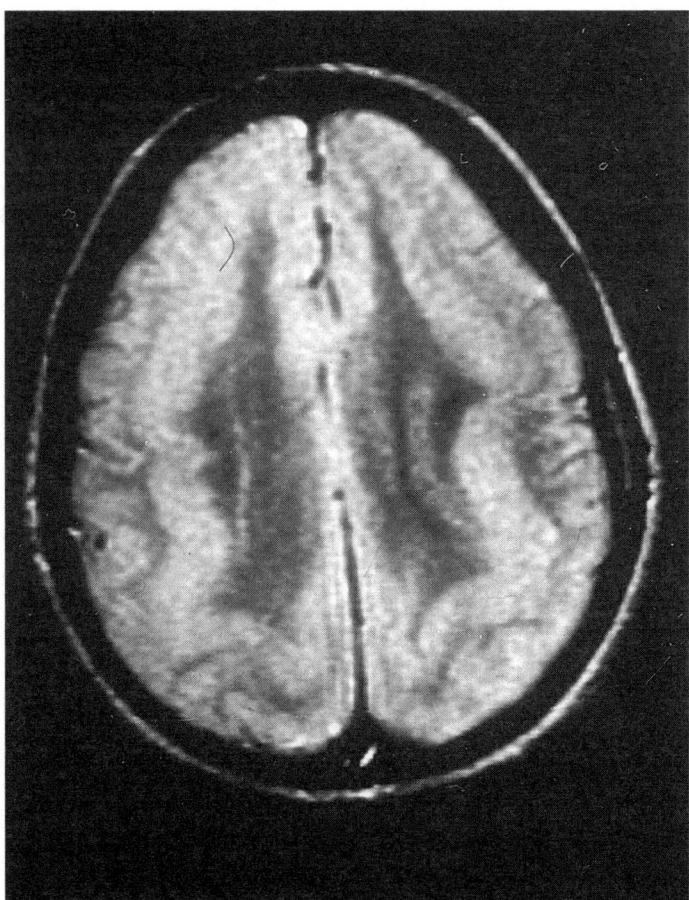

Figure 1. Axial T2-weighted image showing thick laminar heterotopia, with overlying pachygyria, in a 10 year-old girl with severe mental retardation and epilepsy.

Clinical manifestations are mental retardation and epilepsy. Some patients may have normal intelligence. However, most of the patients have mental retardation, ranging from mild to severe, or behavioral problems. Seizures usually begin in childhood or adolescence. Various types of seizure have been observed: partial and generalized tonic or tonic-clonic, atonic, partial complex and atypical absence seizures. Some patients have infantile spasms or Lennox-Gastaut syndrome. Studies on clinical and radiological features showed that the thickness of the heterotopia correlates with the degree of pachygyria. Both of these radiological findings correlate with the clinical characteristics of the patient: precocity of the epilepsy onset, severity of the mental retardation and delay of the motor development [14].

Moutard *et al*. reported 25 female patients with SCLH and peculiar age-related EEG features. These features are non specific and also observed in lissencephaly. Rapid rhythms of high amplitude and frontal alpha rhythms observed during infancy and childhood disappear in adulthood as emerge triphasic slow spikes and waves [7, 15].

Since familial occurrence has been described, genetic origin of subcortical laminar heterotopia is admitted. Different arguments support the hypothesis of a X-linked inheritance. The first one is that sporadic subcortical laminar heterotopia occurs mainly in females. Among 63 known patients with SCLH, 57 are females, including 41 reported distinct patients (cases listed in [7] plus cases reported in [7, 16-19]) and 6 are males, including 3 previously reported [14, 20, 21]. Among another series of 27 patients (including patients mentionned just above), Barkovich reported only 1 male [14]. Clinical and radiological phenotypes appear to be similar in affected males and females. However, the affected gene could cause mainly prenatal lethality or agyria-pachygyria in males as observed in the multiplex families which are the second argument for a X linked inheritance. SCLH and lissencephaly have been reported in 4 families [6-8] in which women with subcortical laminar heterotopia have had daughters with subcortical laminar heterotopia and sons with lissencephaly (Figure 2). In a family, a woman had 3 affected children, 2 girls with SCLH and 1 boy with lissencephaly, each with a different father [6]. Then, this CD varies from SCLH, primarily in females, to pachygyria or agyria in males. The third argument is the description of a girl with lissencephaly and a *de novo* X-autosomal translocation 46, XX, t(X;2)(q22;p25). The gene for SCLH may be located in chromosome Xq22 based on the breakpoint of the X-autosomal translocation. Indeed, in females with balanced X-autosomal translocations, the inactivation of X chromosome (lyonisation) confers a disadvantage on cells with active normal X because of partial functional duplication of the translocated distal part of X chromosome. Thus, cells with the active translocated X predominate over those with the active normal X. If the translocation breakpoint destroys the gene, no functioning protein is produced and a female may have the same disorder as usually observed in males. For the gene of SCLH, male patients with lissencephaly could result from complete absence of functional gene product. In female, SCLH could result from absence of the gene product in cells with inactive normal X, but not in others. Another hypothesis is a partially functional gene product less functional in male than in female.

MRI, EEG and family studies suggested that there are similarities between agyria, pachygyria and SCLH and that they belong to a continuum of brain malformations consequence of a migration defect. However, in a recent pathological study of three epileptic patients with SCLH, pachygyria was not observed. The histological study of the cortex overlying SCLH was normal. This may suggest another explanation. SCLH may result from a failure of normal cell death undergoing in the subplate neurons [19]. Agyria and pachygyria associated with SCLH and due to a same gene could be a consequence of a blocage of the cortical maturation normaly induced by the subplate. The other lissencephalies could have other origins.

Familial lissencephaly

Lissencephaly is caracterized by a thick cortex consisting of two cellular layers separated by a thin sparsed cells layer, and by the absence of surface convolutions with a figure-8 shape on MRI axial sections. The term is often used as synonymous as agyria-pachygyria, spectrum of malformations that includes generalized agyria, mixed agyria-pachygyria and generalized pachygyria [22]. Profound mental retardation, mixed hypotonia and spasticity, intractable epilepsy, infantile spasms or Lennox-Gastaut syndrome, are the main clinical features of this severe brain malformation.

Familial lissencephalies, with mainly male affected patients, were reported in 4 other families distinct from families associating lissencephaly and SCLH [11-13, 23]. One

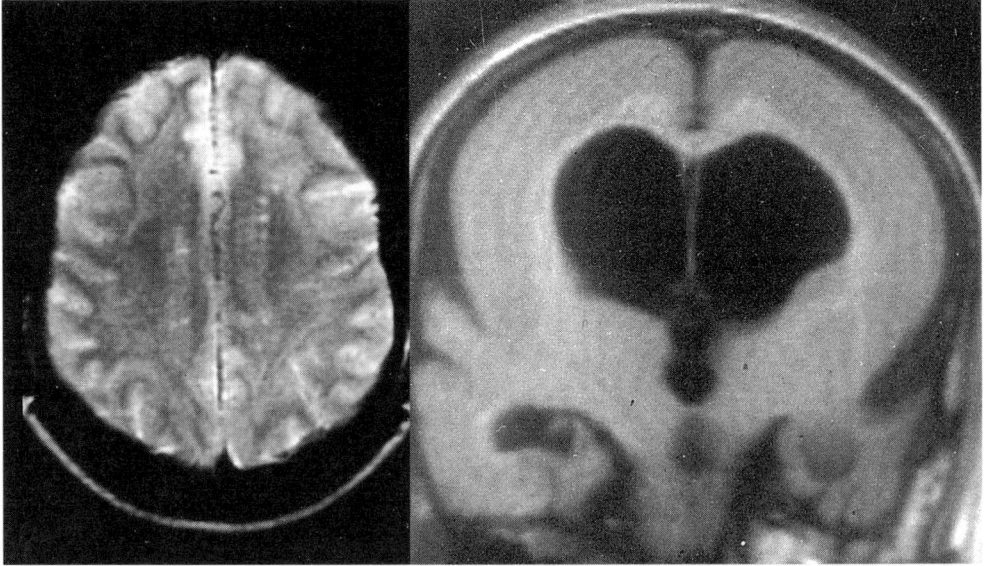

Figure 2. A: Mother : axial T2-weighted image showing subcortical laminar heterotopia. The overlying cortex appears normal. **B:** Son : coronal T1-weighted image showing lissencephaly.

family comprises 1 boy and 4 maternal uncles with lissencephaly and absence of corpus callosum. However, 1 uncle had cardiac malformation. The mother and the maternal grandmother of the proband appeared clinically normal [13]. Pavone reported 3 brothers with lissencephaly. Clinical evaluation of the mother was normal [12]. Barth reported 1 brother and 1 sister with lissencephaly [11]. Zollino described 3 patients (2 males, 1 female) with lissencephaly, congenital microcephaly, facial dysmorphia and genital anomalies. Another affected male patient did not have lissencephaly [23]. Isolated lissencephaly is a heterogenous entity. The last 2 families did not demonstrated arguments for X-linked inheritance. The 2 others might have a same genetic origin as SCLH, or they may be associated to another, X-linked or not, mode of inheritance. Thus, in case of lissencephaly in a male, a precise clinical, EEG and MRI study of the family, overall the family of the mother, is recommended. This could precise the relationship between familial lissencephaly and SCLH.

Bilateral subependymal nodular heterotopia

This other X-linked brain malformation is clearly distinct from SCLH [24]. BSENH is a malformation in which nodular masses of grey matter line the ventricular walls and protrude into the lumen (Figure 3). Nodules may be diffuse, unilateral or focal, contiguous or non-contiguous. On MRI, they have signal intensity similar to that of grey matter. Associated with BSENH, other abnormalities have been described: cerebellar or corpus callosum hypoplasia, areas of cortical dysplasia [25, 26].

Patients with BSENH usually present with normal intelligence and sporadic or familial epilepsy. Seizure may sometimes be difficult to control [9, 24]. However,

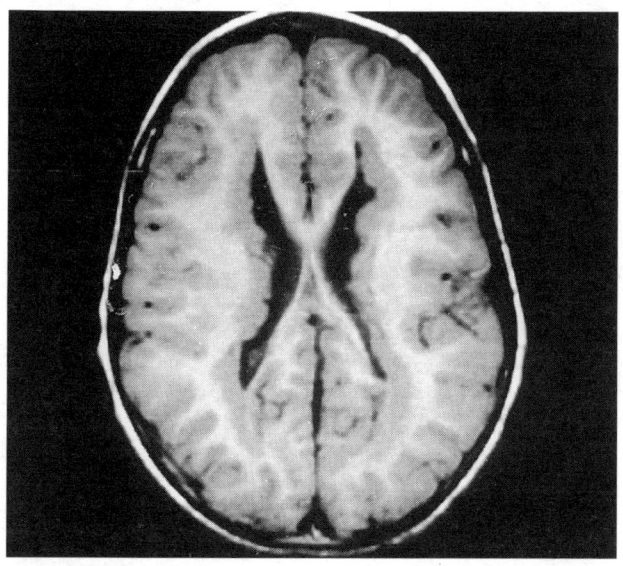

Figure 3. Axial T1-weighted image showing bilateral subependymal nodular heterotopia. Nodules are confluent and protrude into the lumen of both lateral ventricles. The overlying cortex appears normal.

during family evaluations asymptomatic individuals with BSENH have been discovered. Sporadic cases of BSENH occurs in both sexes. However, most of them are female [9, 24, 25]. Among the affected males reported, some have epilepsy with normal intelligence, but others have a severe mental retardation [25].

Several multiplex families have been reported. In 6 families with 18 affected patients, no male is affected [9, 25-28]. In the largest family, six females from four generations are affected, the incidence of miscarriages is increased and the ratio of liveborn sons to daughters is skewed strongly towards daughters [9]. This suggests that most of the miscarriages are males. As for SCLH, this suggests the effects of a gene on the X chromosome with more severe manifestations (or pregnancy loss) in males.

The gene for BSENH has been mapped to chromosome Xq28. Linkage analysis in several of the multiplex families showed positive lod scores (5.37) for markers in distal Xq28 [10]. Genetic hypothesis, similar to thoose suggested for SCLH, may be proposed to explain the clinical and radiological differences between males and females. A somatic mosaicism of brain cells for BSENH gene could explain patients with unilateral subependymal nodular heterotopia.

Conclusion

These brain malformations are a model for the understanding of brain developpement. Genetic analysis will provide tools for this analysis. Recognition of their inherited nature which often results in mild clinical or radiological manifestations in carrier females, is important for genetic counseling.

Abbreviations

BSENH: bilateral subependymal nodular heterotopia
CD: cerebral cortical dysgenesis
SCLH: subcortical laminar heterotopia

References

1. Raymond A, Fish D, Sisodiya S, Alsanjari N, Stevens J, Shorvon S. Abnomalities of gyration, heterotopias, tuberous sclerosis, focal cortical dysplasia, microdysgenesis, dysembryoplastic neuroepithelial tumor and dysgenesis of the archicortex in epilepsy. Clinical, EEG and neuroimaging features in 100 adult patients. *Brain* 1995 ; 118 : 629-60.
2. Dobyns W, Reiner O, Carrozzo R, Ledbetter D. Lissencephaly: a human brain malformation associated with deletion of the LIS1 gene located at chromosome 17p13. *JAMA* 1993 ; 270 : 2838-42.
3. Marchal G, Andermann F, Tampieri D, Robitaille Y, Melanson D, Sinclair B, Olivier A, Silver K, Langevin P. Generalized cortical dysplasia manifested by diffusely thick cerebral cortex. *Arch Neurol* 1989 ; 46 : 430-4.

4. Livingston J, Aicardi J. Unusual MRI appearance of diffuse subcortical heterotopia or "double cortex" in two children. *J Neurol Neurosurg Psychiatr* 1990 ; 53 : 617-20.
5. Palmini A, Andermann F, Aicardi J, Dulac O, Chaves F, Ponsot G, Pinard JM, Goutières F, Livingston J, Tampieri D, Andermann E, Robitaille Y. Diffuse cortical dysplasia, or the "double cortex" syndrome: the clinical and epileptic spectrum in 10 patients. *Neurology* 1991 ; 41 : 1656-62.
6. Pinard JM, Motte J, Chiron C, Brian R, Andermann E, Dulac O. Subcortical laminar heterotopia and lissencephaly in two families: a single X linked dominant gene. *Neurol Neurosurg Psychiatr* 1994 ; 57 : 914-20.
7. Pinard JM, Desguerre I, Motte J, Dulac O, Ponsot G. Hétérotopies laminaires sous-corticales et lissencéphalies : malformations cérébrales à hérédité dominante liée à l'X. *Arch Pediatr* 1995 ; 2 : 493-4.
8. Scheffer I, Mitchell L, Howell R, Fitt G, Syngeniotis A, Saling M, Berkovic S. Familial band heterotopias: an X-linked dominant disorder with variable severity. *Ann Neurol* 1994 ; 36 : 511.
9. Huttenlocher P, Taravath S, Mojtahedi S. Periventricular heterotopia and epilepsy. *Neurology* 1994 ; 44 : 51-5.
10. Eksioglu Y, Scheffer I, Cardenas P, Kuoll S, DiMario F, Ramsby G, Berg M, Kamuro K, Berkovic S, Duyk G, Parisi J, Huttenlocher P, Walsh C. Periventricular heterotopia: an X-linked dominant epilepsy locus causing aberrant cerebral cortical development. *Neuron* 1996 ; 16 : 77-87.
11. Barth P, Reinier M, Stam F, Slooff J. Familial lissencephaly with extreme neopallial hypoplasia. *Brain Dev* 1982 ; 4 : 145-51.
12. Pavone L, Gullotta F, Incorpora G, Grasso S, Dobyns W. Isolated lissencephaly: report of four patients from two unrelated families. *J Child Neurol* 1990 ; 5 : 52-9.
13. Berry-Kravis E, Israel J. X-linked pachygyria and agenesis of the corpus callosum: evidence for an X chromosome lissencephaly locus. *Ann Neurol* 1994 ; 36 : 229-33.
14. Barkovich A, Guerrini R, Battaglia G, Kalifa G, N'Guyen T, Parmeggiani A, Santucci M, Giovanardi-Rossi P, Granata T, D'Incerti L. Band heterotopia: correlation of outcome with magnetic resonance imaging parameters. *Ann Neurol* 1994 ; 36 : 609-17.
15. Moutard ML, Guerrini R, Parain D, Avanzini G, Battaglia G, Dravet C, Franceschetti S, Granata T, Giovanardi-Rossi MP, Parmeggiani A, Pinard JM, Plouin P, Robain O, Ricci S, Vigevano F. Hétérotopies en bandes : aspects électro-cliniques. *Neurophysiol Clin* 1994 ; 24 : 455-6.
16. Tohyama J, Kato M, Koeda T, Inagaki M, Ohno K. The "double cortex" syndrome. *Brain Dev* 1993 ; 15 : 83-4.
17. Miura K, Watanabe K, Maeda N, Matsumoto A, Kumagai T, Ito K, Kato T. Magnetic resonance imaging and positron emission tomography of band heterotopia. *Brain Dev* 1993 ; 15 : 288-90.
18. Bauer J, Elger C. Band heterotopia: a rare cause of generalized epileptic seizures. *Seizure* 1994 ; 3 : 153-5.
19. Harding B. Grey matter heterotopia. In : Guerrini R, Andermann F, Canapicchi R, Roger J, Zilfkin B, Pfanner P, eds. *Dysplasias of cerebral cortex and epilepsy*. Philadelphia-New York : Lippincott-Raven, 1996 : 81-8.
20. Ketonen L, Roddy S, Lannan M. Band heterotopia. *J Child Neurol* 1994 ; 9 : 384 5.
21. Franzoni E, Bernardi B, Marchiani V, Crisanti AF, Marchi R, Fonda C. Band brain heterotopia. Case report and literature review. *Neuropediatrics* 1995 ; 26 : 37-40.
22. Aicardi J. The agyria-pachygyria complex: a spectrum of cortical malformations. *Brain Dev* 1991 ; 13 : 1-8.
23. Zollino M, Mastroiacovo P, Zampino G, Mariotti P, Neri G. New XLMR syndrome with characteristic face, hypogenitalism, congenital hypotonia and pachygyria. *Am J Med Genet* 1992 ; 43 : 452-7.

24. Raymond A, Fish D, Stevens J, Sisodiya S, Alsanjari N, Shorvon S. Subependymal heterotopia: a distinct neuronal migration disorder associated with epilepsy. *J Neurol Neurosurg Psychiatr* 1994 ; 57 : 1195-202.
25. Dubeau F, Tampieri D, Lee N, Andermann E, Carpenter S, Leblanc R, Olivier A, Radtke R, Villemure 1, Andermann F. Periventricular and subcortical nodular heterotopia: a study of 33 patients. *Brain* 1995 ; 118 : 1273-87.
26. Oda T, Nagai Y, Fujimoto S, Sobajima H, Kobayashi M, Togari H, Wada Y. Hereditary nodular heterotopia accompanied by mega cisterna magna. *Am J Med Genet* 1993 ; 47 : 268-71.
27. DiMario F, Cobb R, Ramsby G, Leicher C. Familial band heterotopia simulating tuberous sclerosis. *Neurology* 1993 ; 43 : 1424-6.
28. Kamuro K, Tenokuchi Y. Familial periventricular nodular heterotopia. *Brain Dev* 1993 ; 15 : 237-41.

13

Magnetic resonance in temporal lobe epilepsy

G.D. JACKSON

University of Melbourne, Austin Hospital and Repatriation Medical Centre, Victoria, Australia.

The diagnosis of mesial temporal sclerosis is very important in the context of a patient with epilepsy, and even more so when surgical treatment is contemplated. In the early studies of patients with intractable epilepsy, abnormalities in patients with hippocampal sclerosis were not identified. Most investigators considered that hippocampal sclerosis could not be diagnosed on the basis of visual inspection of the MR, although some studies suggested that severe hippocampal sclerosis (HS) could be diagnosed [1]. Others found that this was possible with high sensitivity and specificity if imaging planes were optimal and diagnostic criteria clearly defined [2, 3]. At the same time quantitative volume measurement studies were developed which gave reliable lateralising information based on relative differences in hippocampal size. These studies have shown that significant asymmetry as measured on MR studies is strongly associated with hippocampal sclerosis, and this has provided useful clinical and research findings. More recent reports [4-9] have confirmed that visual analysis of images is sensitive and specific for diagnosing hippocampal sclerosis if optimised scan acquisition and analysis are performed.

Volumetric techniques have dominated the recent literature. They provide quantitative data which can be used to correlate with other measures of dysfunction in TLE but remain labour intensive and dependant on meticulous technique. Also, despite volume quantitation, only side to side differences have been shown to be reliable, and bilateral disease is still hard to detect. There are two main techniques "other" than volumetric analysis of the hippocampus which have been developed for the diagnosis of hippocampal sclerosis which are the subject of this chapter. These are visual analysis of images, and quantitative T2 relaxometry.

Visual analysis of optimised imaging

Every group has personal experience of visual analysis of MR images as this is the way that clinical studies are typically reported. Often there have been markedly different results between different centres. In experienced centres the rate of diagnosis varies from a low of 30-50% up to 90-95% or even more. There is a developing consensus that it is possible to make this diagnosis based on visual criteria in almost all cases if imaging is optimised and the reporting specialist is experienced in interpreting the sometimes subtle abnormalities which are diagnostic of hippocampal sclerosis [4-10]. It should be emphasised that high sensitivity depends on interpretation of both morphological abnormalities and of signal change with knowledge of the details of hippocampal anatomy and pathology, and a clear understanding of what criteria are sufficient for a definite diagnosis of hippocampal sclerosis.

Factors which influence the ability to make the diagnosis of hippocampal sclerosis are: the orientation of the acquired images, the nature of the imaging sequence, the criteria used to make the MR diagnosis, the precise knowledge of normal and abnormal hippocampal anatomy by the imaging specialist, and confidence that small variations are meaningful information rather than artefacts. We have found asymmetry between sides in 83% of cases, identified signal abnormalities in 89% (77% T2 and 83% T1) and 89% had abnormalities of the internal architecture of the hippocampus. Bronnen recently reported 57 patients with hippocampal sclerosis and showed similar results [4] with visually determined hippocampal atrophy in 55 cases (96%) and signal change in 52 cases (86%) with overall positive diagnosis using both features of 100% in a population of patients where pathological confirmation was possible following temporal lobe resection. Jack [8] also has reported similar rates of diagnostic yield using visual analysis when compared to quantitative analysis in his recent series.

Our recent data comparing visual analysis to quantitative analysis of hippocampal damage suggests that the eye is very sensitive, confident, and reliable in detecting hippocampal asymmetries of greater than 14% between the sides, but may be uncertain if the asymmetry is less than this. Similarly, the eye can reliably detect a signal change on T2 weighted images of more than 10 ms (in our series ≥114 compared to a maximum control value of 107ms) [9]. Values less than this threshold for both volumes and T2 were detected in some cases, but it was not reliable, nor was there complete concordance between observers. In our series no definite diagnostic feature mis-lateralised.

As emphasised by these centres, visual analysis uses more than one parameter for the diagnosis of hippocampal sclerosis. Therefore criteria such as morphologic abnormality and evidence of water content (signal) change may be more diagnostic than either alone. We have found this in our series, and if only one feature alone is relied on (such as side to side cross sectional asymmetry) then the diagnostic yield is not as great or delivered with the same confidence. When all four described features (below) are considered in optimally acquired imaging sequences, then visual analysis appears to be capable of being as sensitive as any other method of analysis, including volumetric analysis, and avoids the occasional mistakes of lateralisation which occur with unusual pathology when relying on volumetrics or T2 relaxometry alone. In centres which specialise in epilepsy it is important that the yield of diagnostic studies approaches this level, and we believe that optimal image acquisition and interpretation is mandatory for this level of visual diagnostic sensitivity and reliability.

Although uncommon, hippocampal sclerosis without detected hippocampal atrophy has been reported where the diagnosis was correctly made on the basis of visual analysis of the signal changes. Similarly we would expect that cases will exist where there is atrophy, but little detectable signal change. While these cases are likely to be uncommon, to avoid occasional misinterpretation of data such as hippocampal volumes or T2 relaxation time values, it is important that they are interpreted in the context of high quality visual analysis. It is becoming increasingly clear that there are occasional cases which are misleading if undue emphasis is placed on a single measure such as hippocampal volume (asymmetry) or T2 relaxation measurement. As in other areas of epilepsy, concordance, and complete description of the abnormality should be a guiding principle.

In the cases in which dual pathology is present, the detection of these regional or focal abnormalities of the temporal lobe or hemisphere in which hippocampal sclerosis is found (probably at least 15% of cases in adults, and even more in children) can only be achieved with visual analysis. This is an example where undue reliance on a single measure such as hippocampal volume measurements or T2 relaxation times would give a misleading impression of the underlying basis of a patient's seizure disorder without the accompanying context of the visual analysis of the entire brain. Conversely, the information provided by these means adds to our understanding of the structural substrates which may be involved in the patients epilepsy condition.

Making the "visual" diagnosis of hippocampal sclerosis

Although visual features were initially considered to be "subtle" and there was a reluctance to attribute diagnostic significance to the findings, it is now clear that knowledge of the hippocampal anatomy, and understanding of MRI artefacts means that the diagnosis of hippocampal sclerosis is easily made in most cases. With experience visual sensitivity for hippocampal sclerosis should approach 95% or better in surgical TLE series where more severe and lateralised abnormality might be expected. It must be emphasised that not all features are seen in all cases. Unequivocal signal change (as long as the hippocampus is not enlarged thereby suggesting a tumor, Figure 1) or atrophy may be accepted as diagnostic of hippocampal sclerosis, with the certainty increased if both are present. The addition of internal structure loss can be very helpful if the abnormality is subtle (Figure 2). Several series which compare blinded visual reports to pathological material have shown beyond doubt that hippocampal sclerosis can be reliably diagnosed by visual analysis. In experienced hands, and with optimised images, high sensitivity and specificity can be achieved. In order to do this, optimised images must be performed and all features of hippocampal sclerosis must be appreciated and searched for [6]. It is our experience that no single feature (such as atrophy) on its own is sensitive enough for reliable routine visual diagnosis in all cases, although some expert centres achieve an accurate diagnosis in over 80% of cases using this feature alone.

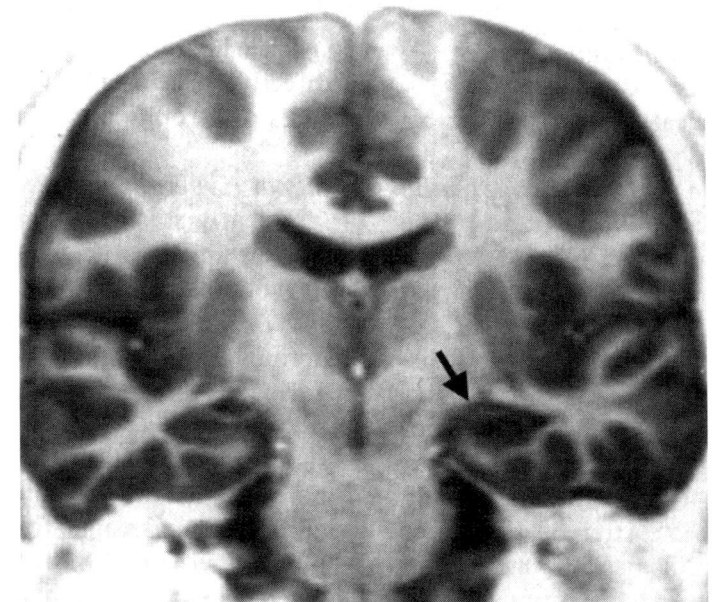

Figure 1. The left hippocampus (arrow) shows decreased signal and disruption of internal structure without the visual feature of atrophy. At operation, hippocampal sclerosis was confirmed.

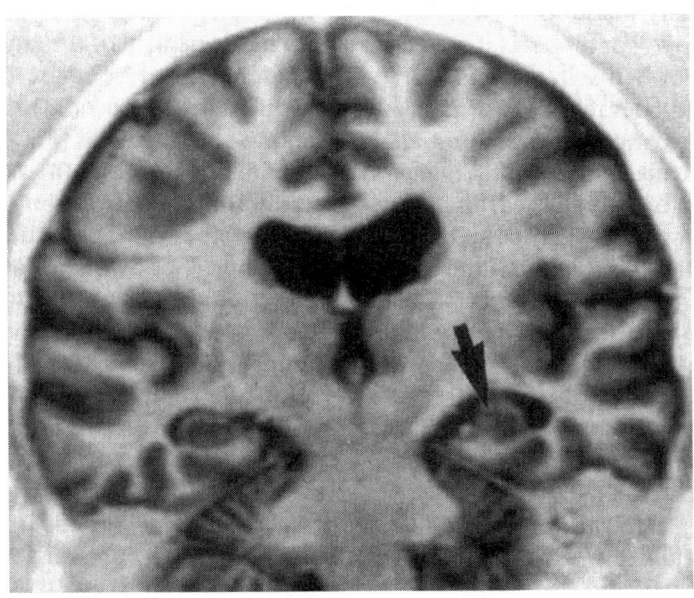

Figure 2. The left hippocampus is smaller with abnormal internal structure. The entire left hemisphere is also atrophic.

Atrophy

The assessment of the cross-sectional size of the hippocampus must be made in images obtained in the modified (tilted) coronal axis that transects the hippocampus at right angles (Figure 3). This axis is essential for coronal imaging, and the axis at right angles to this is essential for axial imaging of the temporal lobe. A smaller hippocampus as detected in this plane either qualitatively or by quantitative methods, reliably predicts the side of the epileptogenic focus in the case of temporal lobe epilepsy but absolute measures of hippocampal size must be interpreted with caution. Quantitation of atrophy (hippocampal volume measurement) is slightly more sensitive than visual assessment of hippocampal size, but with the addition of other visual features of hippocampal sclerosis this difference is less marked, or even reversed. An example of atrophy is shown in Figure 4. For reliable visual diagnosis of hippocampal sclerosis, unless the atrophy is obvious, signal change or internal structure abnormality on optimised imaging is pathognomic of hippocampal sclerosis. In the absence of additional features, the side to side asymmetry is usually accurate, but care must be taken to be aware of the occasional cases where this is misleading.

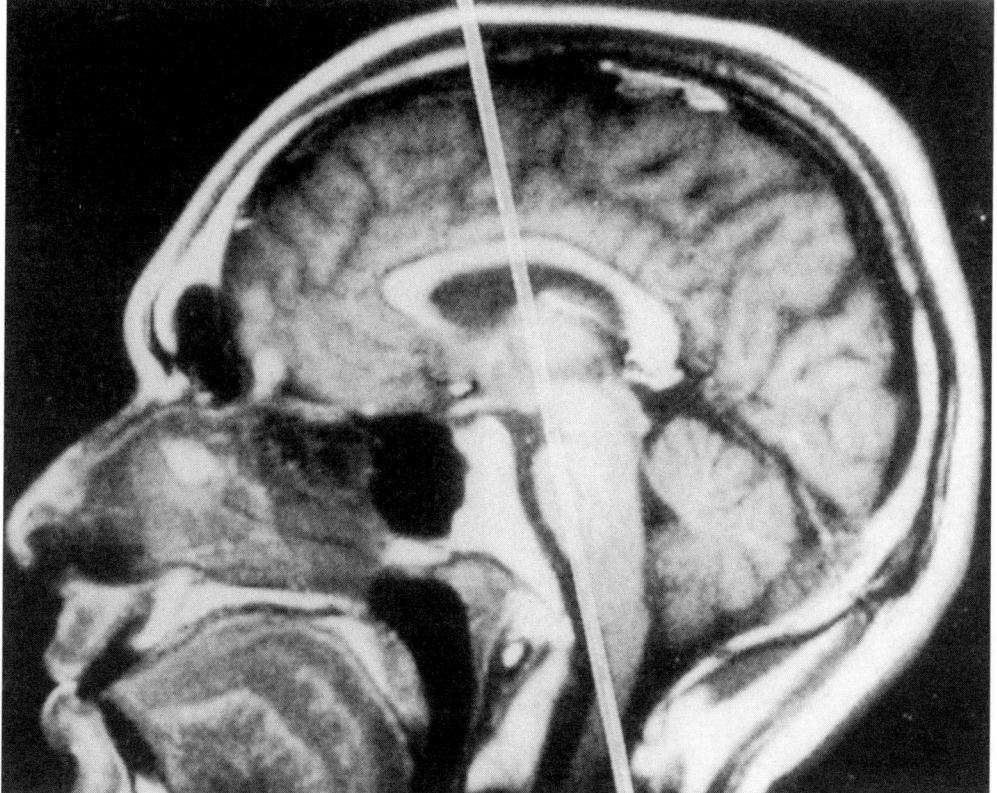

Figure 3. This shows the "temporal lobe" axis for orientation of images using the midline sagittal image. The alternative is to use the hippocampus itself to orient images along it and at right angles to it.

Loss of the normal internal morphological structure of the hippocampus

Normal internal morphological structure (the "architecture") of the hippocampus is produced by the alveus, the molecular cell layer of the dentate gyrus, and the pyramidal cell layer of the cornu ammonis, and can be seen on optimised coronal MR images (Figure 5). In hippocampal sclerosis, the loss of this normal internal structure is a consequence of neuronal cell loss and replacement of normal anatomical layers with gliotic tissue. This feature of hippocampal sclerosis is very important as, with increasing spatial resolution, thinning of the CA1 region of the cornu ammonis may prove to be the most sensitive and specific means of diagnosing hippocampal sclerosis. Attempts have been made to define this with specially designed surface array coils, however, increased resolution which will routinely show this microanatomy is becoming possible using standard equipment. With high field strength, and high resolution imaging, it is probable that analysis of the pattern of the CA1 neuronal loss will be detectable directly. This high resolution "microscopic" MRI will become increasingly important in the diagnosis of subtle abnormalities of the hippocampus and specific histological diagnosis will be able to be made directly, rather that by indirect association with measures of atrophy or signal abnormality.

Signal hyperintensity on T2-weighted images

In early studies increased hippocampal T2 signal was dismissed as due to artefacts of flow, partial volume with CSF, or lateralisation artefact (Figure 6). It is now clear that signal change in the anatomically definite hippocampus is common and can be distinguished from these artefacts with experience and improved imaging techniques. Increased T2 weighted signal when localised imprecisely to the "mesial temporal region" may be due to foreign tissue such as a glioma or hamartoma, to gliotic tissue in the hippocampus, to increased CSF in the atrophied region, to flow artefacts and

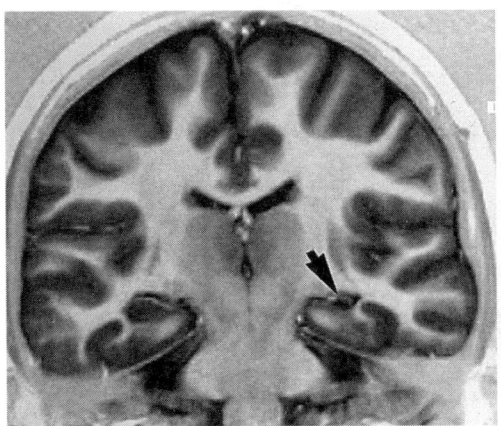
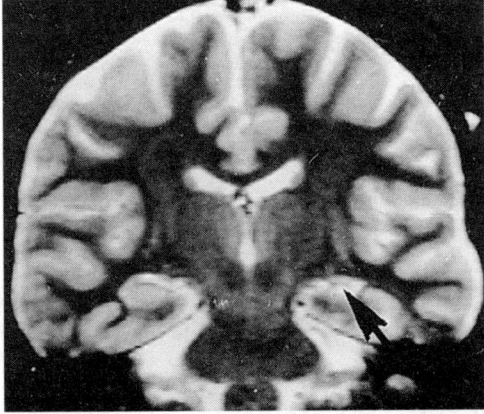

Figure 4. This image shows the classic features of severe hippocampal sclerosis with atrophy, decreased signal and abnormal internal structure in the T1-weighted image (left) and atrophy and increased signal on the T2-weighted image (right).

occasionally from a developmental cyst in the hippocampal head stemming from failure of closure of the lateral aspect of the hippocampal fissure. Careful determination of the exact location of this signal change by detailed examination of the anatomical features enables the correct diagnosis to be made (Figures 4A and 7). It is important to have sufficient knowledge of both the hippocampal anatomy and the easily recognisable artefacts which can occur in this region so that artefacts are not confused with significant signal abnormalities in the hippocampal grey matter.

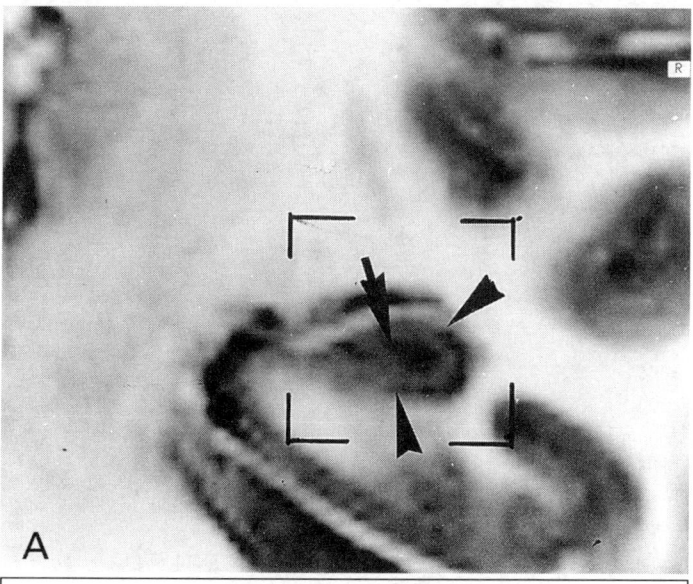

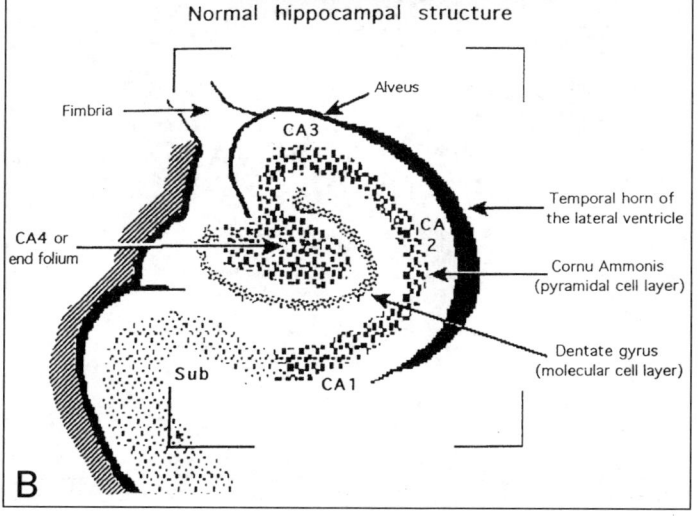

Figure 5. Normal internal structure of the hippocampal body immediately posterior to the amygdala is shown in the T1-weighted inversion recovery image (**A**) and is compared to the diagram (**B**)

Signal hypointensity on T1-weighted IR images

At 1.5 tesla, using a TR of 3500 and a TI of 300ms, a sclerotic hippocampus appears dark, small, and the internal features are obscured (Figure 8). This feature of T1 weighted signal intensity change has been often overlooked as it is rarely prominent in routine T1-weighted sequences. When using a heavily T1-weighted sequence such as

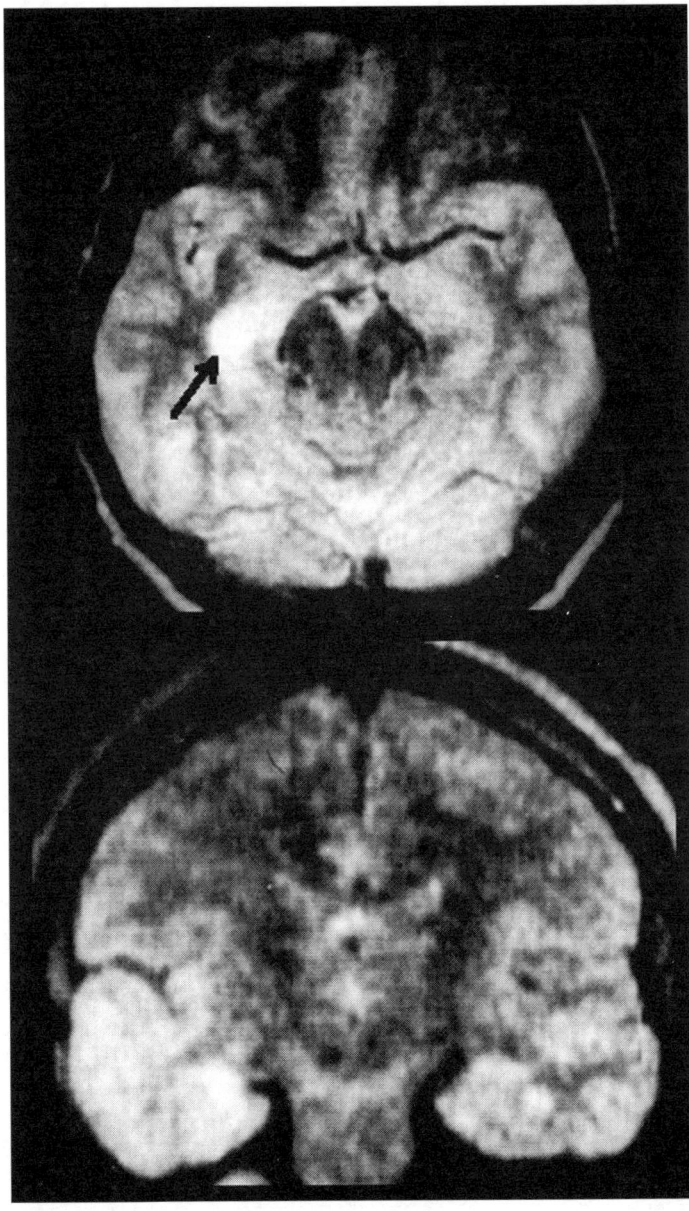

Figure 6. Using a 0.3 tesla system, often signal change was the major visible feature of hippocampal sclerosis seen on T2-weighted images. Note the imprecise localization of the signal to the hippocampal head (upper image) and the associated signal abnormality in the anterior temporal lobe (lower image).

this IR sequence, this is a prominent and common finding which aids in the detection of hippocampal sclerosis. It correlates strongly with the T2 changes, but may be more or less prominent, and more easily seen in the center of the affected hippocampus. The presence of three features in a single coronal image makes the visual diagnosis of hippocampal sclerosis much easier, and makes it possible to detect mild degrees of abnormality.

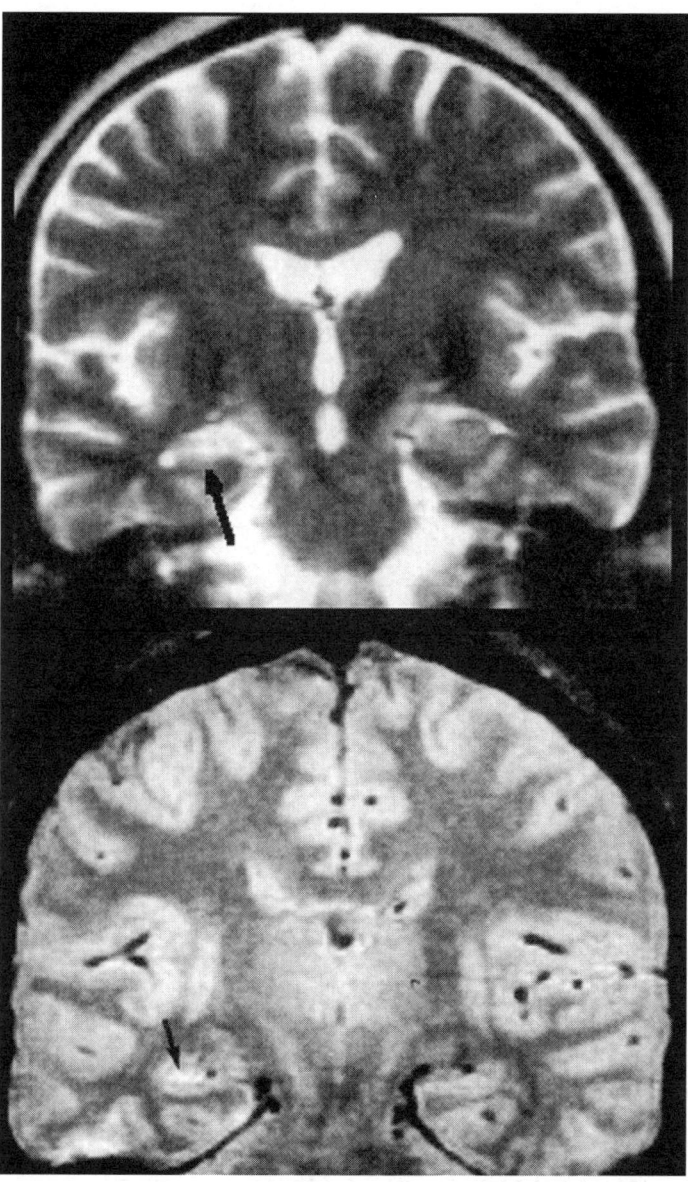

Figure 7. Signal change in the hippocampus is seen in the T2-weighted sequence (upper image) where atrophy can also be appreciated and in a proton density weighted image (lower image). In the case shown in the lower image, no volume asymmetry was present on the quantitative study, but hippocampal sclerosis was confirmed in the surgical specimen.

An abnormal signal on T1 or T2 weighted images arising from an atrophic hippocampus almost always represents hippocampal sclerosis. An abnormal signal arising from an apparently enlarged hippocampus may represent a hamartoma or glioma. If one relied only on a single feature such as atrophy, then these cases of the larger hippocampus being abnormal would be incorrectly lateralised. The principle is that concordance of features makes for more reliable diagnostic certainty.

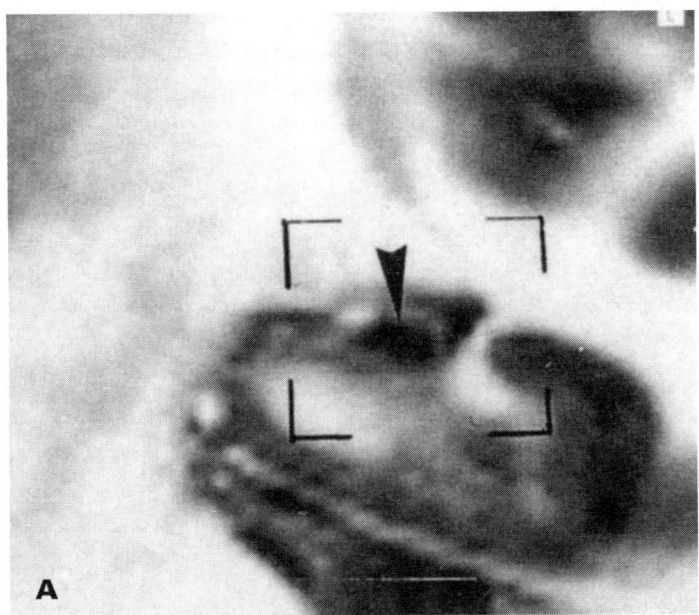

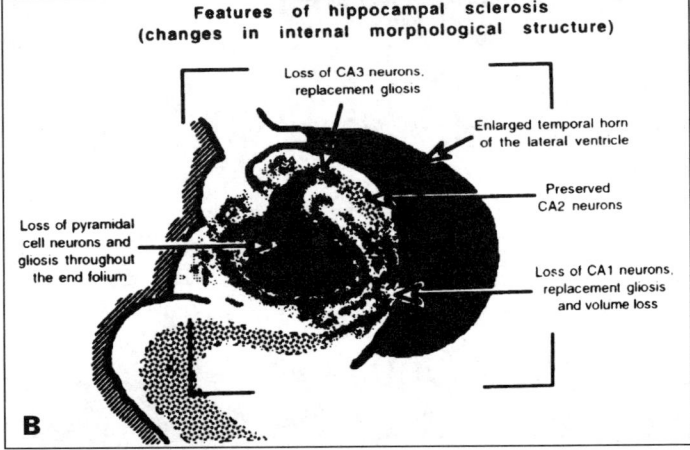

Figure 8. The altered internal structure that is seen on inversion recovery T1-weighted images is shown in **A**, and represented in diagram form in **B**.

Visual analysis
Findings other than hippocampal sclerosis

Regional abnormalities of the temporal lobe

It is clear that hippocampal sclerosis often exists in the context of more regional abnormalities of the temporal lobe. The most common finding is signal change most easily seen in the white matter core of the temporal lobe, although this also may involve the grey matter [11]. This characteristically gives a loss of grey-white matter definition and predominates in the anterior temporal lobe and temporal pole region. Such changes should not simply be dismissed as partial volume effects without considerable care. This has been largely ignored as the focus of attention has been on the hippocampus itself. The amygdala may be involved in a significant number of cases, and regional abnormalities of either the whole or parts of the temporal lobe (such as the entorrhinal area, superior temporal gyrus, and parahippocampal gyrus) may also be commonly found. There have been no systematic studies of these regions in the way that has occurred in the case of the hippocampus. It is our feeling that these findings are less easily distinguished than in the hippocampus, but imaging optimised for this purpose has not been reported. T2 relaxation mapping of the amygdala appears to be a promising technique [9].

Other abnormalities

Detailed analysis of MRI images reveals a high percentage of abnormalities which can be detected in the brains of patients with intractable partial epilepsy. As MR techniques improve, it is becoming clear that most patients with intractable epilepsy have detectable imaging abnormalities. Table I shows the range of abnormalities which were detected in a combined series of patients from several centres. While often, in the past, no cause could be identified for many cases of intractable partial epilepsy, it is now becoming clear that most adults and children with partial epilepsy will have defined brain abnormalities visualised on appropriate optimised imaging [12, 13].

Outcome

The outcome following temporal lobectomy can be predicted prior to operation based on the visual MR findings [14]. It is important to note that the outcome for those patients with hippocampal sclerosis identified as that cause in the preoperative imaging is good, but that occasional seizures continue to occur even many years after successful temporal lobectomy. The cause of these seizures, and why this differs from patients with lesions is not yet clear.

Table I

MRI diagnosis	%	Number/location
Hippocampal sclerosis	57	194
Foreign tissue lesion (glioma, astrocytoma or dysembryoplastic tumor)	13.5	46 (36 temporal, 10 extratemporal)
Cortical dysplasia	10.5	35 (12 temporal, 23 extratemporal)
Vascular malformations (12 cavernous hemangiomas, 2 high flow lesions)	4	14 (6 temporal, 8 extratemporal)
Cystic lesions	1.5	5 (4 temporal, 1 extratemporal)
Miscellaneous	5	17 (5 trauma, 1 tuberous sclerosis, 2 epidermoid, 4 extensive white matter lesions, 1 cerebellar atrophy, 4 uncertain)
No lesion demonstrated	8.5	29
Total	100	340

Quantitative diagnosis of hippocampal sclerosis with T2 relaxation time measurement

There has been a widespread problem in achieving the best results using visual analysis (and routine reporting of MR studies) in the clinical environment. It is clear that the results of visual inspection can be replicated in different centres, and that the findings are specific and sensitive when optimised images are interpreted in expert hands. It is equally clear that this expertise is not always available.

It is also generally not possible to detect bilateral disease of the hippocampus with visual or volume based analysis, as both these techniques rely heavily on side to side comparisons [15, 16]. The quantified features of hippocampal sclerosis are the same as when assessed visually atrophy and signal change. Much initial attention has been given to the quantitation of hippocampal atrophy but we now consider quantitation of signal.

T2 relaxometry

As well as quantifying the hippocampal atrophy, one can quantify the T2 signal in the hippocampus by measuring the T2 relaxation time in the hippocampal grey matter [9, 17, 18]. The T2 relaxation time can be measured quantitatively by measuring the decay in signal intensity at different echo times (TE) in a series of T2 weighted images acquired in the same slice. Each pixel of the resulting T2 map is derived from the intensity in each of these multiple images (in our case 16 images at different TE's, using a specialised pulse sequence) in that same slice.

This objective measurement has a small range of values in normal subjects. The T2 relaxation time appears to be very precise in normal tissue. This enables the detection of pathology without requiring comparison between two hippocampi. Therefore, as well as being sensitive, it permits the detection of pathology in the contralateral hippocampus (Figure 9).

In our experience, the T2 relaxation time within the hippocampus is a robust and reliable objective measurement of hippocampal pathology, providing a means of assessing the hippocampus which is as good as our most skilled visual interpretation of hippocampal abnormality in optimised scans. In contrast to both visual interpretation and volumetric analysis of hippocampal atrophy, the definition of a normal hippocampal T2 relaxation time is very precise. Therefore, T2 quantification has the ability to detect mild degrees of signal abnormality, bilateral abnormalities and can quantitatively evaluate progressive hippocampal abnormalities. Moreover, T2 values can be interpreted in terms of hippocampal pathology even when the other hippocampus is incomplete or distorted, such as when a lesion is present or following temporal lobe surgery [19]. In these difficult cases, pathology of the residual ipsilateral hippocampus and the contralateral hippocampus may still be diagnosed. It has recently been shown that there is a very close correlation between hippocampal atrophy, hippocampal T2 abnormality and pathological findings (Figure 10) [9]. Therefore, findings from hippocampal volume studies (such as outcome, and pathology correlations) should apply to T2 abnormalities, while the latter has the advantage of detecting bilateral disease.

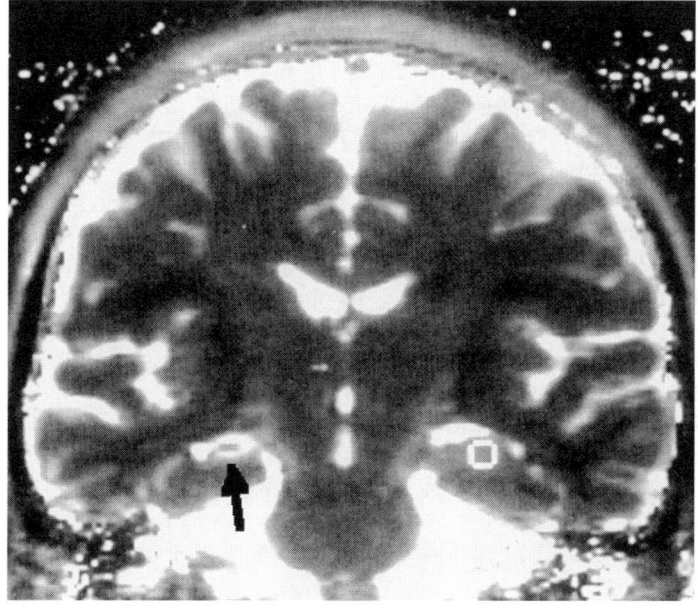

Figure 9. T2 map, where image intensity reflects the measured T2-relaxation time in each pixel. The small hippocampus (arrow) shows increased signal which represents longer T2 relaxation times. The region measured is shown in the left hippocampus.

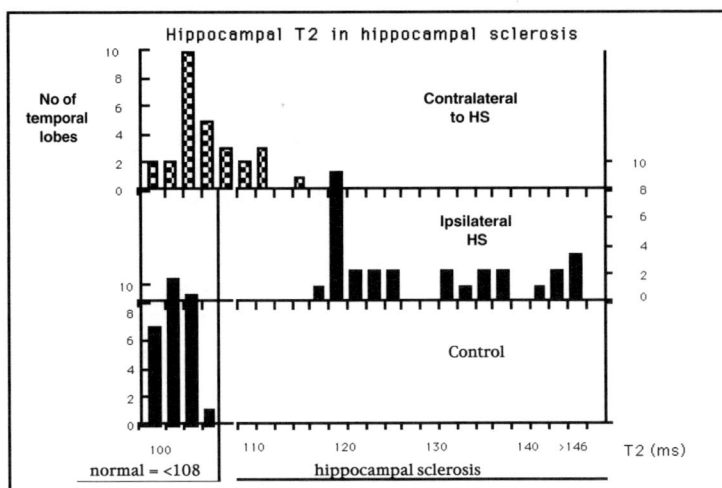

Figure 10. Hippocampal T2 values measured in a consecutive series of surgically treated patients. Contralateral means in the hippocampus opposite to the side resected. Normal control values are shown (open bars).

In general the interpretation of hippocampal abnormalities as measured by volumetric analysis and the clinical correlates of hippocampal asymmetry also applies to T2 relaxation time measurements. The advantages of the T2 method is that analysis after image acquisition takes only a few moments, and the range of normal values is very precise and, in almost all cases, clearly distinct from the values found in hippocampal sclerosis. The precision of normal values means that the diagnosis of hippocampal sclerosis does not depend on using a side to side ratio. Therefore bilateral hippocampal sclerosis can be diagnosed.

Aetiology of HS

There appears to be no significant effect on the T2 relaxation time as a consequence of recent seizures [18], although anecdotes of signal change and progressive damage to the hippocampus following seizures have been reported [20]. The severity of damage can also be accurately assessed even when there is significant bilateral damage, in many cases this will decrease the difference between the sides using conventional volumetric measurements. It would seem apparent that transient events, such as oedema of the hippocampus, or cell swelling for other reasons, should give a prolongation of the T2 signal. Despite studies looking for this occurrence, we have been unable to find significant changes in the hippocampal T2 value following seizures. In all of our cases, the T2 relaxation value appears to reflect chronic changes in the neuronal and glial population of the hippocampus. Recent work comparing quantitative histopathology in resected specimens with T2 relaxation times in the hippocampus has shown that T2 relaxometry correlates with the neuronal loss in CA1-CA4 and with the glial density in CA1 and CA4. Absolute hippocampal T2 values correlates with the ratio of glia to neurons in CA1 ($r=0.83$; $p<0.01$).

The ratio of hippocampal T2 values (left to right) correlates well with volume ratios (left to right) (Figure 10). Therefore measurement of T2 ratios can, in general, be interpreted as being the same as hippocampal volume ratios. T2 relaxometry has the advantage of being able to measure absolute values. Therefore bilateral disease can be detected. In some cases, only a slight asymmetry of left to right hippocampal volume ratios may represent either mild disease, or severe bilateral disease, and the absolute T2 numbers can demonstrate this difference. This could not be determined using visual analysis or volume ratios alone.

The relation of T2 values to outcome has not yet been fully explored. The finding that nearly 30% of all operated cases have an abnormal hippocampus on the other side is important in the context of pathological findings that suggest that bilateral disease is very common (Margerison and Corsellis 1966, Bronen). Despite this, the outcome after temporal lobectomy is generally very good. We have found, in a retrospective study of patients studied 3-17 years after their temporal lobectomy, that the existence of T2 abnormalities in the remaining hippocampus did not predict outcome in terms of seizures, but was important for cognitive outcome [19].

MR spectroscopy

A number of groups are attempting to determine NAA and its ratios to the other metabolites in the hippocampus. Generally the signal to noise requirements means that the volume included in the region of interest is larger than the hippocampus. With recent improvements in technique, and with higher field systems, smaller voxels have been recorded from the mesial temporal regions. This may become a means of detecting hippocampal sclerosis, but it takes a long time of scanning, and this means that spectroscopy may be more important in defining regional abnormalities of the temporal lobe where imaging techniques provide little information [21]. This is particularly so now that hippocampal sclerosis can be reliably and sensitively diagnosed using simpler imaging techniques. The basic observation is that NAA is reduced on in situations of neuronal loss or damage, and that this may give a clue as to the origin of the damage related to the seizures.

Conclusion

All centres with an active interest in epilepsy must have a highly sensitive technique which allows the non-invasive diagnosis of hippocampal sclerosis based on MR images. This can be achieved with a number of techniques including visual analysis of optimised imaging sequences, quantitation of T2 relaxation times in the hippocampus, and measurement of hippocampal volumes. It must be emphasised that all these require modification of imaging technique and acquisition of specialised skills. It should not be assumed that normal imaging excludes hippocampal sclerosis. Preoperative detection of hippocampal sclerosis in patients with intractable epilepsy is essential for patient

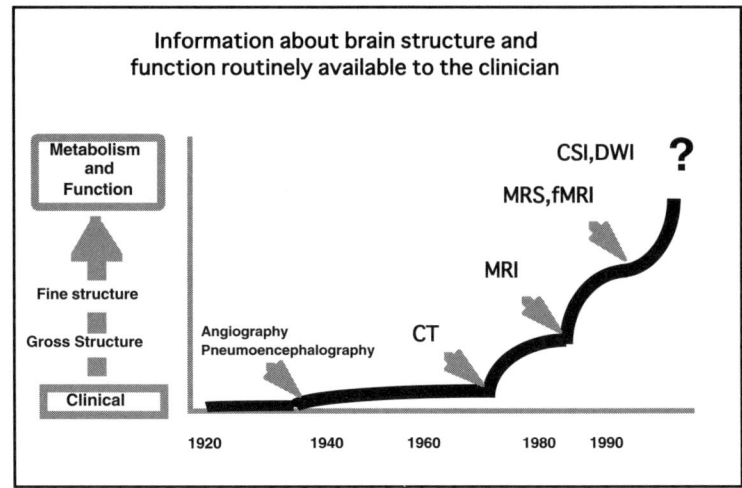

Figure 11. The rapid advances in knowledge of brain structure, metabolism and function routinely available to the clinician.

management and optimal treatment of their condition. A highly sensitive MR method for this diagnosis is now mandatory in all centres which specialise in epilepsy treatment.

Although even recently the detection of abnormality and the determination of the side affected was the sole aim of any of these methods, now increasingly complex questions can be asked, and quantitative techniques should provide more information about the neuropathology of the epilepsy disorder (Table II and Figure 11).

Table II. Summary of questions that can be routinely answered using current techniques for evaluating the hippocampus.

	Visual analysis	Volume ratio	T2 quantitation
Is there hippocampal pathology?	✔	✔	✔
How severe is the hippocampal abnormality?	✘✔	✔	✔
Are the hippocampi definitely normal?	✘	✘	✘✔
Is there bilateral abnormality	✘	✔✘	✔
What is the A-P distribution of the abnormality?	✔	✔	✘
Is the pathology strictly unilateral?	✘	✘	✘✔
Is there pathology outside the hippocampus?	✔	✘	✘

✔ = technique can achieve this
✘ = technique cannot do this
✔✘ = technique can partially do this

Acknowledgements

Many thanks to Jean Aicardi for his inspiration, support and teaching. Portions of this manuscript are reproduced from *Magnetic Resonance Imaging* 1995 ; 13(8) with permission.

References

1. Kuzniecky R, De La Sayette V, Ethier R, *et al.* Magnetic resonance imaging in temporal lobe epilepsy: pathological correlations. *Ann Neurol* 1987 ; 22 (3) : 341-7.
2. Jackson GD, Berkovic SF, Tress BM, Kalnins RM, Fabinyi G, Bladin PF. Hippocampal sclerosis can be reliably detected by magnetic resonance imaging. *Neurology* 1990 ; 40 (12) : 1869-75.
3. Berkovic SF, Andermann F, Olivier A, *et al.* Hippocampal sclerosis in temporal lobe epilepsy demonstrated by magnetic resonance imaging. *Ann Neurol* 1991 ; 29 : 175-82.
4. Bronen RA, Fullbright R, Kim JH, Spencer DD, Spencer SS. MR signal changes associated with pathology proven hippocampal sclerosis. *Epilepsia* 1994 ; 35 (suppl 8) : 22.
5. Kuzniecky R, Cascino GD, Palmini A, *et al.* Structural imaging. In : Engel JJ, ed. *Surgical treatment of the epilepsies,* 2nd edition. New York : Raven Press, 1993 : 197-200.
6. Jackson GD, Berkovic SF, Duncan JS, Connelly A. Optimising the diagnosis of hippocampal sclerosis using magnetic resonance imaging. *Am J Neurorad* 1993 ; 14 : 753-62.
7. Jackson GD, Kuzniecky RI, Cascino GD. Hippocampal sclerosis without detectable hippocampal atrophy. *Neurology* 1994 ; 44(1) : 42-6.
8. Jack C. MRI-based hippocampal volume measuremnts in epilepsy. *Epilepsia* 1994 ; 35 (suppl 6) : 14-9.
9. Van Paesschen W, Sisodiya S, Connelly A, *et al.* Quantitative hippocampal MRI and intractable temporal lobe epilepsy. *Neurology* 1995 ; 45 (in press).
10. Grattan-Smith JD, Harvey AS, Desmond PM, Chow CW. Hippocampal sclerosis in children with intractable temporal lobe epilepsy: a clinical and MRI correlative study. *Epilepsia* 1993 ; 34(6) : 127.
11. Meiners LC, Valk J, Jansen GH, Luyten PR. Magnetic resonance of epilepsy: three observations. In : Shorvon SD, Fish DR, Andermann F, Bydder GM, Stefan H, eds. *Magnetic resonance scanning and epilepsy.* New York : Plennum, 1994 : 79-82.
12. Cross JH, Jackson GD, Neville BGR, *et al.* Early detection of abnormalities in partial epilepsy using magnetic resonance. *Arch Dis Child* 1993 ; 69 : 104-9.
13. Cook MJ, Fish DR, Shorvon SD, Straughan K, Stevens JM. Hippocampal volumetric and morphometric studies in frontal and temporal lobe epilepsy. *Brain* 1992 ; 115 : 1001-15.
14. Berkovic SF, McIntosh AM, Kalnins RM, *et al.* Preoperative MRI predicts outcome of temporal lobectomy: an actuarial analysis. *Neurology* 1995 ; 45 (in press).
15. Bergin PS, Raymond AA, Free SL, Sisodiya SM, Stevens JM. Magnetic resonance volumetry. *Neurology* 1994 ; 44 : 1770-1.
16. Jack CJ, Bentley MD, Twomey CK, Zinsmeister AR. MR imaging-based volume measurements of the hippocampal formation and anterior temporal lobe: validation studies. *Radiology* 1990 ; 176 (1) : 205-9.
17. Jackson GD, Connelly A, Duncan JS, Grünewald RA, Gadian DG. Detection of hippocampal pathology in intractable partial epilepsy: increased sensitivity with quantitative magnetic resonance T2 relaxometry. *Neurology* 1993 ; 43 : 1793-9.
18. Grünewald RA, Jackson GD, Connelly A, Duncan JS. MR detection of hippocampal pathology in epilepsy: factors influencing T2 relaxation time. *Am J Neurorad* 1994 ; 15 : 1149-56.
19. Incisa della Rocchetta A, Connelly A, Gadian DG, *et al.* Verbal memory impairment after right temporal lobe surgery: the role of contralateral damage as revealed by 1H MRS and T2 relaxometry. *Neurology* 1995 ; 45(4) : 797-802.
20. Nohria V, Lee N, Tien RD, *et al.* Magnetic resonance imaging evidence of hippocampal sclerosis in progression: a case report. *Epilepsia* 1994 ; 35 : 1332-9.
21. Connelly A, Jackson G, Duncan J, Gadian D. Magnetic resonance spectroscopy in temporal lobe epilepsy. *Neurology* 1994 ; 44(8) : 1411-7.

14

Congenital muscular dystrophies: an overview

Y. FUKUYAMA [1,2], M. OSAWA [1], K. SAITO [1]

1. Department of Pediatrics, Tokyo Women's Medical College, Tokyo, Japan.
2. Child Neurology Institute, Tokyo, Japan.

The term "congenital muscular dystrophy" (CMD) was first coined by Howard [1] in 1908 to describe a floppy infant with joint contractures, although descriptions of similar conditions had appeared sporadically in Europe [2, 3]. The basic concept of investigators in those early days was to recognize a condition in a baby suffering from generalized weakness, hypotonia and often joint contractures since birth, resulting in more or less severe motor developmental delay, associated with a disability that appeared nonetheless to be non-progressive. Deep tendon reflexes were usually retained, a finding which facilitated distinguishing this condition from neurogenic muscular atrophies. Congenital myopathy was strongly suspected, but as no good laboratory examinations were as yet available, the concept of congenital primary myopathy could not at that time be substantiated. Coinciding with the introduction of another benign condition called "amyotonia congenita" by Oppenheim, virtually simultaneously, the ill-defined concept of CMD was abandoned as an uninteresting area of investigation for many years, while heated debate concerning the identity of amyotonia congenita *versus* infantile spinal muscular atrophy dominated the thinking of most investigators during the first half of the 20th century [4].

After a long period of silence, CMD began to receive the attention of mainly German-speaking neuropediatricians in the 1960s. They produced a series of excellent landmark publications on CMD in German [5-9].

Curiously, however, these studies did not provoke appropriate interest in other spheres, probably due to the language barrier.

The ignorance and confusion which surrounded CMD in the international arena until the end of the 1970s is well illustrated in the famous textbook by R.D. Adams, *Diseases of muscle* (3rd edition) published in 1975 [10], which read that congenital muscular dystrophies consist of two groups: (1) established progressive muscular dystrophy at birth or infancy, and (2) congenital myopathy of unidentified type. The former group conforms with the strict definition of progressive muscular dystrophy and includes Duchenne muscular dystrophy, the facioscapulohumeral type of Landouzy-Dejerine and the myotonic dystrophy of Steinert. In contrast, the latter group includes variable conditions which do not necessarily fit with the definition. Thus, there is no trace of the knowledge we now have concerning CMD in the 3rd edition of Adams' book. In 1979, Lazaro *et al.* [11] wrote in their article on CMD that this disorder is a vanishing category or a simple misnomer.

On the other hand, CMD research in Japan followed a completely different path from that in Western countries. Fukuyama *et al.* presented their observations on 15 cases of CMD at a local meeting of the Japan Neurology Society, on December 12, 1959 and published a short paper entitled: "A peculiar form of congenital progressive muscular dystrophy" in 1960 [12]. This report was rather rapidly accepted by many Japanese investigators, and numerous supportive reports followed. The clinical spectrum as well as laboratory findings, including high CK levels, EMG and muscle histology, are so unique and more or less pathognomonic that the condition was easily recognizable to any attentive clinician. A rather high prevalence rate of the condition in Japan also facilitated the propagation of knowledge on this newly described condition among medical staff throughout the country. Consequently, there is no one in Japan who doubts the existence of CMD as a disease entity, and furthermore, many Japanese physicians once tended to believe that all CMD patients are of the so-called Fukuyama type (FCMD). Currently, of course, the greater understanding of Japanese physicians regarding CMD in Japan has led to steady progress in improving the recognition of CMD cases which do not fit the clinical picture of FCMD. Thus, a subclassification of CMD patients into FCMD or nonFCMD is now widely accepted in Japan.

Turning to the rest of the world, a similar system of subclassifying CMD into FCMD and nonFCMD was also adopted in principle by the ICD-10 NA of WHO in 1991, which contains two groups of CMD in the category of muscular dystrophy (G71.0); that is, G 71.084-CMD with CNS abnormalities (Fukuyama) and G71.085-CMD without CNS abnormalities.

It would probably not be an overemphasis to state that the history of CMD research in the world actually started with the discovery and establishment of the entity of FCMD. It should be pointed out that the original work of Fukuyama *et al.* was quickly and fully appreciated inside Japan, but was not recognized for many years outside Japan. The enlightenment of Western investigators took about 20 years or even longer, because the first paper by the Fukuyama group appeared, though in English, in a local, not widely read journal and because the condition newly described was seen as existing almost exclusively in Japan. Tenacious efforts were necessary to disseminate this knowledge in the international sphere, but there were several momentus activities which merit specific mention: these include the publications of good papers by Kamoshita *et al.* (1975) [13], Nonaka and Chou (1979) [14] and Fukuyama *et al.* (1981) [15] in either an influential journal or an internationally popular handbook. A number of free papers on FCMD were impressively presented at the first International Congress of Child Neurology (ICCN), in Toronto, in October of 1975. Fukuyama presented a lecture on FCMD in a symposium at the 2nd ICNC, in Sydney, in November of 1979. Moreover, Fukuyama gave lectures on FCMD at various institutions and societies worldwide, by invitation, 38 times from 1977 through 1994. Through these unwavering activities, knowledge of FCMD spread worldwide, gradually at first and then explosively in recent years. Finally, FCMD was first registered under the number M 253800 in the 7th edition of McKusick's *Mendelian inheritance in man* in 1986. Subsequently, it was first included formally as an independent subtype of muscular dystrophy in the 10th revision of the *Neurological adaptation of the international classification of diseases* in 1991, as mentioned above. Figure 1 shows the chronological trend in world publications of original articles specifically focusing on CMD (including both FCMD and nonFCMD), illustrating well the dramatic globalization of research on CMD-associated issues.

As shown in Table I, 1,103 infants and children with various neuromuscular disorders were treated at the specialized clinic of the Department of Pediatrics, Tokyo Women's Medical College during the last 23 years 2 months period (January 1971- February 1994). The majority of the patients was occupied by those with disorders of muscle (710 out of 1103 patients, 64.4%). The breakdown of the latter by disorder is shown in Table II. A special attention may be called upon the unusually large proportion of CMD patients among the population of progressive muscular dystrophy (PMD), that is, 117 CMD among 337 PMD patients (34.7%). CMD was the second largest subtype of PMD, only after Duchenne muscular dystrophy (DMD), and the relative ratio between FCMD and DMD was 1.00:1.44 in our hospital. This high figure for FCMD in our hospital clearly reflects the nature of clinical service offered by our tertially referral special clinic, but still it will be helpful to understand how often Japanese physicians encounter with FCMD patients.

Clinical features of FCMD

In 1960, Fukuyama *et al.* [12] summarized the clinical features of 15 cases, as shown in Table III, and these original descriptions are still largely valid and no major amendments are necessary. Generally speaking, clinical pictures of FCMD typically mimick those of the floppy infant syndrome in infancy (Figure 2), and later, after the age of 2 years, resemble those of congenital multiple arthrogryposis (Figure 3). Owing to more than 30 years' experience after the first report, however, there emerged a certain aspect which appears to merit supplemental addition to the previously acquired knowledge.

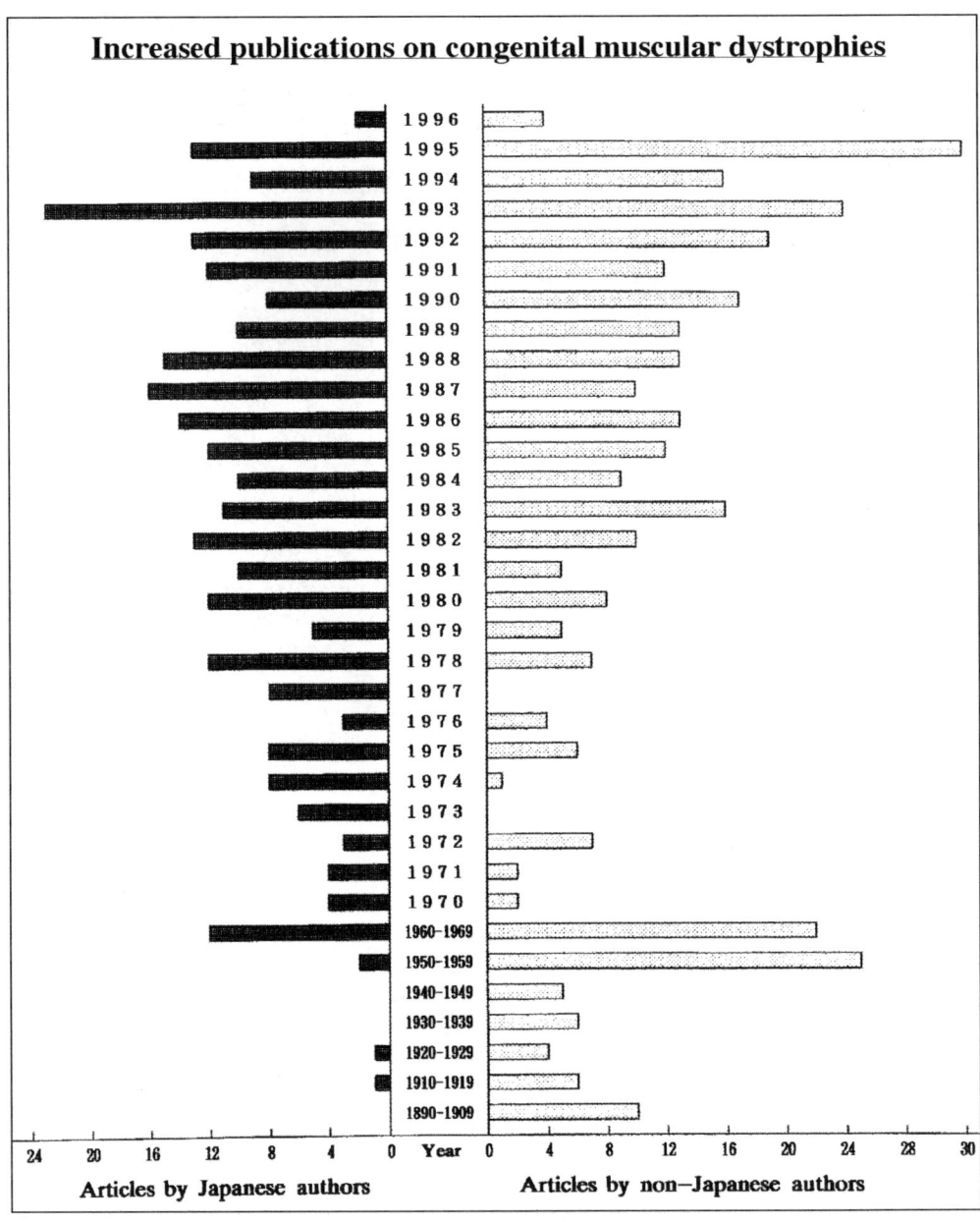

Figure 1. Chronological trend in publications of original articles on congenital muscular dystrophies. Original articles, reviews and case reports which appeared in various journals have been included, but books (or chapters), proceedings of research committees and abstracts were excluded from the count and do not appear in the figure.

CONGENITAL MUSCULAR DYSTROPHIES

Table I. Patients with neuromuscular disorders seen at the Department of Pediatrics, Tokyo Women's Medical College during the period from January 1971 through February 1994.

Grand total of outpatients		82,385	
Total cases with neuromuscular disorders		1,103	1.3%
Motor neuron diseases		103	9.3%
Spinal muscular atrophies			
Werdnig-Hoffmann I, II, III	66		
Kugelberg-Welander	13		
Fazlo-Londe	1		
Amyotrophic lateral sclerosis	6		
Spino-cerebellar degeneration	10		
Hereditary spastic paraplegia	4		
Cord injury due to birth trauma	2		
Others	1		
Peripheral neuropathies		45	4.1%
Charcot-Marie-Tooth	14		
Guillain-Barre syndrome	14		
Mono/poly-neuritis	9		
Others			
Disorders of N-M junction		103	9.9%
Myasthenia gravis			
Ocular type	82		
Generalized type	27		
Others	0		
Disorders of muscle		710	64.4%
CNS disorders		136	12.3%
Cerebral hypotonia	87		
Cerebral palsy (hypotonic type)	8		
Down syndrome	19		
Prader-Willi syndrome	22		

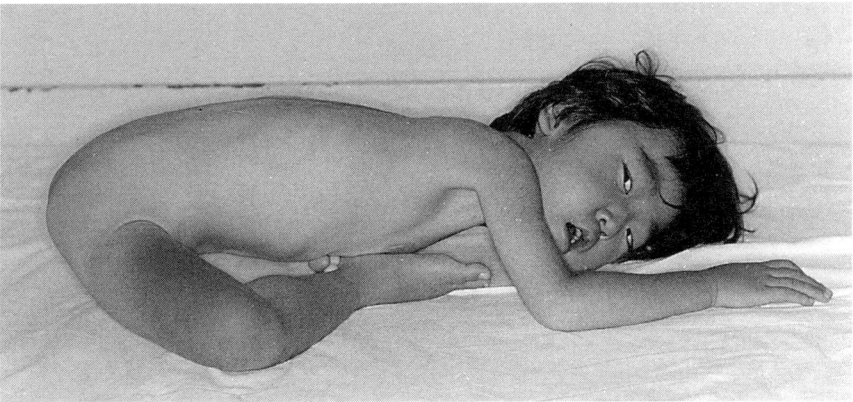

Figure 2. A three-year-old female with FCMD. The child was posed, so as to illustrate the typical double folding posture without difficulty, due to generalized hypotonia and weakness.

Table II. Patients with disorders of muscle seen at the Department of Pediatrics, Tokyo Women's Medical College, during the period from January 1971 through February 1994.

Cases with neuromuscular disorders			1,103	
Cases with disorders of muscle			710	64.4%
Progressive muscular dystrophy			337	47.5%
Duchenne		169		
Becker		15		
Limb-girdle		16		
Facioscapulohumeral		9		
Scapuloperoneal		3		
Autosomal recessive in childhood		6		
Congenital		117		
Symptomatic Duchenne carrier		2		
Myotonias			21	3.0%
Myotonic dystrophy		16		
Myotonia congenita		5		
Inflammatory disorders			49	6.9%
Viral myositis		24		
Dermatomyositis		16		
Polymyositis		9		
Congenital myopathies			29	4.1%
Nemaline		4		
Central core		4		
Minicore		3		
Myotubular		2		
Congenital fiber type disproportion		4		
Others(unclassifiable)		12		
Metabolic myopathies			127	17.9%
Mitochondrial				
CCO deficiency		14		
PDH deficiency		4		
MELAS (unknown origin)		3		
Kearns-Sayre syndrome		2		
Others (with lactic acidosis)		69		
Lipid storage myopathy				
Glycogen storage myopathy		9		
Others				
OTC deficiency		1		
Methylmalonic acidurla		1		
Thyrotoxic myopathy		2		
Malignant hyperthermia		5		
Hoffmann syndrome		1		
Periodic paralysis			4	0.6%
Benign congenital hypotonia (Walton)			24	3.6%
Floppy infant syndrome, unclassifiable			88	12.4%
Arthrogryposis multiplex congenita			5	0.7%
Others (hyper CKemia)			24	3.4%

CONGENITAL MUSCULAR DYSTROPHIES

Table III. Clinical characteristics of FCMD according to its original description in 1960 [l2].

1. Early onset, usually before 9 months
2. Hypotonia and weakness in early infancy
3. Later development of muscle wasting and joint contractures
4. Involvement is diffuse and extensive, but most prominent proximally
5. Myopathic facies in nearly all cases, pseudohypertrophy present in half of cases
6. Mental and speech retardation in nearly all cases, febrile or afebrile convulsions in half of cases
7. EMG, CK and muscle biopsy findings characteristic of muscular dystrophy
8. Course is either slowly progressive or stationary
9. Autosomal recessive inheritance

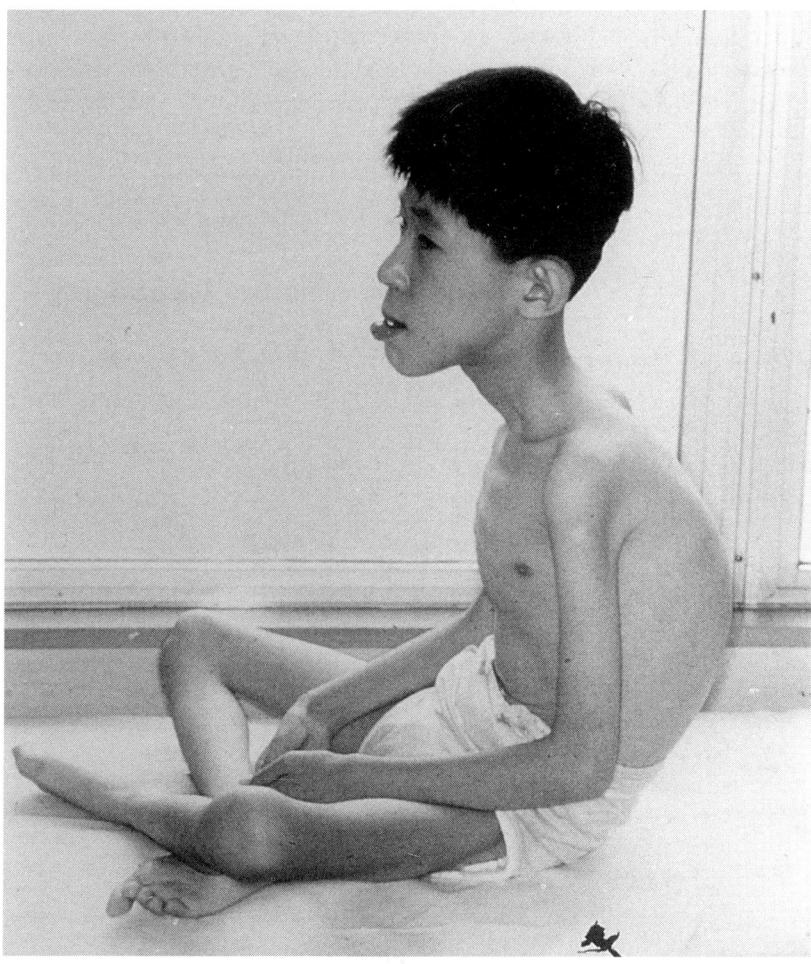

Figure 3. A 7-year-old-boy with FCMD. Extreme thinness is evident at the neck, shoulders and upper arms. Thoracic deformity with increased antero-posterior diameter, multiple joint contractures, and prognathism are remarkable.

First, the clinical onset of the disease may be at any time during the first 9 months of life, but is most often between 3 and 6 months of age. Some abnormalities are occasionally noticeable in the neonatal period, but such cases are rather rare and usually less severe, in contrast to those with other congenital myopathies such as X-linked myotubular myopathies, neonatal nemaline myopathies, congenital COX deficiency, etc.

Second, without exception, deep tendon reflexes are barely elicitable or abolished.

Third, although it can appear to be stationary, the clinical course is always slowly progressive, as evidenced by our long-term follow-up study carried out using a functional grading system which was developed by Ueda et al. [16] to specifically evaluate motor function in FCMD (Figure 4). Motor functions of FCMD patients initially improve, reaching a maximum level of development at around 5 years of age, and thereafter gradually deteriorate. The maximum level attained by the vast majority of patients was level 4, which corresponds to sliding along the floor on the buttocks. Only a few reach level 7 or higher, *e.g.* independent walking. Our recent molecular

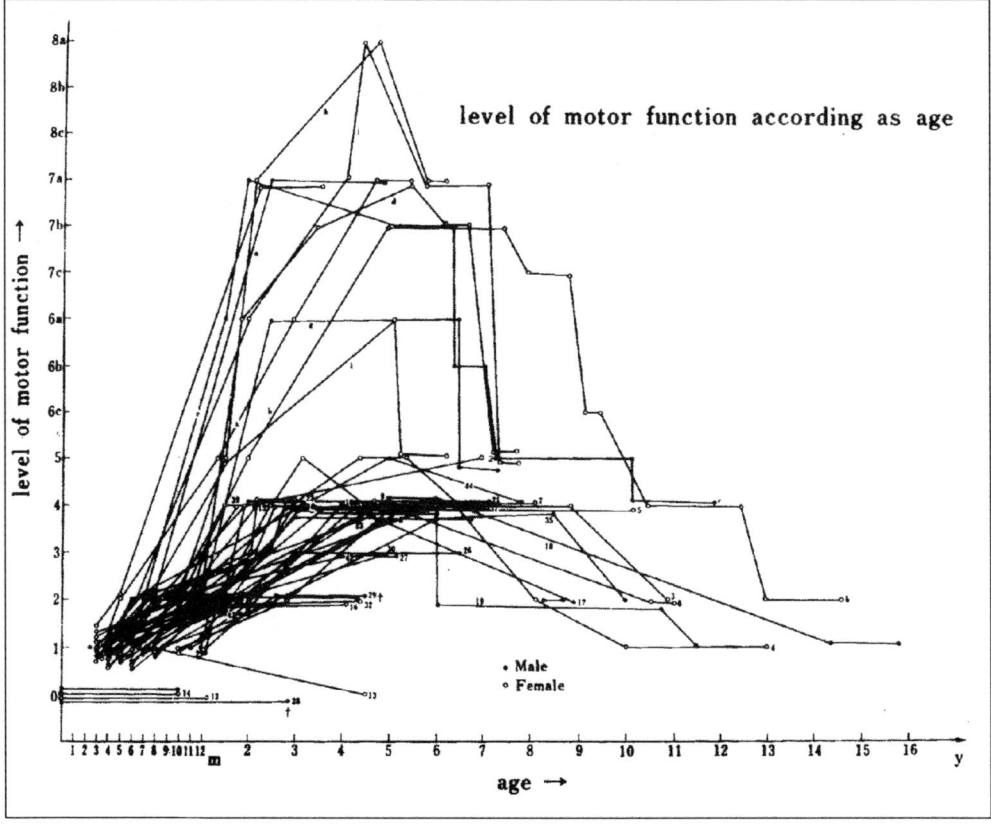

Figure 4. Chronological motor functional grade changes of patients with FCMD. Motor function level was evaluated according to the modified Ueda system [16].

genetic study demonstrated that these ambulant subjects share exactly the same haplotype at nine marker loci spanning 23.3cM surrounding the FCMD locus, suggesting a broad spectrum of clinical phenotype of FCMD (Kondo et al., in press).

Fourth, seizure disorders in FCMD patients were recently studied in detail by our group [18]. Eighty-six typical and 13 atypical FCMD patients were followed up for various periods, the majority being observed for more than 5 years, as to the presence or absence of seizure episodes of any kind. It was revealed that 19.2% of typical FCMD patients had experienced afebrile seizures once or more, 37.3% had isolated or recurrent episodes of seizures consistently associated with fever, and the remaining 43.4% never developed seizures (Figure 5). The study on 13 atypical cases yielded a similar result.

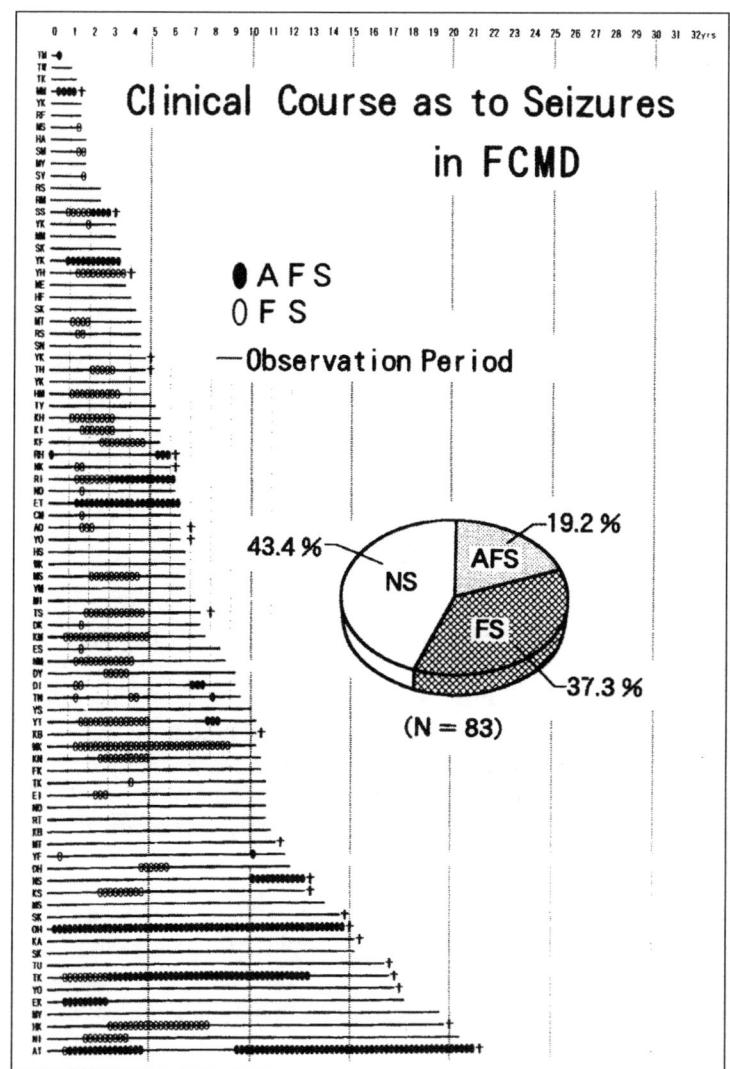

Figure 5. Clinical course of 86 typical FCMD patients in terms of seizure episodes. Febrile seizures occurred most frequently in the 1 to 5 year age range, but tended to persist, though at a lower frequency, after 5 years of age.
FS = febrile seizure, AFS = afebrile seizure, NS = no seizure

The most common seizure type was a generalized, non-focal, tonic-clonic convulsion of less than a few minutes duration. Seizures in FCMD were usually infrequent, responded well to medication, and appeared to be rather self-limited in nature, although a proportion of exceptional cases had frequent, intractable seizures. On repeated EEG examinations, epileptiform discharges were detected only in 22 out of 71 cases (31.0%) (Table IV). Epileptic complications in FCMD seem to have a relatively low incidence and are mild, in view of the severe brain malformations which constitute the *sine qua non* of FCMD at autopsy or on neuroimaging studies.

Table IV. Paroxysmal EEG activities in FCMD.

Epileptiform discharges	Seizures(+) n=46	Seizures(-) n=25
Absent	29 (63%)	20 (80%)
Present	17 (37%)	5 (20%)
Focal spikes	6 (13%)	5 (20%)
Diffuse sp-W	2 (4%)	0
Focal + diffuse	7 (15%)	0
Hypsarhythmia	2 (4%)	0

Laboratory examinations in FCMD

Laboratory examinations utilizing different modalities (biochemical, physiological, morphological and radiological) invariably indicate the nature of muscle lesions to be primarily myopathic, while neuroimaging studies, together with EEG as mentioned above, demonstrate the presence of central nervous system abnormalities.

Biochemical studies

Serum CK activity is always markedly elevated and tends to decrease as the patient ages. Ikenaka [19] from our department reported the results of her analysis of serum CK activities in 68 typical FCMD patients according to which serum CK values correlated well with patient age (in years) and the following equation was derived: CK = 3723.55–232.19 x age (in years) (Figure 6). The youngest baby studied was a 4-month-old boy, who showed a CK level of 4,348 mU/ml, about half of the peak CK activity attained at the age of 4 years. The average CK value for 15 infants under one year of age was about 3,800 mU/ml.

Serum ALT, AST, LDH, aldolase and carbonic anhydrase III activities were also found to be 1.5-3 times higher than the normal upper limit. Myoglobinemia was confirmed in 4 out of 13 patients with FCMD using a counter-immunophoresis technique. However, measurements of serum enzymes and myoglobin are not helpful in detecting healthy carriers among relatives of the proband.

Physiological studies

A routine EMG study revealed low amplitude potentials during contraction, and a reduction in functioning motor units in the later stage of the disease. Motor nerve conduction velocity in FCMD cases is within normal range. Likewise, evoked potential studies (BAEP, VEP, SSEP) are normal, although minor abnormalities in VEP have been described. EEG findings were already shown (Table IV).

Histology of biopsied muscle

Histologically, advanced connective tissue infiltration into the endomysium and perimysium enlarges the interfibrillar space and the basic structure of the fiber bundle

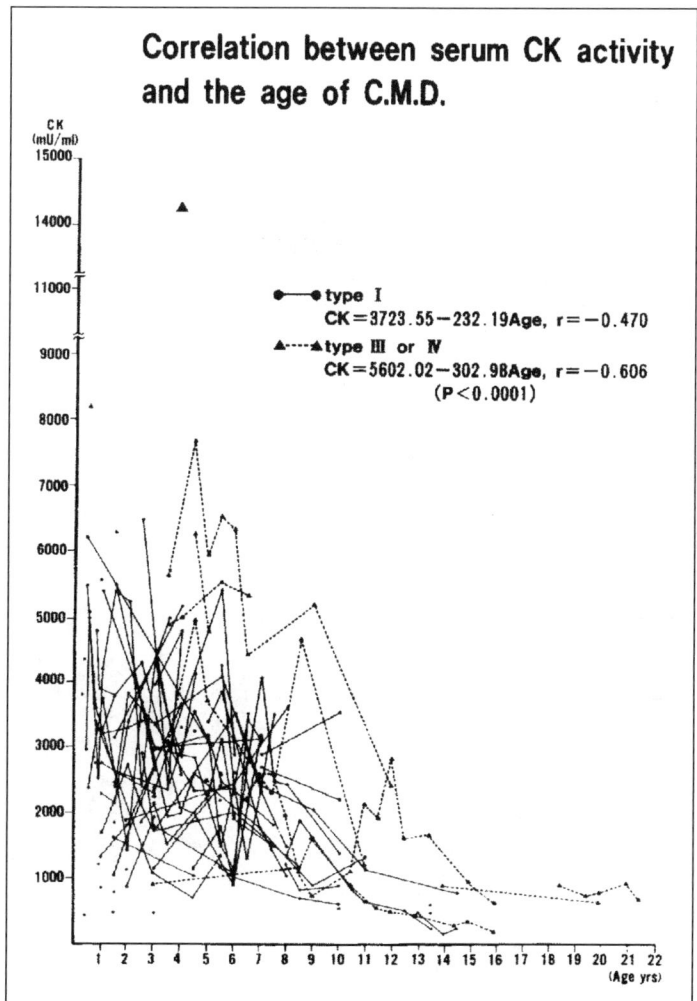

Figure 6. Sequential measurements of serum creatine kinase activity in 68 typical (type I) and 11 atypical (type III/IV) FCMD cases. The upper normal limit in our laboratory is 130 mU/ml.

is destroyed (Figure 7). Generally, fat infiltration tends to be less severe than connective tissue infiltration. In the later period of pathological change, only small round fibers remain as islands or are scattered diffusely in an enormous amount of connective tissue and fat (Figure 8). Although increases in the number of sarcolemmal nuclei and connective tissue nuclei are recognizable in the interfibrillar space and connective tissues, inflammatory cell infiltration is not generally seen. Muscle fiber sizes may differ, but are primarily small and round in shape. Hypertrophic fibers are remarkably rare.

In addition to fibers with central nuclei, phagocytosis, hyaline degeneration and fiber splitting, degenerative findings include sarcoplasmic reticulum degeneration and loss of striation. However, these degenerative findings were not as marked as those in Duchenne muscular dystrophy (DMD). Regenerative fibers were also present in significant numbers (Figure 7).

Classic histochemical stainings revealed degenerative findings such as ring fibers, sarcoplasmic reticulum degeneration, moth-eaten-like enzyme deficiency and snake coils. These changes were seen to randomly affect both type I and II fibers, and there was no fiber type-specificity in the distribution of muscle fiber diameters.

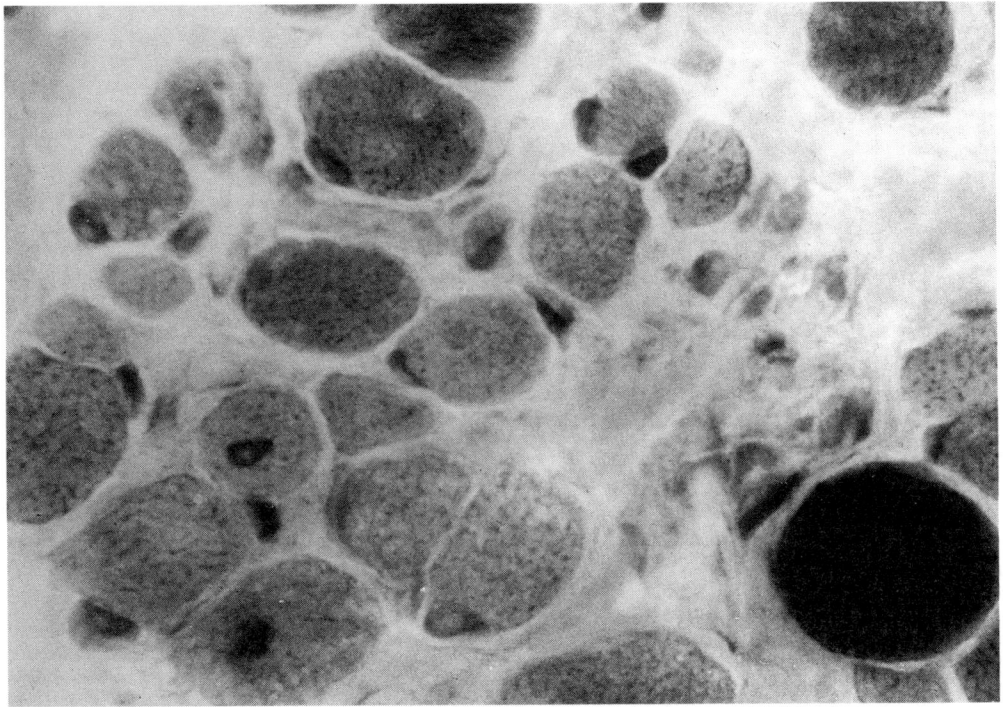

Figure 7. Histology of biopsied musle in FCMD. Specimen was obtained from M vastus medialis. Modified Gomori-trichrome staining. A conglomerate of regenerating fibers and darkly stained fibers (opaque fiber) is seen.

As a whole, the muscle histology in FCMD resembles mainly the dystrophic muscular changes found in DMD, but there are certain characteristics that are more specific to FCMD. They are: 1) a greater degree of connective tissue infiltration; 2) muscle fiber diameters are more uniform, *i.e.* hypertrophic fibers are fewer, small-sized fibers being predominant.

A number of detailed electron microscopic studies have been published by Japanese investigators, notably Miike and his group [20, 21], and Wakayama *et al* [22, 23]. According to these studies, the ultrastructural abnormalities of FCMD are consistent with those of DMD and are demonstrable in the T system [20], intramuscular vascular endothelial cell [21], caveolae, the orthogonal array [22] and cholesterol in the plasma membrane [23] of FCMD muscle.

An immunochemical analysis of connectin (titin) performed by Matsumura *et al.* [24] also revealed a similar type of abnormality in both DMD and FCMD.

Arahata *et al.* [25, 26] analyzed the immunoperoxidase staining patterns for dystrophin and spectrin (a membrane-associated cytoskeletal protein) in biopsied

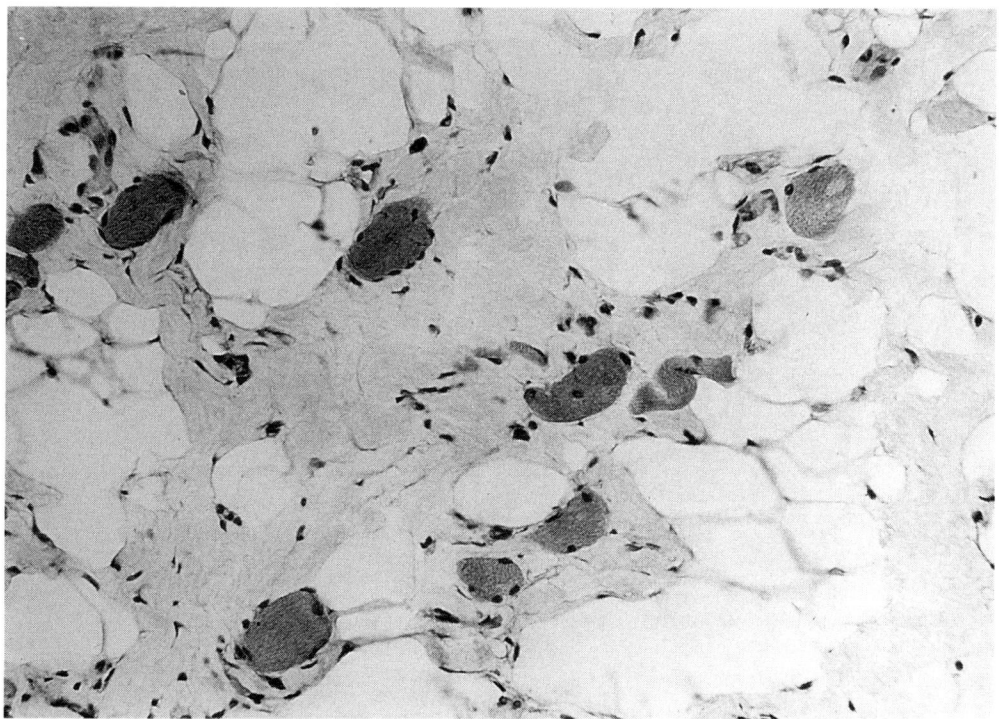

Figure 8. End stage histology of biopsied muscle. Muscle tissue degradation is so severe that only a few scattered muscle fibers, compressed by increased interstitial tissue, are seen. Not only connective tissue, but also fatty tissue is extremely increased in this case, though fatty tissue proliferation is usually of a modest degree in the majority of FCMD patients.

muscle specimens from 34 FCMD patients and compared the findings with those in nonFCMD, SMA and DMD patients. In contrast with DMD, in which dystrophin was absent, FCMD muscle showed an unusual heterogeneous immunostaining pattern, 28% of fibers being negatively or abnormally stained (Figure 9). Abnormally immunostained fibers for spectrin were also increased in FCDM muscles (25%). Hayashi *et al.* [27] and Matsumura *et al.* [28] both reported a marked reduction of laminin subunits (particularly laminin 2) in most muscle fibers in FCMD. Based upon these findings, both groups of researchers speculated as to the presence of intrinsic factor(s) responsible for an abnormality of the plasma membrane and basal lamina of FCMD muscle.

Radiological studies

Muscle CT scan

Using CT scans, Arai [29] from our department evaluated the spatial distribution of diseased muscle *in situ* at the trunk, thigh and calf levels in 18 FCMD patients, and also followed the evolution of imaging abnormalities over time in a portion of the subjects.

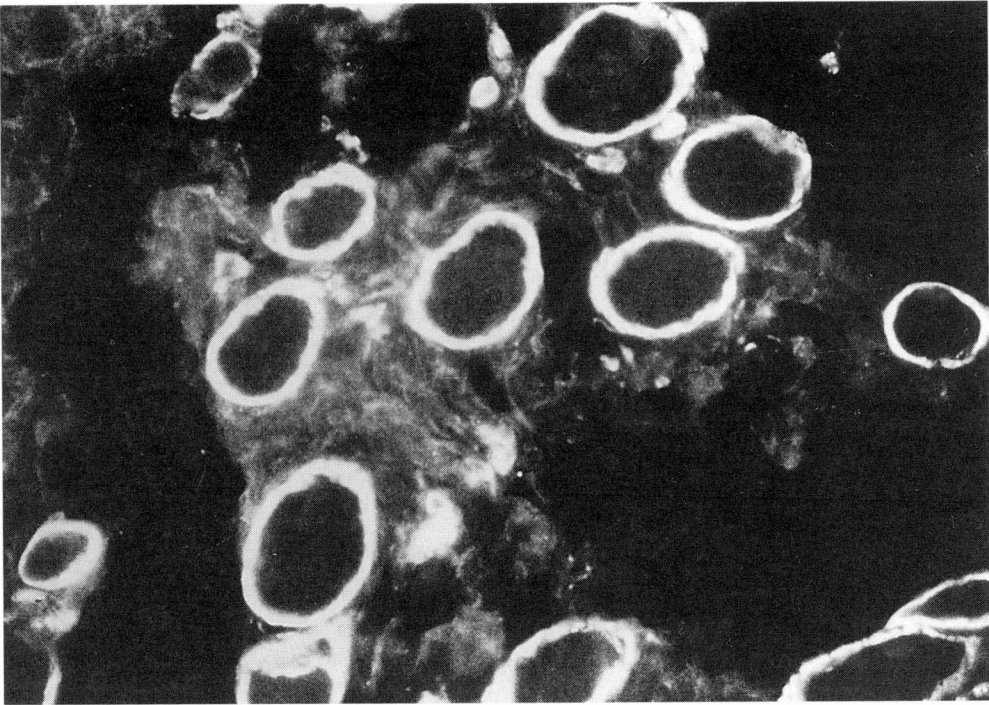

Figure 9. Monoclonal anti-dystrophin antibody immunostaining of FCMD muscle. Many fibers show normally positive immunostaining, but there are also a few fibers with faintly positive or negative stainings in the picture.

CONGENITAL MUSCULAR DYSTROPHIES

Progressive degeneration and atrophy were clearly recognized on visual inspection of CT scans, and the rate of progression was far more rapid in FCMD than in DMD (Figure 10). Regression lines derived from the CT numbers of muscles and ages of the subjects showed a progressive decline with time in all muscles examined. The slopes of regression lines were far steeper in FCMD than in age-matched DMD patients.

Brain MRI and CT

It is now well known that neuroimaging modalities such as brain MRI and CT greatly facilitate characterization of the brain involvement in patients with primary myopathy. The first trial of this neuroradiological approach was undertaken by ourselves in 1976 [30] when we conducted cranial CT scannings on 50 PMD cases including 22 FCMD and 5 nonFCMD cases, and quite unexpectedly found a striking abnormality, *i.e.* a

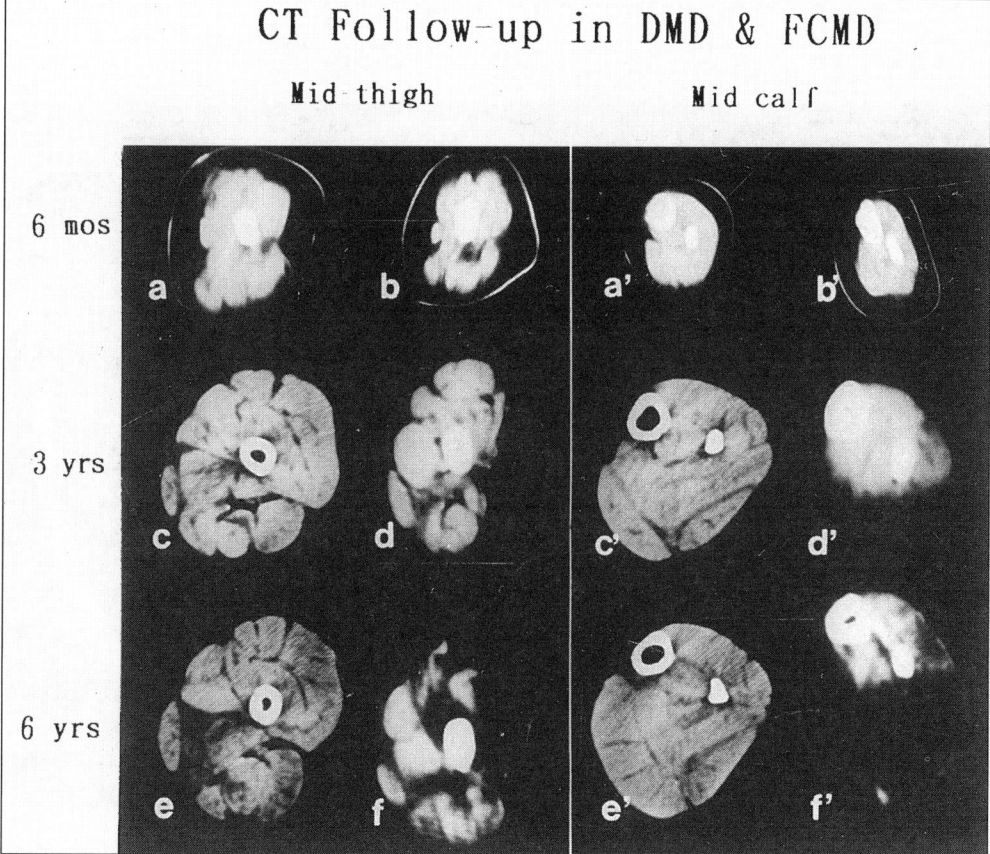

Figure 10. Cross-sectional CT scans of the mid-thigh and mid-calf in patients with Duchenne muscular dystrophy (DMD) and FCMD at the ages of 6 months, 3 years and 6 years. Reduced muscle mass and radiodensity changes are more profound and appear earlier in FCMD than in DMD. Scans a, a',c,c',e,e' are of DMD patients, while scans b,b',d,d' f and f' are of FCMD patients.

leukodystrophy-mimicking widespread white matter low density in about 40% of cases, in addition to the findings of essentially non-specific brain deformation (usually plagiocephalic) and atrophic changes (subarachnoid space widening) (Figure 11). The cause of this white matter hyperlucency remains unknown. Lysosomal enzyme measurements ruled out leukodystrophies of common types. Consecutive follow-up CT scans revealed a tendency for normalization with age (Figure 12). Delayed myelination or dysmyelination was suggested as a plausible mechanism for this neuroimaging feature.

Unfortunately, the CT scanner at our hospital was not sensitive enough to detect abnormal cortical structures in FCMD patients. A full appreciation of MRI's superb capability of demonstrating abnormal cortical gyrations (polymicrogyria, pachygyria) in FCMD was first realized in the mid-1980s, when a 3rd generation 1.5T scanner was introduced at our hospital. Three dimensional MR imaging was reported to be highly effective in visualizing brain surface anomalies in FCMD [31].

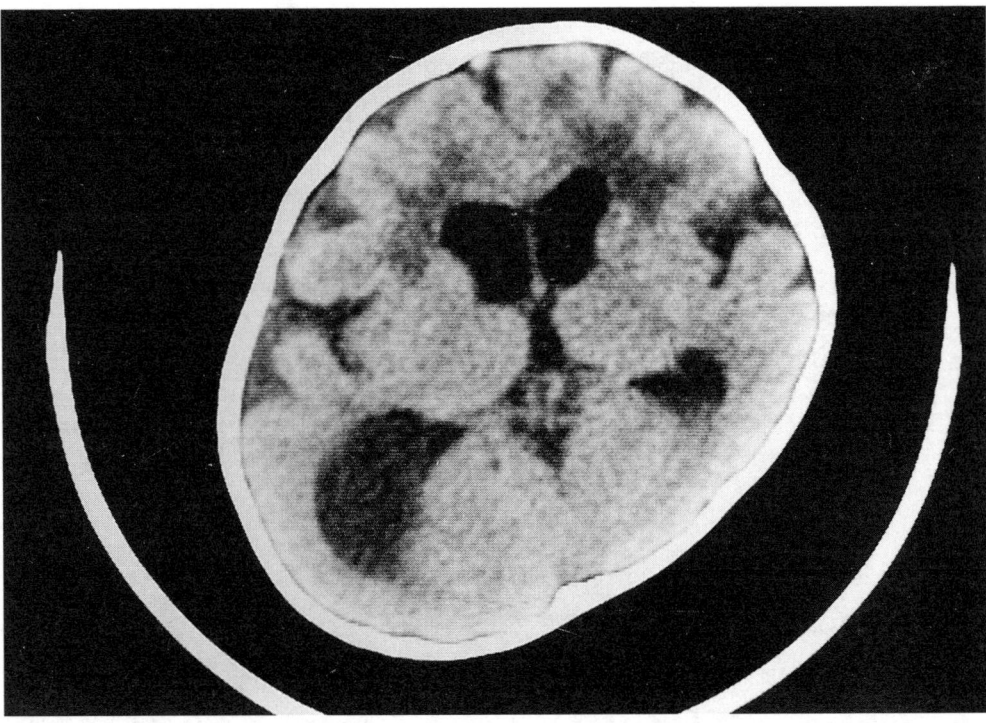

Figure 11. Axial T1-weighted MRI of the brain in a one-and-half-year-old FCMD patient. Plagiocephalic deformation of the skull, moderate enlargement of the lateral ventricles, prominent posterior horn dilatation (colpocephalic), marked reduction of gyral formation in the anterior half of the brain, absent gyration in the posterior half of the brain (pachygyria), thickened cortical zones, widened Sylvian fissures, and hyperlucency of bilateral frontal subcortical white matter are evident.

Autopsy: neuropathology of the FCMD brain

In 1981, Fukuyama et al. [15] summarized the neuropathological findings of brains obtained from 24 autopsied patients (Figures 13-17). Since then, more than 25 autopsy cases have additionally been accumulated and registered by the research committee sponsored by the Ministry of Health and Welfare. Autopsy information collected from about 50 cases to date revealed the remarkable fact that a unique brain malformation (polymicrogyria and pachygyria) is present in all cases without exception. The brain malformation characteristic of FCMD is a form of neuroblast migrational disorder, and

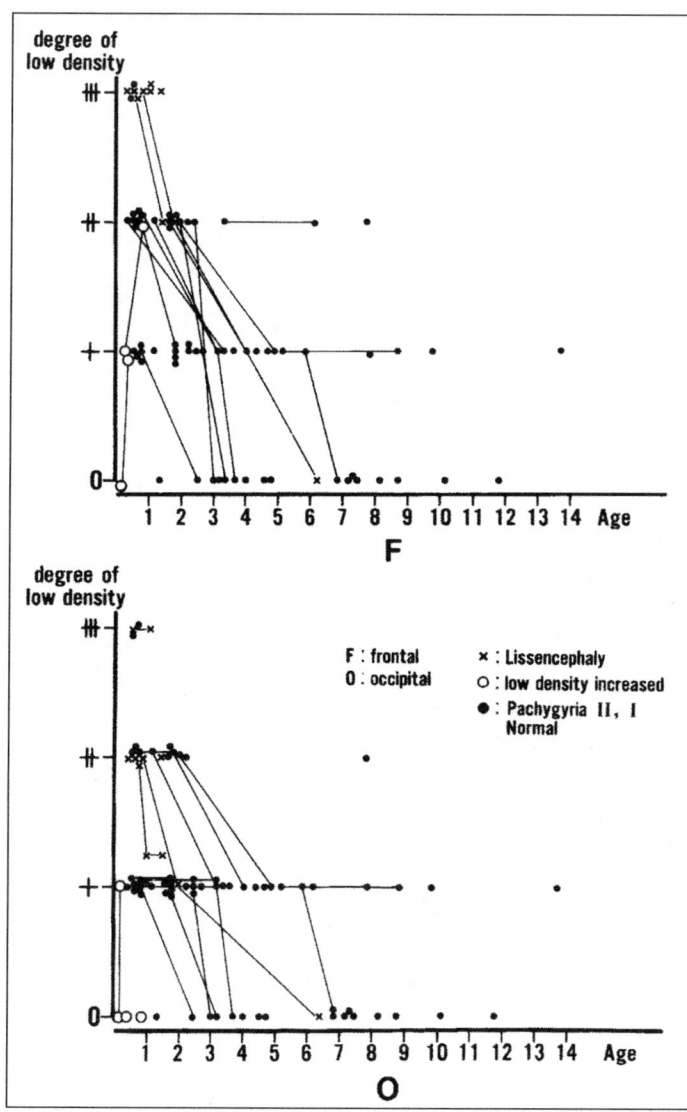

Figure 12. Evolution of white matter low density with age. The degree of low density was evaluated by visual inspection of T1-weighted MRI. The lines connecting two or three points represent cases in which MR imagings were carried out twice or three times. The abnormal white matter low density became less distinctive in most cases, and even disappeared in some patients.

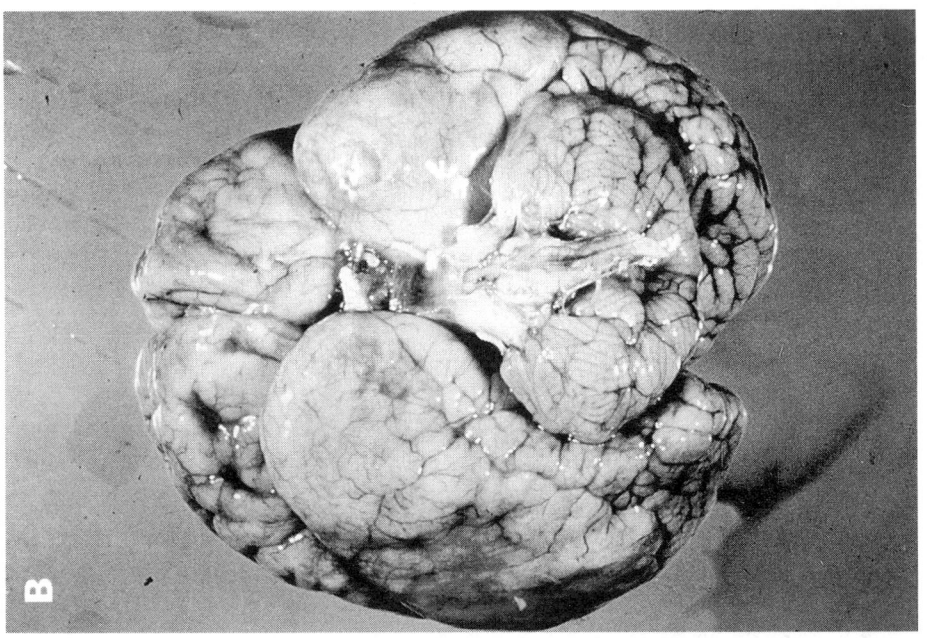
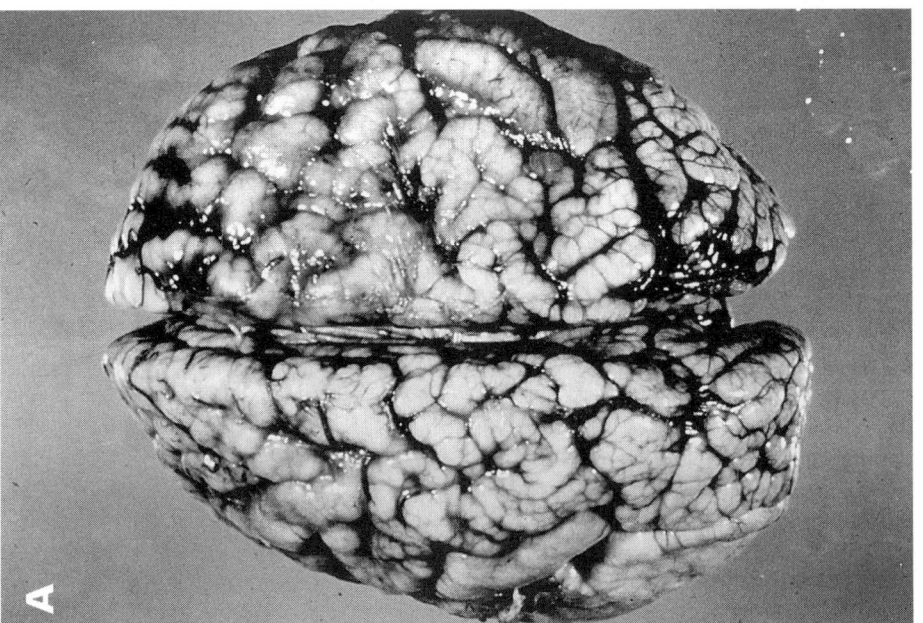

Figure 13. The FCMD brain shows a distinct cobblestone appearance at the vertex (A), while the broad smooth surfaces of the bilateral temporal lobes are striking in the basal view (B).

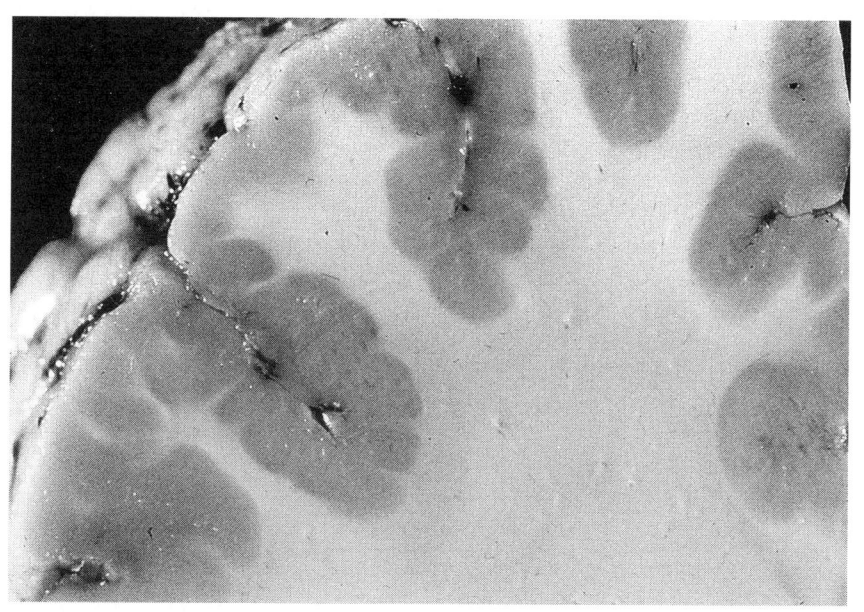

Figure 15. Coronal section of the brain. The cortex is thick, each gyrus being broad and consisting of several microgyri. Microsulci are often obliterated by multiple fused portions.

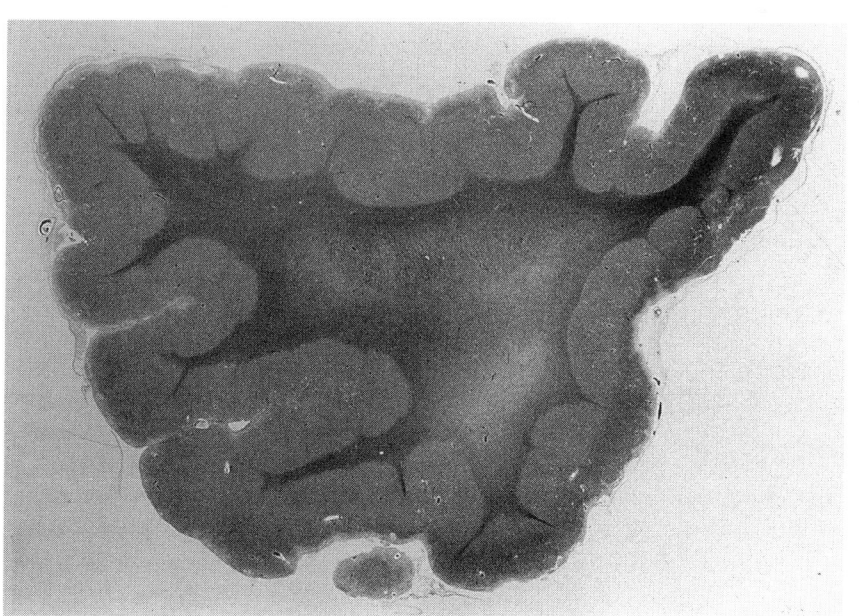

Figure 14. Coronal section of the FCMD brain clearly shows an extreme thickness and simplified winding of the cerebral cortex, as well as a broad area of pallor in the white matter (Kluver-Barrera stain).

has been called by various names, such as status verrucosus deformis [32], pachygyre Mikropolygyrie [33], type II lissencephaly [34], and cobblestone lissencephaly [35]. The most detailed neuropathological findings ever reported are those described in Takada's two papers [36, 37].

Epidemiology and genetics of FCMD

Prevalence rates of FCMD were obtained from three population-based and one hospital-based studies, as shown in Table V. The two studies conducted in the 1970s both showed similarly higher rates (5.6×10^{-5} and $6.2\text{-}11.9 \times 10^{-5}$) than those from the two studies done in the 1980s which showed much smaller figures (1.0×10^{-5} and 2.1×10^{-5}). The two groups of studies were carried out approximately 10 years apart. The authors of the latter two studies attributed the difference in prevalence rates to the difference in consanguinity rates between the two groups of studies, although it is somewhat unlikely that this is the only cause.

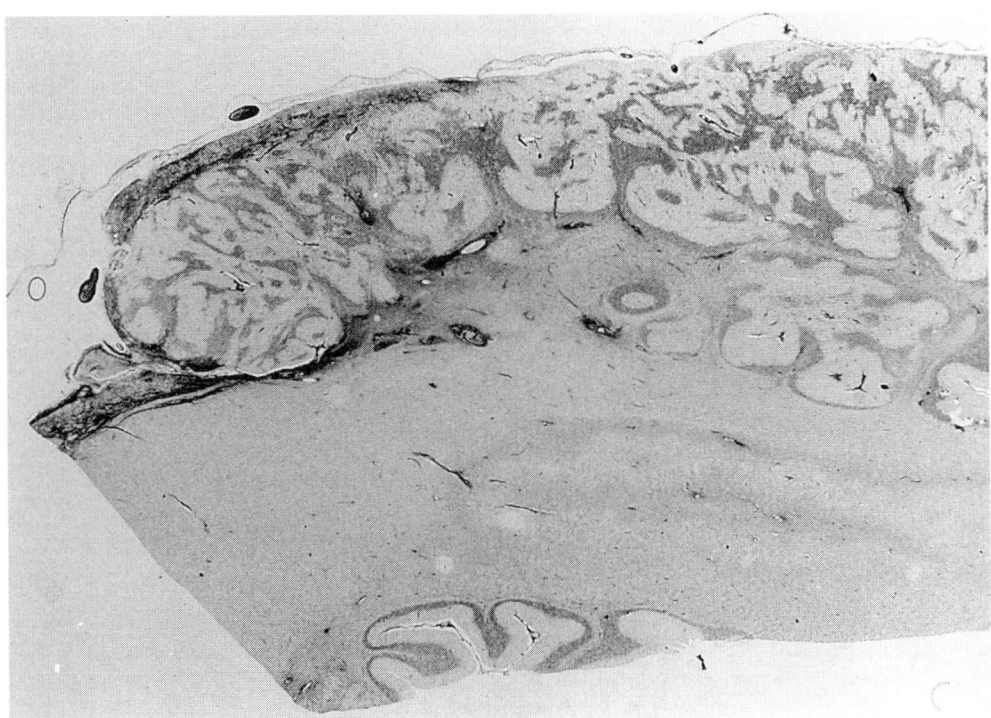

Figure 16. Cerebellar polymicrogyria showing disorganized molecular and granular layers and Purkinje cells.

Interestingly, Takeshita *et al.* [38] conducted another epidemiological study in 1993 on the same geographic area (San-in distict) as that in their 1975 study, and found a remarkable decreasing trend in the FCMD prevalence from 5.6×10^{-5} in the 1956-1960 period to 2.1×10^{-5} live births in the 1986-1990 period.

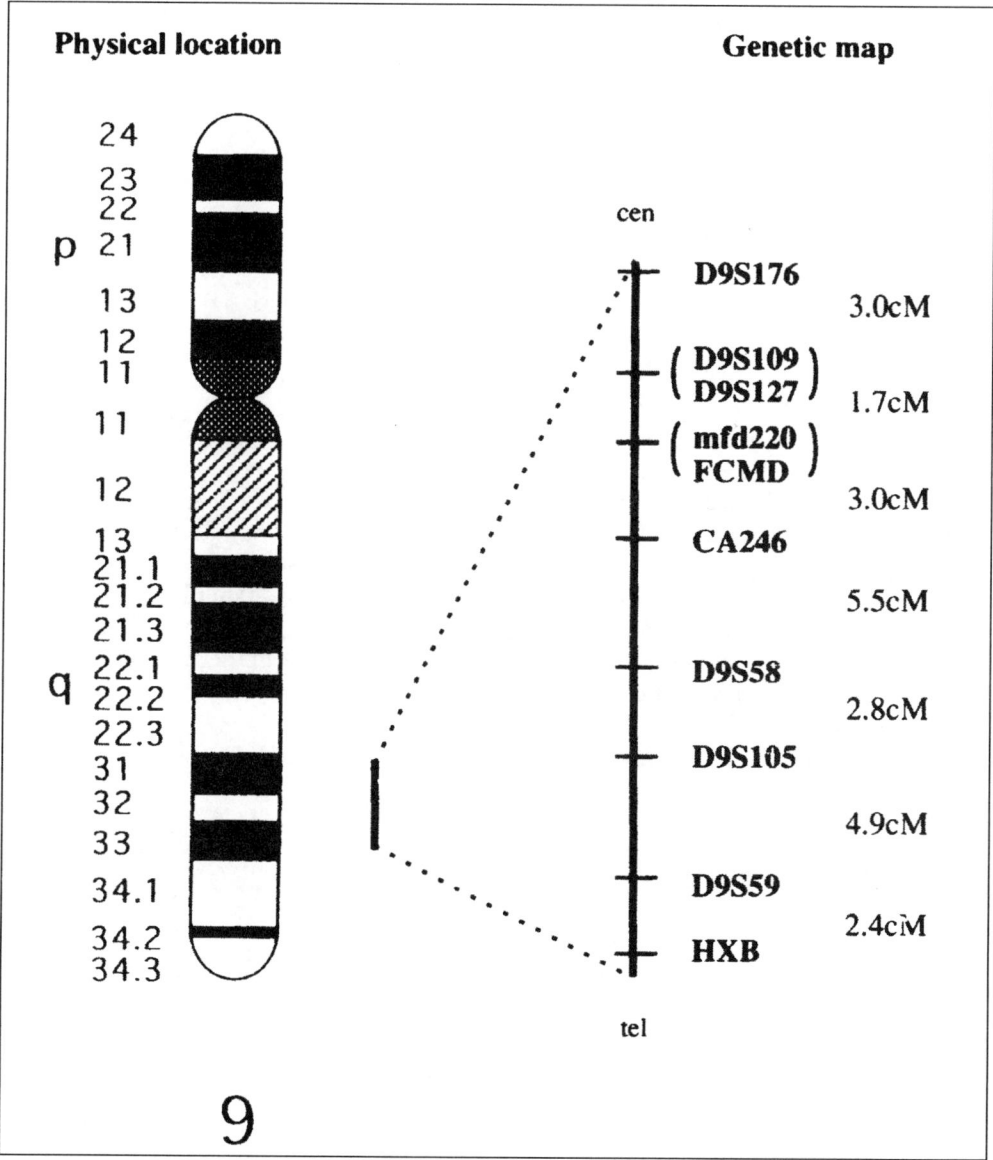

Figure 17. Physical and genetic locations of markers on chromosome 9q. Toda *et al.* identified the location of the FCMD gene which lies within a distance of a few hundred kilobases from the *mfd220* locus, and more recently, this group further narrowed the locus to a region of less than 100 kb containing J12 (this marker is not depicted in the figure).

Table V. Prevalence rates of FCMD in Japan.

Authors (year)	Year of survey	Area of survey	Method of survey	Age	Size of population	Patients ascertained	Prevalence rate ($\times 10^{-5}$)	Consanguinity rate (%)
Takeshita et al. (1977)	1975	Shimane prefecture	Population-based	Under 20	178,457	11	5.6	29.6
Osawa (1978)	1976	ns Majority in Kanto	Hospital-based	Unlimited	ns	153	6.2•11.9	26.8
Oshiro et al (1989)	1985	Okinawa prefecture	Population-based	Unlimited	1,010,000	10	1.0 (?)	0
Hirayama et al (1992)	1988	Tokyo	School-based	6 - 14	1,227,000	26	2.1	ns

ns = not specified

The annual incidences of FCMD and non FCMD in the 1974-1978 period in Japan were calculated to be 1.11×10^{-5} and 0.35×10^{-5}, respectively, based upon the data collected in a nationwide multi-institutional collaborative survey conducted by the research committee sponsored by the Ministry of Health and Welfare (Table VI). It was speculated that these figures represent the minimum rate, because it was likely to be biased by partial participation of the institutions involved in the survey, resulting in incomplete recruitment of patients.

Table VI. Annual incidence ($\times 10^{-5}$) of FCMD and NFCMD in Japan.

Year of birth	Live-born babies	FCMD		NFCMD		TOTAL	
		Patients	Incidence	Patients	Incidence	Patients	Incidence
1974	2.029,989	22	1.08	9	0.44	31	1.53
1975	1,901,440	22	1.16	4	0.21	26	1.37
1976	1.832.617	17	0.93	7	0.38	24	1.31
1977	1,755,100	22	1.25	3	0.17	25	1.42
1978	1.708,643	19	1.11	9	0.53	28	1.64
Total	9, 227.789	102	1. 11	32	0.35	134	1.45

Whether FCMD occurs in populations of non-Japanese ethnicity, or is strictly limited to the Japanese, is an important and yet unsolved problem. It is safe to state that two reported Korean patients and two Chinese families (3 babies [39]) had and have been suffering from FCMD, because I had an opportunity to examine the patients or pertinent materials myself, and in particular, the diagnosis of two Taiwanese sibs was confirmed through a molecular genetic analysis in our laboratory [39].

As to other cases reported in papers from various countries, I cannot be certain yet whether they really represent a true case of FCMD or of another entity with a similar phenotype.

As to the mode of inheritance, we convincingly established that FCMD is an autosomal recessively inherited disorder [40].

Molecular genetics of FCMD

Despite numerous attempts, over many years, to locate the chromosomal region harboring the gene responsible for causing FCMD, neither positive data nor even a hint as to the location were obtained until recently. In 1993, however, a dramatic breakthrough took place when Toda *et al.* [41] succeeded in mapping the FCMD gene to chromosome 9q31-33 by means of genetic linkage analyses with six polymorphic microsatellite markers, involving 21 Japanese families, in 13 of which the parental marriage was consanguineous. A hint as to which location to probe was provided by a FCMD patient from consanguineous family which was also affected with group A xeroderma pigmentosum (XP), which has been localized to chromosome 9q34.1. As no other siblings were affected with either FCMD or XP, Toda *et al.* [41] assumed the co-existence of FCMD and group A XP to be attributable to homozygosity by descent in this individual. In this first report from Toda's group, the most probable location of the FCMD gene was said to lie within a 7.7 cM interval between D9S58 and D9S59.

Subsequently, in 1994, Toda *et al.* [42] further narrowed the locus to a region of - 5cM between loci *D9S127* and *CA246* by homozygosity mapping in patients born to consanguineous parents and by recombination analysis in other families. They also found strong evidence of linkage disequilibrium between FCMD gene and a polymorphic microsatellite marker, mfd220, and suggested that the FCMD gene could lie within a few hundred kilobases of the mfd220 gene.

More recently, Toda *et al.* [43] developed five new CA repeat markers from YAC contigs containing mfd220, and demonstrated that the FCMD gene could lie within a region of less than 100 kb containing J12 (the distance between the FCMD gene and marker J12 is presumed to be 30 kb).

Prenatal diagnosis of FCMD

The identification of the FCMD gene at chromosome 9q31 by Toda et al. opened a new avenue for reliable prenatal diagnosis of this as yet incurable disease.

Kondo et al. [44], from our group, reported a successful prenatal diagnosis conducting for two unrelated FCMD families using polymorphism analysis with nine microsatellite CA repeat markers flanking the FCMD locus (Figure 18) and calculated the fetal phenotype probabilities for both families using the Linkage package of a computer program. The fetus in family 1 showed a 99% probability of being healthy, either as a normal homozygote or a carrier, and was born without signs of FCMD. In family 2, an at least 86% probability of the fetus being affected led the parents to terminate the pregnancy and the abortus showed brain malformations characteristic of a FCMD fetus.

Other forms of CMD

As FCMD was better delineated over time, it became more clear that there are other forms of CMD which do not fit well clinically with FCMD. At first, a major difference as a distinguishing hallmark was recognized in terms of intellectual development. Contrary to FCMD which always accompany mental retardation, the vast majority of European CMD cases presents age-corresponding normal mental development, and they were called by some as the classical or pure or occidental form of CMD. It has become recently clear that more than 40% of European CMD patients have a laminin α 2-chain (alpha 2 subunit of laminin-2 or merosin) deficiency, and the disease is now referred to as merosin-negative or merosin-deficient CMD [45-47].

Clinically, merosin-negative CMD shows rather homogeneous features with marked elevation of serum CK levels, severe neonatal hypotonia and delayed motor miletones, respiratory insufficiency and abnormal MRI/CT scans, but normal intellectual development. In most cases [48], neuroimaging abnormality in the merosin-deficient CMD is characteristically localized to white matter, which diffusely shows an abnormal, increased signal intensity on T2-weighted MRI, but no abnormal gyral pattern, heterotopia or other migration abnormalities are noticeable [49].

On the other hand, the merosin-positive CMD is considered by Fardeau et al. [49] as a heterogeneous group of CMDs which are only poorly delineated but usually affected clinically in a milder degree in comparison to the merosin-negative CMD patients. Nonaka et al. [50], however, pointed out a possibility that the merosin-positive CMD may constitute a single disease, because of its clinico-pathological uniformity.

The Walker-Warburg syndrome (WWS) is an another extreme of CMDs, with severest brain malformation, eye involvement and a very short life span. There are many common clinicopathological features between FCMD and WWS, as do the

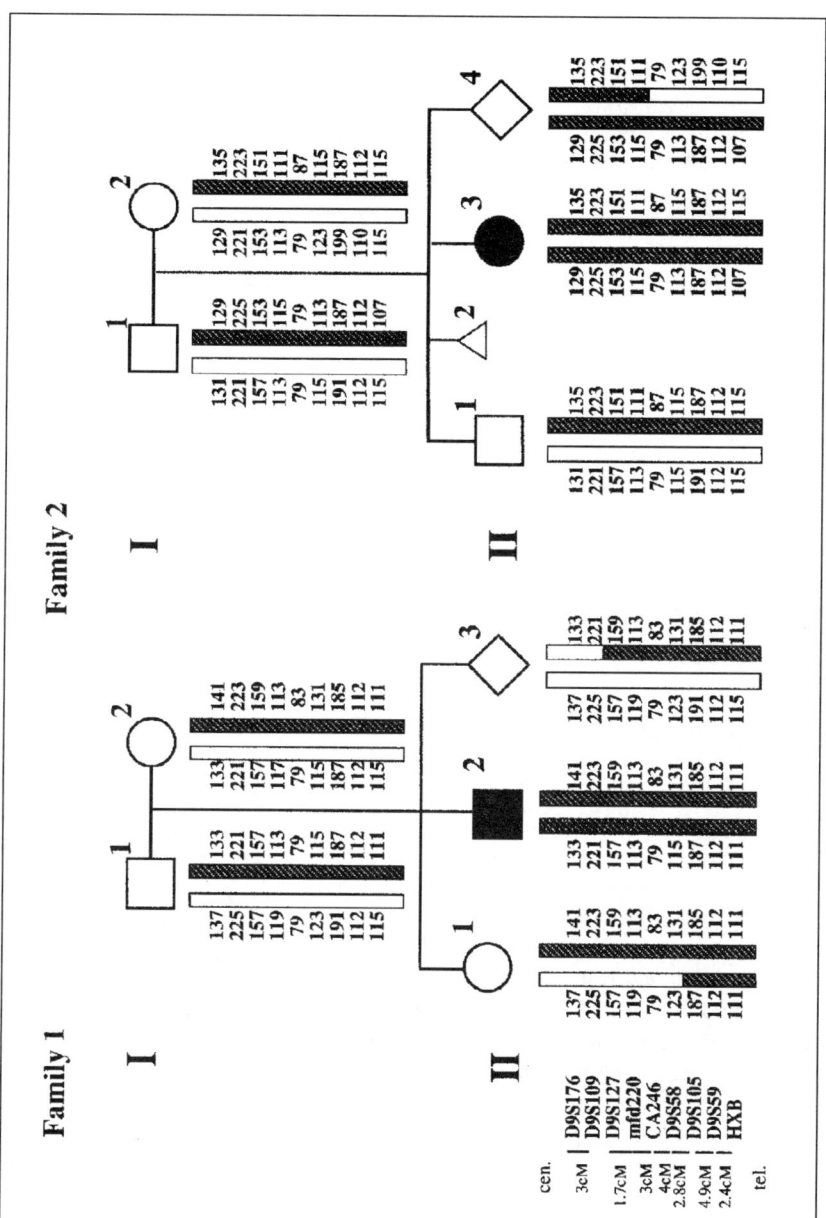

Figure 18. Genotypes of the two pedigrees. Nine-loci genotypes from members of the two pedigrees. The FCMD gene is presumed to lie between *D9S127* and *CA246* loci. The *mfd220* is the closest marker. Values shown as haplotypes are PCR-product sizes. Shaded and unshaded columns depict the regions carrying the mutant and wild-type FCMD alleles, respectively. In the fetus (II-3) of family 1, the paternally-derived chromosome carries the wild-type allele, while the maternally-derived chromosome carries the mutant allele, irrespective of occurrence of a cross-over at a site proximal to DgS127. The fetus (II-4) in family 2 inherited a paternal allele carrying the mutation. In the maternal allele, a crossover was identified between loci *mfd220* and *CA246* (reproduced from [42] with permission of the publisher).

difference as well. There appeared a report claiming the genetic identity of both conditions [51], but other reports on more many cases do not support the claim [52].

The nosological relation of WWS with muscle-eye-brain (MEB) syndrome advocated by Santavuori *et al.* is still controversial, but most investigators momentarily agree to leave the two conditions as an independent entity each other until a more definite evidence becomes available [35].

Based upon the information currently available, the author proposes to subclassify CMD into 5 subtypes as shown in Table VII, although there will be rare cases which are elusive from any of subtypes listed in Table VII.

Table VII Classification of congenital muscular dystrophies.

Subtype	Muscle	PNS	CNS WM	CNS GM	Eye	Gene locus
Pure form	++	-	-	-	-	?
Merosin-deficiency	++	+	++	-	-	6q2
FCMD	++	-	+	++	-	9q31-52
MEB	+	-	+	++ Giant VEP	+	?
WWS	+	-	++	++	+	?

FCMD : Fukuyama type congenital muscular dystrophy
MEB : Muscle-eye-brain syndrome
WWS : Walker-Warburg syndrome
PNS : Peripheral nervous system
CNS : Central nervous system
WM : White matter
GM : Grey matter
VEP : Visual evoked potential

Conclusion

It is amazing to observe a dramatic advance of medical knowledge on a single disease or syndrome like CMD which occurred in the last decade or so. Detailed clinical observations coupled with an application of cell biology/molecular genetics techniques greatly contributed to the establishment of the current realms of CMD [53], although there are undoubtedly so many things to be done. It is anticipated, however, that the progress in research will be further accelerated and bring out a solution of elucidating the pathogenesis and a substantial measure for curing the disease and preventing its occurrence in near future.

References

1. Howard R. A case of congenital defect of the muscular system (dystrophia musculorum congenita) and its association with congenital talipes equino-varus. *Proc R Soc Med* 1908 ; 1 (3) pathol section : 157-66.
2. Haushalter P. Trois nouveaux cas d'amyotrophie primitive progressive dans l'enfance. *Rev Med* 1898 ; 18 : 445-60.
3. Batten FE. Three cases of myopathy, infantile type. *Brain* 1903 ; 26 : 147-8.
4. Brandt S. *Werdnig-Hoffmann's infantile progressive muscular atrophy. Clinical aspects, pathology, heredity and relation to Oppenheim's amyotonia congenita and other morbid conditions with laxity of joints or muscles in infants.* Copenhagen : Munksgaard, 1950.
5. Vassella F, Mumenthaler M, Rossi E, Moser H, Wiesmann U. Die kongenitale Muskeldystrophie. *Dtsch Z Nervenheilk* 1967 ; 190 : 349-74.
6. Rotthauwe HW, Kowalewski S, Mumenthaler M. Kongenitale Muskeldystrophie. *Z Kinderheilk* 1969 ; 106 : 131-62.
7. Otto HF, Lucking T. Congenitale Muskeldystrophie. Licht- und elektronenmikroskopische Befunde. *Virchows Arch Abt A Pathol Anat* 1971 ; 352 : 324-39.
8. Lucking T, Otto HF. Kongenitale Muskeldystrophie. *Z Kinderheilk* 1971 ; 110 : 59-73.
9. Ketelsen UP, Freund-Molbert E, Beckmann R. Klinische und ultrastrukturelle Befunde bei kongenitaler Muskeldystrophie. *Msch Kinderheilk* 1971 ; 119 : 586-92.
10. Adams RD. *Diseases of muscle: a study in pathology.* 3rd ed. Hagerstown : Harper and Row, 1975 : 245.
11. Lazaro RP, Fenichel GM, Kilroy AW. Congenital muscular dystrophy: case reports and reappraisal. *Muscle Nerve* 1979 ; 2 : 349-55.
12. Fukuyama Y, Kawazura M, Haruna H. A peculiar form of congenital progressive muscular dystrophy. Report of fifteen cases. *Paediatr Universitat Tokyo* 1960 ; 4 : 5-8.
13. Kamoshita S, Konishi Y, Segawa M, Fukuyama Y. Congenital musuclar dystrophy as a disease of the central nervous system. *Arch Neurol* 1975 ; 33 : 513-6.
14. Nonaka I, Chou SM. Congenital muscular dystrophy. In : Vinken PJ, Bruyn GW, eds. *Handbook of clinical neurology. Vol 41.* Amsterdam : North Holland, 1979 : 27-50.
15. Fukuyama Y, Osawa M, Suzuki H. Congenital progressive muscular dystrophy of the Fukuyama type. Clinical, genetic and pathological considerations. *Brain Dev Tokyo* 1981 ; 3 : 1-29.
16. Ueda S, Eto F, Kikuchi N. Rehabilitation of congenital muscular dystrophy (Fukuyama type). Clinical analysis of 50 patients (in Japanese). *Sogo Rehabilit Tokyo* 1975 ; 3 : 51-64.
17. Osawa M, Suzuki H, Fukuyama Y. Congenital musuclar dystrophy (in Japanese). *Adv Neurol Sci Tokyo* 1980 ; 24 : 702-17.
18. Sumida S, Osawa M, Arai Y, et al. Clinical and electroencephalographic study on seizures in congenital muscular dystrophy (in Japanese). *Tokyo Joshi Ikadaigaku Zasshi* 1993 ; 63 Suppl : S36-42.
19. Ikenaka H. Serum enzyme activities in progressive muscular dystrophies: part 2. Serial changes of serum GOT, GPT, LDH and CK activities in congenital muscular dystrophy (in Japanese). *Tokyo Joshi Ikadaigaku Zasshi* 1992: 62 : 1185-96.
20. Miike T, Ohtani Y, Tamari H, Ishitsu T, Nonaka I. An electron microscopical study of the T-system in biopsied muscles from Fukuyama type congenital muscular dystrophy. *Muscle Nerve* 1984 ; 7 : 629-35.
21. Miike T, Ohtani Y. Vascular endothelial cell injury and platelet embolism in Fukuyama type congenital muscular dystrophy (abst). *Brain Dev Tokyo* 1987 ; 9 : 242.

22. Wakayama Y, Kumagai T, Jimi T. Small size of orthogonal array in muscle plasma membrane of Fukuyama type congenital muscular dystrophy. *Acta Neuropathol* 1986 ; 72 : 130-3.
23. Wakayama Y, Kumagai T, Jimi T, Shibuya S. Freeze-fracture analysis of cholesterol in muscle plasma membrane of Fukuyama type congenital muscular dystrophy. *Acta Neuropathol* 1987 : 75 : 46-50.
24. Matsumura K, Shimizu T, Sunada Y, *et al.* Degradation of connectin (titin) in Fukuyama type congenital muscular dystrophy: immunochemical study with monoclonal antibodies. *J Neurol Sci* 1990 ; 98 : 155-62.
25. Arikawa E, Ishihara T, Nonaka I, Sugita H, Arahata K. Immunocytochemical analysis of dystrophin in congenital muscular dystrophy. *J Neurol Sci* 1991 ; 105 : 79-87.
26. Arahata K, Hayashi YK, Mizuno Y, Yoshida M, Ogawa E. Dystrophin-associated glycoprotein and dystrophin co-localisation at sarcolemma in Fukuyama congenital muscular dystrophy. *Lancet* 1993 ; 342 : 623-4.
27. Hayashi YK, Engvall E, Arikawa-Hirasawa E, *et al.* Abnormal localization of laminin subunits in muscular dystrophies. *J Neurol Sci* 1993 ; 119 : 53-64.
28. Matsumura K, Nonaka I, Campbell KP. Abnormal expression of dystrophin-associated proteins in Fukuyama type congenital muscular dystrophy. *Lancet* 1993 ; 341 : 521-2.
29. Arai Y. Characteristics of muscle involvement evaluated by CT scans in early stages of progressive muscular dystrophy: comparison between Duchenne and Fukuyama types (in Japanese). *Tokyo Joshi Ikadaigaku Zasshi* 1993 ; 63 : 1089-103.
30. Fukuyama Y, Maruyama H, Hirayama Y, *et al.* Neuroradiological analysis of central nervous system abnormalities in congenital muscular dystrophy (in Japanese). In : Okinaka S, ed. *The 1976 annual report of the research committee on the pathogenesis of progressive muscular dystrophy*, sponsored by the Ministry of Health and Welfare. Tokyo, 1977 : 116-8.
31. Toda T, Watanabe T, Matsumura K, *et al.* Three-dimensional MR imaging of brain surface anomalies in Fukuyama-type congenital muscular dystrophy. *Muscle Nerve* 1995 ; 18 : 508-17.
32. Bertrand I, Grunec J. The status verrucosus of the cerebral cortex. *J Neuropathol Exp Neurol* 1955 ; 14 : 331-47.
33. Ogasawara Y, Ito K, Murogushi K. Neuropathological studies on two cases of congenital muscular dystrophy, with special reference to morphological characteristics of micropolygyria found in the cerebral and cerebellar cortex. *Brain Nerve (Tokyo)* 1976 ; 28 : 451-7.
34. Dobyns WB, Kirkpatrick JB, Hittner HM, Roberts RM, Kretzer FL. Syndromes with lissencephaly. II. Walker-Warburg and cerebro-oculo-muscular syndromes and a new syndrome with type II lissencephaly. *Am J Med Genet* 1985 ; 22 : 157-95.
35. Dobyns WB, Truwit CL. Lissencephaly and other malformations of cortical development: 1995 update. *Neuropediatrics* 1995 ; 26 : 132-47.
36. Takada K, Nakamura H, Tanaka J. Cortical dysplasia in congenital muscular dystrophy with central nervous system involvement (Fukuyama type). *J Neuropathol Exp Neurol* 1984 ; 43 : 395-407.
37. Takada K. Fukuyama congenital muscular dystrophy as a unique disorder of neuronal migration: a neuropathological review and hypothesis. *Yonago Acta Med* 1988 ; 31 : 1-16.
38. Takeshita K, Takahashi K, Ishii S, Otani I, Eda T, Kisa T. The changing panorama of various types of muscular dystrophy in San-in district, Japan, 1956-1990: epidemiological trends in incidence and prevalence (abstract). *Muscle Nerve* 1994 ; Suppl 1 : S169.
39. Jong YJ, Liu GC, Chiang CH, Wang PJ, Shen YZ. Fukuyama type congenital muscular dystrophy. Two Chinese families (abstract). In : Fukuyama Y, Osawa M, eds. *The abstracts of International Symposium on Congenital Muscular Dystrophies*, Tokyo, July 7-8, 1994. Tokyo, 1994 : 36.
40. Fukuyama Y, Osawa M. A genetic study of the Fukuyama type congenital muscular dystrophy. *Brain Dev Tokyo* 1984 ; 6 : 373-90.

41. Toda T, Segawa M, Nomura Y, et al. Localization of a gene for Fukuyama type congenital muscular dystrophy to chromosone 9q31-33. *Nat Genet* 1993; 5 : 283-6.
42. Toda T, Ikegawa S, Okui K, et al. Refined mapping of a gene responsible for Fukuyama-type congenital muscular dystrophy: evidence for strong linkage disequilibrium. *Am J Hum Genet* 1994 ; 55 : 946-55.
43. Toda T, Miyake M, Mizuno K, Nakagome Y, Nakahori Y. Linkage disequilibrium of a gene for Fukuyama-type congenital muscular dystrophy (abstract). *Jpn J Hum Genet Tokyo* 1996 ; 41 (1) : 41.
44. Kondo E, Saito K, Toda T, Osawa M, Fukuyama Y. Prenatal diagnosis in Fukuyama type congenital muscular dystrophy by polymorphism analysis. *Am J Med Genet* 1996 (in press).
45. Tome FMS, Evangelista T, Leclerc A, et al. Congenital muscular dystrophy with merosin deficiency. *CR Acad Sci Paris (III)* 1994 ; 317 : 351-7.
46. Hillaire D, Leclerc A, Faure S, et al. Localization of merosin-negative congenital muscular dystrophy to chromosome 6q2 by homozygosity mapping. *Hum Mol Genet* 1994 ; 3 : 1657-61.
47. Dubowitz V, Fardeau M. Workshop report: proceedings of the 27th ENMC sponsored workshop on congenital muscular dystrophy. *Neuromusc Disord* 1995 ; 5 : 253-8.
48. Philpot J, Sewry C, Pennock J, Dubowitz V. Clinical phenotype in congenital muscular dystrophy: correlation with expression of merosin in skeletal muscle. *Neuromusc Disord* 1995 ; 5 : 301-5.
49. Fardeau M, Tome FMS, Helbling-Leclerc A, et al. Dystrophie musculaire congénitale avec déficience en mérosin : analyse clinique, histopathologique, immunocytochimique et génétique. *Rev Neurol* 1996 ; 152 ; 11-9.
50. Nonaka I, Kobayashi O, Osari S. Clinico-genetic analysis on non-Fukuyama (classical) form of congenital muscular dystrophy (abstract). *Jpn J Hum Genet Tokyo* 1996 ; 41 : 26.
51. Toda T, Yoshioka M, Nakahori Y, Kanazawa I, Nakamura Y, Nakagome Y. Genetic identity of Fukuyama type congenital muscular dystrophy and Walker-Warburg syndrome. *Ann Neurol* 1995 ; 37 : 99-101.
52. Ranta S, Pihko H, Santavuori P, Takvanainen E, de la Chapelle A. Muscle-eye-brain disease and Fukuyama type congenital muscular dystrophy are not allelic. *Neuromusc Disord* 1995 ; 5 : 221-5.
53. Arahata K, Ishii H, Hayashi YK. Congenital muscular dystrophies. *Cur Op Neurol* 1995 ; 8 : 385-90.

15

Molecular genetics of spinal muscular atrophy

J. MELKI, A. MUNNICH

Unité de Recherches sur les Handicaps Génétiques de l'Enfant, INSERM Unité 393, IFREM, Hôpital Necker-Enfants Malades, Paris, France.

Spinal muscular atrophies (SMA) are characterized by degeneration of the anterior horn cells of the spinal cord leading to progressive symmetrical limb and trunk paralysis associated with muscular atrophy. SMA represents the second most common, fatal, autosomal recessive disorder after cystic fibrosis (1 in 6 000 new borns, [1-4]). Childhood SMA is classically subdivided into three clinical groups on the basis of age of onset and clinical course [5]. The acute form of Werdnig-Hoffmann disease (type I, [6, 7]), is characterized by severe, generalised muscle weakness and hypotonia at birth or within the next 3 months. Death, from respiratory failure, usually occurs within the first two years. This disease may be distinguished from the intermediate (type II) and juvenile (type III, Kugelberg-Welander disease, [8]) forms. Type II children are able to sit, although they cannot stand or walk unaided, and survive beyond 4 years. Type III patients have proximal muscle weakness, starting after the age of two. The underlying biochemical defect(s) remain(s) unknown.

Identification and characterization of a spinal muscular atrophy- determining gene

By means of linkage analysis we, and others, have shown that all three forms of spinal muscular atrophy map to chromosome 5q11.2-q13.3 suggesting that they are allelic disorders [9-12]. Various yeast artificial chromosome (YAC) contigs of the 5q13 region spanning the disease locus have been constructed and the presence of low copy-repeats in this region demonstrated [13-15]. Inherited or *de novo* deletions were observed in SMA patients. In addition, deletion events were statistically associated with the severe form of SMA (type I, [15]).

The characterization of the smallest critical SMA region was established by a combination of genetic and physical mapping in SMA patients. This critical region suggested a precise location for the SMA gene and, therefore, a limited region within which to search for candidate genes. We identified a duplicated gene in the 5q13 region, one of which, the SMN gene encoding an hitherto unknown protein of 294 amino acids, was located within the critical region [16]. This gene was lacking in 213/229 (93%) or interrupted in 13/229 (5,6%) SMA patients. In patients where the SMN gene was neither lacking nor interrupted (3/229, 1,4%), the presence of deleterious mutations provided strong evidence that this gene, termed the survival motor neuron (SMN) gene, is a SMA-determining gene [16-18]. Recently, analysis of 54 unrelated Spanish SMA families has detected a 4bp deletion in SMN exon 3 of 4/54 unrelated patients. This deletion which results in a frameshift and a premature stop codon was found on the background of a same haplotype suggesting that a single mutational event is involved in the four families. The other patients showed either deletions of the SMN gene (49/54) or a gene conversion event changing SMN exon 7 into its highly homologous copy (^{C}BCD541, 1/54). This observation gave strong support to the view that mutations of the SMN gene were responsible for the SMA phenotype as it was the first frameshift mutation hitherto reported in SMA [19].

Large scale deletions of the 5q13 region are specific to Werdnig-Hoffmann disease

Taken together, these data suggest the SMN gene is a SMA-determining gene. However, no genotype- phenotype correlation between the gene defect and the type of SMA was observed, as the SMN gene was absent or truncated in 98,6% of SMA cases independent of the type of SMA. Recently, a second gene, XS2G3 or the highly homologous neuronal apoptosis inhibitory protein gene (NAIP) have been found to be more frequently deleted in type I than in the milder forms (types II and III, [20]). We investigated the correlation between the clinical phenotype and the genotype at these loci. A total of 106 patients were classified into type I (44), type II (31) and type III (31) and analysed using SMN, markers C212 and C272, and NAIP mapping upstream and downstream from SMN respectively. The combined analysis of all markers showed that a large proportion of type I patients (43%) carried deletions of both SMN and its flanking markers (C212/C272 and NAIP exon 5), as compared with none of the patients suffering type II or III SMA. The presence of large scale deletions involving these loci is specific to Werdnig-Hoffmann disease (type I) and allow one to predict the severity of the disease in our series [21].

It is tempting to hypothesize therefore that NAIP along with other genes mapping close to SMN modify the SMA phenotype thus accounting for the different clinical subtypes of the disease. However, smaller rearrangements can still result in a severe phenotype as 23% of SMA type I patients lacked the SMN gene but not C212-C272 or NAIP loci, suggesting that other genetic mechanisms might be involved in the severe form of the disease. Elucidating the function of the gene products will be important for the understanding of the pathogenesis of SMA [21].

SMN gene deletion in variants of spinal muscular atrophy

Clinical diagnosis is confirmed by the absence or interruption of the SMN gene in the majority of typical SMA patients [16-18]. Yet, variants of infantile SMA with cerebellar hypoplasia, pontocerebellar degeneration, multiple long bone fractures at birth or congenital heart defects (CHD) with or without joint contractures have been described [22]. The question of whether these SMA variants represent separate genetic entities or stem from allelic mutations remained unanswered. We have recently found deletions of the SMN gene in the SMA-CHD association suggesting that this group was allelic to SMA [23]. The SMN gene was also lacking in 6/12 patients with arthrogryposis multiplex congenita (AMC) and spinal muscular atrophy. Neither point mutation in the SMN gene nor evidence for linkage to chromosome 5q13 were found in the other patients. These data strongly suggest that AMC of neurogenic origin is genetically heterogeneous, with a subgroup being allelic to SMA. Absence or interruption of the SMN gene in the AMC-SMA association will make the diagnosis easier and genetic counselling will now become feasible [24].

Our ability to detect 98,6% of SMA patients by analysis of exon 7 of the SMN gene will greatly facilitate genetic counselling by eliminating the need for complex linkage analysis. Further, it will extend the option of prenatal diagnosis to families in which affected individuals are not available to establish genetic phase.

Conclusion

Although the exact nature of the genetic mechanisms resulting in SMA remains to be clarified, this study provides important clues to the unravelling of this complex puzzle and forms a base from which to explore the molecular biology, biochemistry and cell biology of this devastating disease. Furthermore, this work will contribute to the fundamental understanding of the survival of motor neurons.

Abbreviations

AMC: arthrogryposis multiplex congenita
CHD: congenital heart defects
NAIP: neuronal apoptosis inhibitory protein

SMA: spinal muscular atrophy
SMN: survival motor neurone

Acknowledgements

We thank the patients, families and doctors who have contributed to this work and without whom this study would not have been possible. This work was supported by INSERM, the Association Française contre les Myopathies (AFM), the Groupement de Recherches et d'Études sur les Génomes, the Fondation de France and the Assistance Publique, Hôpitaux de Paris.

References

1. Roberts DF, Chavez J, Court SDM. The genetic component in child mortality. *Arch Dis Child* 1970 ; 45 : 33-8.
2. Pearn J. The gene frequency of acute Werdnig-Hoffmann disease (SMA type I). A total population survey in North-East England. *J Med Genet* 1973 ; 10 : 260-5.
3. Pearn J. Incidence, prevalence, and gene frequency studies of chronic childhood spinal muscular atrophy. *J Med Genet* 1978 ; 15 : 409-13.
4. Czeizel A, Hamula J. A Hungarian study on Werdnig-Hoffmann disease. *J Med Genet* 1989 ; 26 : 761-3.
5. Munsat TL. Workshop report: international SMA collaboration. *Neuromusc Dis* 1991 ; 1 : 81.
6. Werdnig G. Die fruhinfantile progressive spinale Amyotrophie. *Arch Psychiatr* 1894 ; 26 : 706-44.
7. Hoffmann J. Uber die hereditare progressive spinale Muskelatrophie im Kindesalter. *Muenchen Med Wschr* 1900 ; 47 : 1649-51.
8. Kugelberg E, Welander L. Heredo-familial juvenile muscular atrophy simulating muscular dystrophy. *Arch Neurol Psych* 1956 ; 75 : 500-9.
9. Brzustowicz LM, Lehner T, Castilla LH, Penchaszadeh GK, Wilhelmsen KC, Daniels RJ, Davies KE, Leppert M, Ziter F, Wood D, Dubowitz V, Zerres K, Hausmanova-Petrusewics I, Ott J, Munsat TL, Gilliam TC. Genetic mapping of chronic childhood-onset spinal muscular atrophy to chromosome 5q11.2-q13.3. *Nature* 1990 ; 344 : 540-1.
10. Melki J, Abdelhak S, Sheth P, Bachelot MF, Burlet P, Marcadet A, Aicardi J, Barois A, Carriere JP, Fardeau M, Fontan D, Ponsot G, Billette T, Angelini C, Barbosa C, Ferriere G, Lanzi G, Ottolini A, Babron MC, Cohen D, Hanauer A, Clerget-Darpoux F, Lathrop M, Munnich A, Frézal J. Gene for proximal spinal muscular atrophies maps to chromosome 5q. *Nature* 1990 ; 344 : 767-8.
11. Melki J, Sheth P, Abdelhak S, Burlet P, Bachelot MF, Lathrop M, Frézal J, Munnich A, and the French spinal muscular atrophy investigators. Mapping of acute (type I) spinal muscular atrophy to chromosome 5q12-q14. *Lancet* 1990 ; 336 : 271-3.
12. Gilliam TC, Brzustowicz LM, Castilla LH, Lehner T, Penchaszadeh GK, Daniels RJ, Byth BC, Knowles J, Hislop JE, Shapira Y, Dubowitz V, Munsat TL, Ott J, Davies KE. Genetic homogeneity between acute and chronic forms of spinal muscular atrophy. *Nature* 1990 ; 345 : 823-5.

13. Kleyn PW, Wang CH, Lien LL, Vitale E, Pan J, Ross BM, Grunn A, Palmer DA, Warburton D, Brzustowicz LM, Kunkel LM, Gilliam TC. Construction of a yeast artificial chromosome contig spanning the SMA disease gene region. *Proc Natl Acad Sci USA* 1993 ; 90 : 6801-5.
14. Francis MJ, Morrisson KE, Campbell L, Grewal PK, Christodoulou Z, Daniels RJ, Monaco AP, Frischauf AM, McPherson J, Wasmuth JJ, Davies KE. A contig of non-chimaeric YACs containing the spinal muscular atrophy gene in 5q13. *Hum Mol Genet* 1993 ; 2 : 1161-7.
15. Melki J, Lefebvre S, Bürglen L, Burlet P, Clermont O, Millasseau P, Reboullet S, Bénichou B, Zeviani M, Le Paslier D, Cohen D, Weissenbach J, Munnich A. De novo and inherited deletions of the 5q13 region in spinal muscular atrophies. *Science* 1994 ; 264 : 1474-7.
16. Lefebvre S, Bürglen L, Reboullet S, Clermont O, Burlet P, Viollet L, Bénichou B, Cruaud C, Millasseau P, Zeviani M, Le Paslier D, Frezal J, Cohen D, Weissenbach J, Munnich A, Melki J. Identification and characterization of a spinal muscular atrophy-determining gene. *Cell* 1995 ; 80 : 155-65.
17. Rodrigues NR, Owen N, Talbot K, Ignatius J, Dubowitz V, Davies KE. Deletions in the survival motor neuron gene on 5q13 in autosomal recessive spinal muscular atrophy. *Hum Mol Genet* 1995 ; 4 : 631-4.
18. Van der Steege, Grootscholten PM, Van der Vlies P, Draaijers TG, Osingo J, Cobben JM, Scheffer H, Buys CHCM. PCR-based DNA test to confirm clinical diagnosis of autosomal recessive spinal muscular atrophy. *Lancet* 1995 ; 345 : 985-6.
19. Bussaglia E, Clermont O, Tizzano E, Lefebvre S, Bürglen L, Cruaud C, Urtizberea JA, Colomer J, Munnich A, Baiget M, Melki J. A frame-shift deletion in the survival motor neurone gene in Spanish spinal muscular atrophy patients. *Nature Genet* 1995 ; 11 : 335-7.
20. Roy N, Mahadavan MS, McLean M, Shutler G, Yaraghi Z, Farahani R, Baird S, Besner-Johnston A, Lefebvre C, Kang X, Ioannou P, Crawford TO, de Jong P, Surh L, Ikeda J, Korneluk RG, MacKenzie A. The gene for neuronal apoptosis inhibitory protein (NAIP), a novel protein with homology to baculoviral inhibitors of apoptosis is partially deleted in individuals with type 1, 2 and 3 spinal muscular atrophy (SMA). *Cell* 1995 ; 80 : 167-78
21. Burlet P, Burglen L, Clermont O, Lefebvre S, Viollet L, Munnich A, Melki J. Large scale deletions of the 5q13 region are specific to Werdnig-Hoffmann disease. *J Med Genet* 1996 ; 33 : 281-3.
22. Emery AEH. *Diagnostic criteria for neuromuscular disorders.* Barn, The Netherlands : ENMC, 1994 : 48-54.
23. Bürglen L, Spiegel R, Ignatius J, Cobben JM, Landrieu P, Lefebvre S, Munnich A, Melki J. SMN gene deletion in a variant of infantile spinal muscular atrophy. *Lancet* 1995 ; 346 : 316-7.
24. Bürglen L, Amiel J, Viollet L, Lefebvre S, Burlet P, Clermont O, Raclin V, Landrieu P, Verloes A, Munnich A, Melki J. SMN gene deletion in the arthrogryposis multiplex congenita-spinal muscular atrophy association (submitted).

16

Rett syndrome: recent clinical and biological aspects

B. HAGBERG

Department of Pediatrics, East Hospital, Gothenburg, Sweden.

Rett syndrome (RS), first described in 1966 [1] in German language and for long overlooked by the medical profession, mainly affects small girls at age 1-3 years. In Sweden cases have been observed since 1960 but under another provisional eponym. RS is an enigmatic condition clinically and biologically. What causes an initially seemingly normal developing little girl to stop playing with toys, no longer using previously acquired purposeful hand skills, stop expressing already learned words, and not acquiring new communication skills? These are still unsolved questions 12 years after the 1983 publication [2] of a pooled French-Portuguese-Swedish series of 35 RS girls which started the present intensive international attention and research, recently reviewed [3, 4]. The prevalence of classic RS is in many European countries around 1/15 000 girls. When additionally traced new variants are added, 1/10 000 is indicated. Thus next to Down syndrome, RS might be the second most prevalent single specific cause behind severe mental retardation in females. The Swedish series at present comprises 185 RS females (October 1995) in ages 2-54 years.

The clinical presentation and subsequent course of classic RS, from infancy to middle age, follows a characteristic pattern with a unique long-term disease profile. A staging system was presented from Sweden in 1986 [5] and has later been further elaborated [3, 5, 6], as illustrated in Table I. Through the last decade atypical RS presentations have become increasingly actual. Thus different variant RS forms have now been described and are of increasing actuality for systematic delineation [3, 4].

Table I. The four clinical stages of classic Rett syndrome.

Original staging system [3, 5]	Added points [6]
Stage I: early onset stagnation	
Onset age: 6 months to 1.5 year	Onset from 5 months of age
Developmental progress delayed	Early postural delay
Developmental pattern still not significantly abnormal	Dissociated development
Duration: weeks to months	"Shufflers"
Stage II: rapid developmental regression	
Onset age: 1–3 or 4 years	Loss of acquired skills:
Loss of acquired skills/ communication	fine finger, babble/words, active playing
Mental deficiency appears	Seldom "quite out"
Duration: weeks to months, possibly 1 year	Eye contact preserved
	Breathing problems yet modest
	Seizures only in 15%
Stage III: pseudostationary period	
Onset: after passing stage II	"Wake up" period
Some communicative restitution	Prominent hand apraxia/dyspraxia
Apparently preserved ambulant ability	
Inapparent, slow neuromotor regression	**Stage III/IV introduced**
Duration: years to decades	The non-ambulant group
Stage IV: late motor deterioration	
Onset: when stage III ambulation ceases	**Subgrouping introduced**
Complete wheelchair dependency	Stage IV A: previous walkers,
Severe disability: wasting and distal distorsions	now non-ambulant
Duration: decades	Stage IV B: never ambulant

In the absence of a diagnostic laboratory marker a battery of clustered remarkable RS behavioral and other clinical oddities can be of considerable help [7]. In addition to the classic stereotyped hand wringings such peculiarities are: the breathing irregularities with episodic hyperventilation, the remarkable air swallowing with bloating, the creaking type of teeth grinding (like "slowly uncorking a wine bottle"), the bursts of sudden unexpected laughing, also during night, the terrible screaming spells as of utmost horror or pain, the characteristic communication through using intense eye pointing and first appearing with age in so many RS girls, the slowly developing intricate neurodeviations of secondary type (*e.g.* dystonic plantar positioning of the toes). By applying clusters of such complex phenomenology in a diagnostic system [7] our actual series now comprises $\approx$ 70% of classic RS and $\approx$ 30% of RS variants among those today aged 12 years and over (Table II).

The actual diagnostic dilemmas for the clinician (Table III) rather have increased in later years. One is now not seldom expected to set or to exclude a RS diagnosis even in very small girls with not yet clearly chiselled developmental deviations. Another diagnostic riddle, difficult to solve, is the old presumptive RS lady in a final frozen rigidity and with only, if any, fragmentary data known from early history. An accurate laboratory diagnostic test is indeed highly needed but not yet available.

Table II. Clinical types of Swedish Rett syndrome females aged 12 years and older (1995)*.

	n	%
Classic Rett syndrome	88	70
Formes fruste variants	27	22
Late regression variants	7	6
Other variants	3	2
Total	125	100

* Those with an early seizure onset history have not been particularly kept apart

Table III. Rett syndrome — Diagnostic problem cases.

The very young	1-2 year-old
The "very old"	"Inveterated" "Frozen"
The "very good"	"Simple mental retardation"
The "very bad"	"Congenital" Immobile
The "very odd"	"Neuropsychiatric"

The genetic basis for RS is now indisputable. Twin studies reveal concordance in identical female twins, discordance in non-identical [3]. A woman with classic RS has given birth to a girl, now aged 6 years and with classic RS [3, 4]. The genetic transmission occurs both over maternal and paternal lines and indicates recessive traits, so far unsolved as to biological type [8]. The consanguinity rate three generations back is on a ten times raised level [8, 9]. Half of the Swedish RS series can be traced back to a restricted number of small rural "Rett areas", often even the same homestead, and unevenly spread over the country [8, 9].

The biology of RS is mysterious. Nosologically, RS is neither a neurodegenerative nor a traditional neurometabolic condition but is indicated to be a neurodevelopmental disorder. Huge efforts to trace deviating biologic parameters of primary importance — metabolic derangements, hormonal deficiencies, chromosomal aberrations — have all been in vain. Specific diagnostic markers are still lacking. However, the deceleration of skull growth starting in early infancy, the impressive brain hypoplasia (mainly grey matter) and its specific localisation at quantitative and volumetric neuroimaging investigations, the remarkable hypoplastic brain pathology with few and likely secondary degenerative traits, altogether support either a lack of a specific brain growth factor or a defect in the arrest of programmed normal neuronal cell death. Of these alternatives, a deficiency of a neurodevelopmental factor acting in a specific window of early CNS development seems more likely [4]. Recent findings of various types of dendritic architectural derangements of pyramidal neurons in different cortices support a postneonatal age-limited deficiency of such a decisive factor for normal infantile brain development [10, 11].

References

1. Rett A. *Ueber ein Cerebral-atrophisches Syndrom bei Hyperammonämie.* Vienna : Brüder Hollinek, 1966.
2. Hagberg B, Aicardi J, Dias K, Ramos O. A progressive syndrome of autism, dementia, ataxia and loss of purposeful hand use in girls: Rett's syndrome: report of 35 cases. *Ann Neurol* 1983 ; 14 : 471-9.
3. Hagberg B. Rett syndrome; clinical and biological aspects. London : Mac Keith Press : Clinics in Developmental Medicine n° 127, 1993.
4. Hagberg B. Rett syndrome: clinical pecularities and biological mysteries. *Acta Paediatr* 1995 ; 84 : 971-6.
5. Hagberg B, Witt Engerström I. Rett syndrome: a suggested staging system for describing impairment profile with increasing age towards adolescence. *Am J Med Genet* 1986 ; 24 : 47-59.
6. Witt Engerström I. Rett syndrome in Sweden. *Acta Paediatr Scand* 1990 ; suppl 369.
7. Hagberg B, Skjeldal OH. Rett variants: a suggested model for inclusion criteria. *Pediatr Neurol* 1994 ; 11 : 5-11.
8. Åkesson H-O, Hagberg B, Wahlström J, Witt Engerström I. Rett syndrome: a search for gene sources. *Am J Med Genet* 1992 ; 42 : 104-10.
9. Åkesson HO, Wahlström J, Witt Engerström I, Hagberg B. Rett syndrome: potential gene sources; phenotyical variability. *Clin Genet* 1995 ; 48 : 169-72.
10. Armstrong D, Dunn K, Antalffy B, Trivedi T. Selective dendritic alterations in the cortex of Rett syndrome. *J Neuropathol Exp Neurol* 1995 ; 54 : 195-201.
11. Belichenko PV, Oldfors A, Hagberg B, Dahlström A. Rett syndrome: 3-D confocal microscopy of cortical pyramidal dendrites and afferents. *Neuro Report* 1994 ; 5 : 1509-13.

Table IV. Essential tremor. Doubtful familial observations.

Obs	S	Age	F-Up	Tremor		Familial data	Handicap	Treatment	Other
D-1	M	18	<2	Post	Arm>left, tongue eyelid, leg	Paternal grandfather: tremor ageing, father: slight tremor	Writing, drinking	Flunarizine	Chronic motor tic
D-2	M	23	3	Post	Arm>left	Maternal grandfather maternal uncle ET (mother 45 Y: no ET)	Writing Eating	No	
D-3	F	21	3	Post inten	Arm>left	Sisters consang.	Writing	Primidone	
D-4	F	15	2.5	Post	Arm	maternal uncle:ET	Writing	Primidone	
D-5	M	14	<2	Post	Arm, tongue	Maternal uncle:ET	Writing		Syncopes
D-6	M	9	<2	Post	Arm>left	Father: tremor stress	Writing, eating	No	
D-7	F	5	2	Post	Arm, tongue	Father: slight tremor	Writing, task precision	No	

* in years   S= sex   F-up= follow-up   Und= undetermined   Post= postural

Table V. Essential tremor. Sporadic observations.

Obs	S	Age	F-up	Tremor		Handicap	Neuroimg (age)	Byochemic	Treatment	Other
S-1	M	19	2	16	Post action	Arm, leg, head	No	CT, RMI (15)	Cu, AA, Berry	Propanolol flunarizine	Chronic tic
S-2	M	23	16	7.3	Post action	Arm>right		CT (6)		Primidone, propanolol	Behavioral disorder
S-3	M	21	5	11	Post action	Arm>left	Drinking, eating		Cu, AA, VC, EEG	Primidone, propanolol, flunarizine	Alcohol responsive
S-4	F	17	Und	5	Post action	Arm>right	Writing, eating drinking	TC (1) RMI (15)	Low IgA	No	ADDH
S-5	M	26	8	9	Post action	Arm>left	Writing drinking	Rx Cran	Cu, T3-T4	PRM	
S-6	M	24	Und	8	Post	Arm>left	Drinking	RMI		No	
S-7	M	35	Und	21	Post	Arm	Writing, drinking	RX-cran	Cui, ACTH	Primidone propanolol	Syncope
S-!	M	15	<2	2	Post	Arm	Writing carrying obj	RMi (13)	Cu	No	

* in years   S= sex   F-up= follow-up   Und= undetermined   Post= postural

ESSENTIAL TREMOR IN CHILDHOOD

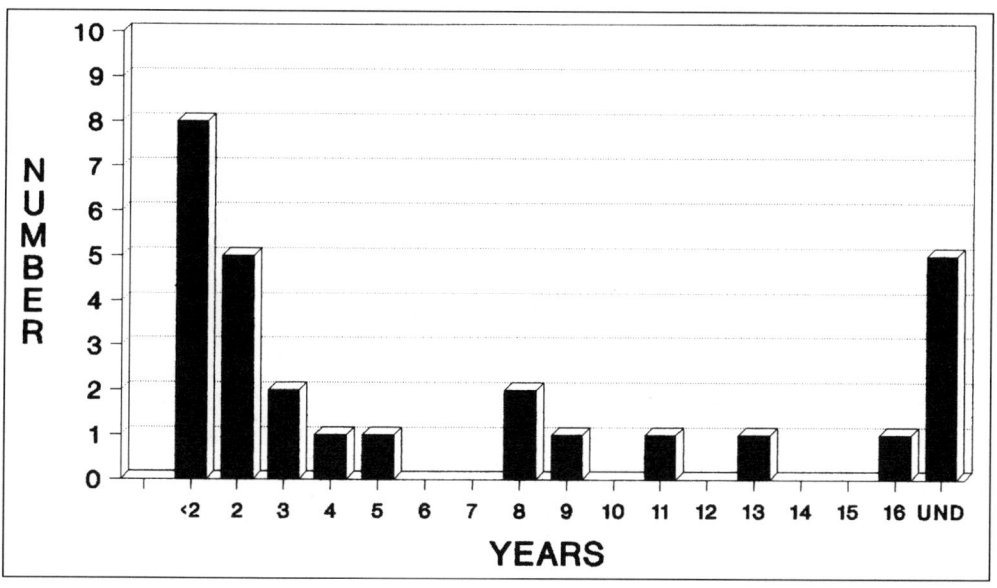

Figure 1. Essential tremor; age of onset (n = 28).

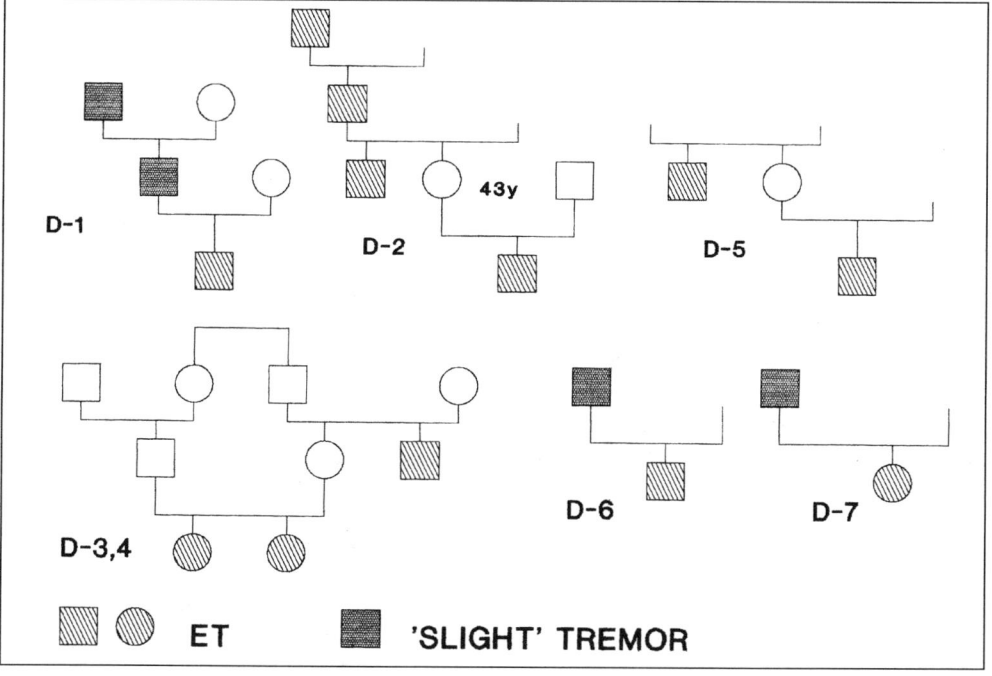

Figure 2. Atypical familial essential tremor.

Table VI. Esential tremor (n = 28) Upper extremities.

Asymmetrical	17
Dominant hand	4
Non-dominant hand	13
Symmetrical	11

Discussion

ET is transmitted as an autosomal dominant character [4], although penetrance and expressivity are quite variable. Sporadic cases have been widely reported [5, 6]. Their proportion varies depending on different studies [7, 8]. From this small series, some conclusions can be drawn. Autosomal dominant inheritance is very probable in 13 (45%) out of the 28 ET cases of this series. Eight (25%) cases were sporadic but in the remaining 7 cases, the dominant inheritance was the most probable although atypical. These are interesting cases: in case D-2 ET was obvious in the maternal branch (great-grandfather, grandfather and an uncle) but the mother at the age of 43 was tremor-free suggesting a skipping generation. Larsson and Sjogren [9] did not encounter families with missed generations but Critchley [10] and Rautakorpi et al. [7] recorded such pedigrees. Because the age of onset is very variable within the same family [9] and can be as late as 75, the occurrence of missed generations could easily be only apparent. More confusing is the condition of two sisters (D-3, D-4) whose parents were consanguineous and moreover one maternal uncle had ET. In three other cases, the affected parent (always the father) had a slight tremor with characteristics similar to the enhanced physiological tremor. Anticipation in ET has been suggested [10] but negated by others [7, 9]. These cases argue to the anticipation but obviously more studies in children are necessary.

Another point to be considered in this series is the male predominance. Whether we consider only ET cases or all the patients (ET and "doubtful ET"), the relation male/female is 3:1. Sex distribution is predominantly in males in Scandinavian studies (female/male ratios of 0.5 and 0.71 respectively) whereas predominant females involvement was found in the USA [11]. The explanation of this inconsistence between the results of our series and the reported adult series is not easy. If future studies confirm this finding, this may be related to an earlier occurrence of ET in males reported by Borges [12] or a transient childhood form predominating in males.

"Probable ET" cases are also an interesting group. Two cases (P-1, P-4) developed postural upper extremities tremor some years after an infancy neurological condition: spontaneous subdural bilateral effusion and opsoclonus-myoclonus syndrome but in both cases, there was a close family member affected by ET. One speculation is that the expressivity of the supposed ET gene is increased by the previous neurological condition. Case P-2 has Alpert disease but his clinical signs are typical of ET, and moreover nerve conduction velocities are normal. A similar situation occurs in P-5 with elevation of T3 as the only endocrinological abnormality and moreover without any signs of clinical hyperthyroidism. Finally, in one case tremor was obvious only in the morning (episodic) and, in another case, for some years (transient).

The impairment resulting from ET is variable. It is negligible in some children, limited to irregularities in handwriting and to some "insecurity" in fine movements. In others, it is marked interfering with everyday life, for example drinking out of a glass. Impairment varies according to the amplitude of the tremor but is often made worse by the anticipation of awkward situations. One patient had to renounce going to restaurants because he would then spill the content of his glass, which did not occur at home.

In conclusion, ET is a very interesting pediatric neurological condition, but, unfortunatelly, clinical studies of this population are scarce. As our knowledge of ET in childhood is mainly provided by studies on adult patients, many specific pediatric questions remain unanswered.

References

1. Elsasser G. Erblicher tremor. *Fortschr Erbpath* 1941 ; 5 : 117-35.
2. Bain PG, Findley LJ, Thompson PD, Gresty MA, Rothwell JC, Harding AE, Marsden CD. A study of hereditary essential tremor. *Brain* 1994 ; 117 : 805-24.
3. Paulson GW. Bening essential tremor in childhood. *Clin Ped* 1976 ; 15 : 67-70.
4. Critchley Mc D. Observations on essential (heredofamilial) tremor. *Brain* 1949 ; 72 : 113-39.
5. Hubble JP, Busenbark KL, Koller WC. Essential tremor. *Clin Neuropharmacol* 1989 ; 12 : 453-82.
6. Koller WC, Busenbark K, Gray C, Hassanien RS, Dubinsky R. Classification of essential tremor *Clin Neuropharmacol* 1992 ; 15 : 81-7.
7. Rautakorpi I, Takala J, Martila RJ, Sievers K, Rinne UK. Essential tremor in a Finnish population. *Acta Neurol Scand* 1982 ; 66 : 58-67.
8. Rajput AH, Offord KP, Beard CM, Kurland LT. Essential tremor in Rochester, Minnesota: a 45-year study. *J Neurol Neurosurg Psychiatr* 1984 ; 47 : 466-70.
9. Larsson T, Sjogren T. Essential tremor: a clinical and genetic population study. *Acta Psychiatr Neurol Scand* 1960 ; 36 (Suppl 144) : 1-176.
10. Critchley E. Clinical manifestations of essential tremor. *J Neurol Neurosurg Psychiat* 1972 ; 35 : 365-72.
11. Haerer AF, Anderson DW, Schoenberg BS. Prevalence of essential tremor. Results from the Copiah county study. *Arch Neurol* 1982 ; 39 : 750-1.
12. Borges V. Tremor essencial: caracteriçao clínica de uma amostra de 176 pacientes. Tese Sao Paulo, 1993.

18

Dopa-sensitive progressive childhood dystonia (Segawa's syndrome). From symptom to gene. A 20 years history

T. DEONNA

Pediatric Department, Neuropediatric Unit, CHUV, Lausanne, Switzerland.

At the first ICNA conference in Toronto in 1975, during an almost empty late-evening poster session held in the basement of a big international hotel, I met a lonely Japanese colleague (Masaya Segawa) standing in front of his panel. I did not realize at this moment that I was facing one of the most extraordinary neuropediatric condition whose recognition was to change the life of a number of children throughout the world and add much to our understanding of neurotransmitter function and basal ganglia diseases. Two years later in 1977, we admitted a 13 year-old girl for work-up of progressive gait difficulties. The student who first examined her in the morning found little abnormal and wondered if this was not a functional disorder. We thought we were smarter because we found later in the day that she had a slight asymmetrical dystonia of the lower extremities and wondered if this was not an incipient "progressive dystonia musculorum deformans", but the girl did not return for follow-up. Learning and getting convinced can be a slow and painful process. At the EFCNS meeting in Oxford in 1981, Goutières and Aicardi gave me a booster injection when they presented a case of fluctuating childhood dystonia responsive to L-Dopa. On my return, I pulled our girl's record, looked at the movie made 5 years before, called the family and this time insisted that they come back which they had not wanted before. She had clearly worsened and diurnal fluctuation of symptoms was evident.

It needed a personal letter and pressing insistence on my part to have the family accept treatment with L-Dopa which had been declared immediately as poisonous by the "doctor" who had the family and girl under his control.

Fortunately, L-Dopa worked quickly enough (within two weeks but not immediately) to persuade the girl and her parents to continue. She is now a 30 year-old kindergarten teacher, married with two healthy children and is asymptomatic on low doses of L-Dopa.

Our girl's condition had indeed been first recognized and published as a probable separate entity in Japan by Segawa in 1971 as "Childhood basal ganglia disease with remarkable response to L-Dopa, hereditary basal ganglia disease with marked diurnal fluctuation". Response to L-Dopa in isolated cases of childhood dystonia had been occasionally reported before and also cases with fluctuations. A new disease can always be found to have several fathers. Nygaard, who has toured the world trying to see each reported case in the mideighties has an interesting historical review on that [1].

In 1983, I had the priviledge to conduct for the EFCNS a questionaire survey on Dopa-sensitive childhood dystonia [2]. Colleagues from 7 European countries, some of which are present at this meeting, participated and this allowed to describe 20 new cases. It confirmed that HPD (hereditary progressive dystonia as abbrevated by Segawa) was not so rare and was present probably world-wide. I can't help quoting the description of the case proposed by the famous tandem Goutières-Aicardi (in various orders!) for this survey which in its usual simplicity and precision describes in a particulaly spectacular fashion the severe cases with marked fluctuations: "In the morning, she can get up alone, wash herself and walk downstairs holding on the bannister. After breakfast, she can not walk alone to the car. At school, she sits on her chair and can not walk anymore the whole day. At 4 pm., she cannot hold her pencil anymore. At dinner, she cannot bring her fork to her mouth and cannot hold her head straight. She must be carried into her bed where she cannot turn around anymore." (free translation T.D.).

Although widely written about in the last 15 years and now known to most neurologists and neuropediatricians, HPD can still be sometimes a tricky condition to recognize for several reasons. It can start at any age, progress very variably, be severe or mild and may present itself as "fatigue", "cramps" or bizarre gait. It can be misdiagnosed as a functional disorder, congenital spastic diplegia or progressive spastic paraplegia, among many other labels. The variability of symptoms and their evolution as well as the previous diagnosis received can be particularly well observed in large families when several affected members from different generations are discovered with HPD. Progression to and overlap with "Parkinsonism" was initially recognized from the study of such a family by Nygaard [3] and this problem has led to lively debates about the relation between HPD and JP (juvenile Parkinson's disease) which are now seen as separate entities.

Remarkably, regardless of age and severity, very small doses of L-Dopa reverse all or almost all symptoms without "escape" or "on-off phenomena" and the treatment remains apparently effective throughout life (unlike Parkinson's disease). A new family with HPD was recently found in Switzerland by my colleague Dr J. Ghika and treatment with L-Dopa started at almost the same time in 3 women of 20, 50 and 70 years. The existential change brought about by the rapid cure (too rapid?) was narrated to us by two of these very articulate women and their story is breathtaking. It involves not only a motor change: "it does not only change the body". I hope that R. will have finished writing her experience in details (as I insisted she should do) so that I can tell you more about it at the meeting. I had never heard or thought before about some of the things she has explained me.

The fluctuations of symptoms in HPD, the total and sustained reponse to L-Dopa and the increased incidence and severity of the disease in females (although it is clearly a dominantly inherited disorder) have raised many exciting physiopathological questions. These have recently received new answers.

Rajpur *et al.* reported the pathological and biochemical observation of a 20 year-old woman who accidentally died. They found no evidence of a degenerative process in the striatum and concluded that "disturbed dopamine synthetic capacity or a reduced arborization of striatal dopamine terminals may be the major disturbance in Dopa-responsive dystonia" [4]. Positron-emission tomography (PET) using the tracer 6-L (F) fluorodopa to investigate the nigrostriatal pathway has given normal results in HPD (as opposed to what one has found in classical Parkinson's disease and more recently in cases of juvenile Parkinsonism) giving support to the idea that there is only a "functional" deficit of L-Dopa.

It has been recently found that the gene for hereditary progressive dystonia with marked diurnal fluctuation maps to chromosome 14q [5]. Shortly thereafter, it was determined that the gene locus of the GTP cyclohydrolase I is within the region containing the HPD/DRD locus. The mutational analysis of genomic DNA of HPD patients revealed mutations in the GTP cyclohydrolase I gene. This enzyme is involved in the synthesis of tetrahydrobiopterins, itself a necessary co-factor for tyrosine hydroxylases [6].

As noted by Segawa in his introduction to a book which he has edited and which has just been published (1995) on *Age-dependant dopamine disorders* [1]: "This is the first discovery of the causative gene for inherited dystonia and may lead to a breakthrough in clarifying the biochemical components of the basal ganglia disorders. Furthermore, this cyclohydrolase I in normal subjects has higher activity in males than females, which might play a role in the gender difference in the dopamine neuron."

What has been learned in the last 25 years from the time HPD was recognized as a special clinical entity (with the simultaneous finding of an empirically effective treatment) to discovery of the causative gene is indeed remarkable. However, there is still a gap to understand how a biochemical deficit relates to the complex neurological symptoms and signs of this disease.

A last personal note. In 1990, Segawa organized a satellite meeting to the ICNA conference in Tokyo on HPD and asked me what was the situation with HPD in Europe. For that occasion, I reviewed the litterature and bothered again colleagues with a questionaire, this time adressed to the members of the SNI (Société Européenne de Neurologie Infantile). Among the new questions which interested me were the following: writer's cramp as an isolated, initial or main symptom? (7/17 yes); variability of symptoms other then diurnal? (4/17 yes; exercice: 3; infection: 1).

This was precisely the problem of Anik. She complained of fatigue and writing problems. Dystonia could be seen clearly only in the evening when she had exercized or had an infection. All symptoms disappeared with L-Dopa (the most disturbing one was "the writing and the fatigue") which has been stopped and restarted on several occasions. Her mother was found to have mild Parkinsonism and she says the main reason she takes L-Dopa and never wants to stop it is her "fatigue".

I do not want to imply that measuring the GTP cylohydrolase activity will be the new way to approach the clinical challenge of the child presenting with fatigue, writing problems or bizarre gait!

On the contrary, clinicians will always be needed to help find the rare (not so rare maybe?) cases of HPD who hide behind these frequent and unspecific complaints and see if the spectrum of symptoms and undiagnosed cases are more numerous than imagined. I do not want to say either that we lack L-Dopa when we are tired, but that the very striking effect on this symptom in some patients with HPD could also give us some insight on some of the components of this multifaceted and devastating feeling.

Anik's case also raises a medico-philosophical question. Does she have a "threshhold" disease? It is invisible or apparent depending on a combination of factors (holidays, evening, stress, infection, physical effort) or with a very special activity (writing!). Yet, she was very troubled by it, suffered in school (because of the writing) and saw many physicians.

I had not realized, when I proposed to speak on HPD for the meeting in the honor of Jean Aicardi that he had, as with so many other new diseases in neuropediatrics, been in the frontline with this one also! I guess this is the best compliment and thank you note I can give him.

References

1. Segawa M, Nomura Y. Age-related Dopamine-dependent disorders. Karger, 14. Monographs in Neural Sciences, 1995.
2. Deonna T, *et al*. Dopa-sensitive progressive dystonia of childhood with fluctuations of symptoms- Segawa's syndrome and possible variants. *Neuropediatrics* 1986 ; 17 : 81.

3. Nygaard TG, *et al.* Dopa-responsive dystonia. The spectrum of clinical manifestations in a large North-American family. *Neurology* 1990 ; 40 : 66-9.
4. Rajput, *et al.* Dopa-responsive dystonia: pathological and biochemical observations in a case. *Ann Neurol* 1994 ; 35 : 396-402.
5. Tanaka, *et al.* The gene for hereditary progressive dystonia with marked fluctuation maps to chromosome 14q. *Ann Neurol* 1995 ; 37 : 405-8.
6. Ichinose H, *et al.* Hereditary progressive dystonia with marked diurnal fluctuation caused by mutations in the GTP cyclohydrolase I gene. *Nature Genet* 1994 ; 8 : 236-42.
7. Deonna T, *et al.* Dopa-sensitive childhood dystonia. A "forme fruste" with writer's cramp triggered by exercice. Abstract (french) Societé Européenne de Neurologie Infantile, Genève, 1992; *Dev Med Child Neurol* 1996 (in press).

19

Alternating hemiplegia of childhood. A report of 29 cases and a review of the literature

M. BOURGEOIS

Neurological Unit, Department of Pediatrics, Hôpital des Enfants Malades, Paris, France.

Alternating hemiplegia of childhood (AHC) was first described in 1971 by Verret and Steele [1]. Subsequent reports have further delineated the clinical features of the condition and emphasized the importance of stereotyped paroxysmal manifestations that include tonic and dystonic attacks, nystagmus and other oculomotor abnormalities, respiratory and autonomic changes [2, 3]. The secondary emergence of developmental retardation and of non-paroxysmal neurological symptoms, especially ataxia and choreoathetotic movements, is a constant feature.

We report 29 cases of AHC, some of the clinical data on cases 1 through 22 have been previously reported [4-6]. The average duration of the disease before last examination was 8 years 6 months (range 2 to 19 years, median 5, 9 years). There were 15 girls and 14 boys aged 3 weeks to 11 months at first examination. None had a family history of a similar disorder. In only seven was a family history of common migraine or of epilepsy. The first manifestations clearly related to AHC appeared in all cases before age 6 months and in 14 before 3 months and are usually tonic or dystonic attacks (16/29) and paroxysmal nystagmus (5/29) rather than hemiplegias (6/29) and these appear early in life, sometimes even in the neonatal period. Bilateral tonic attacks occurred in some patients with arching of the back, upward gaze deviation and extreme misery. They were sometimes followed by hemiplegia on the same side and these manifestations are often interpreted as seizure followed by Todd's paralysis. Hemiplegic attacks appeared before 18 months and progressively became during the first year of life the predominant paroxysmal phenomenon. They had obvious characteristics: hemiplegias could begin abruptly or progress within minutes, often precipitated by emotional triggers, fatigue, bright lights, cold or hot weather... and be preceded by screaming; they varied in intensity from one moment to the next; they were usually flaccid. The frequency and duration of hemiplegias varied widely. Brief episodes lasted from a few minutes to about one hour. Long attacks could last from several hours to several days, up to two weeks, the average duration being 8 days. Both sides were always affected in alternance but 13 patients had a clear predominance of left hemiplegia, while 5 had more right-sided attacks and 11 had an approximately equal distribution. The hemiplegias could shift from one side to the opposite within the same episode, usually following a period of bilateral weakness but occasionally in an abrupt manner. During some attacks, ten children had a disturbance of verbal production, apparently of motor origin, irrespective of the side involved. Consciousness was preserved during bouts of hemiplegia but some children appeared quite sleepy while others were fretful and miserable or even cried out as if in pain.

Episodes of double hemiplegia or quadriplegia occurred in all 27 patients for whom a complete history was available. In 26 patients they were seen at the time a hemiplegia was shifting from one side to the opposite. Eighteen patients had episodes of bilateral paralysis from the start, without previous hemiplegia. During this period, which could last from one hour to over one day, the condition of the patients deteriorated. Swallowing difficulties, dribbling, choking, slurred speech were prominent in 20 children and only mild in 7. Misery and apparent pain were considerably more intense than in unilateral attacks. Paroxysmal dyspnea was present in 15 cases. Some such attacks were quite prolonged, up to three weeks in three cases. During protracted bouts, waves of transient improvement could occur and all children were free of paralysis during sleep, as well as during a brief period following awakening. Several parents took advantage of this period to feed their child without risk of choking and aspiration. At the end of such generalized attacks, the patients appeared exhausted and a severe regression of their motor and cognitive abilities was common and lasted up to several weeks.

Another remarkable feature of AHC is the constant effect of sleep. All parents volunteered that as soon as their child fell asleep, there was resumption of symmetrical movements. In long-lasting attacks, paralysis would reappear in same location 10 to 20 minutes after awakening. Even a short nap resulted in remission of the hemiplegia. Sleep has an analogous role in others disorders: in some migraine syndrome, Segawa's dystonia, attacks cease during sleep. The attacks of some AHC also resemble cataplectic attacks. Howeuver, patients with AHC show a normal pattern of sleep [7] in contrast to the abnormal patterns found in patients with narcolepsy or cataplexy.

Other paroxysmal manifestations as dyspneic episodes and abnormal eye movements were frequently present. Episodes of monocular isolated nystagmus were observed in 15 children, however complex oculomotor disturbance ressembling internuclear ophtalmoplegia may also be found .

Epilepsy is a very common misdiagnosis for AHC. Moreover, true seizures occur in some patients with AHC [2, 7]. Epileptic seizures were reported in 8 of our patients but never observed directly. Seizures were described as generalized in six patients and as simple partial in two. They occurred only at the peak of a bilateral episode in four children and independently of hemiplegic attacks in the others. In our experience, these have been mostly clonic in type. Occasional patients with interictal paroxysmal EEG abnormalities have been reported but repeated recording of attacks of AHC have not shown any paroxysmal discharge [7, 8]. Preservation of consciousness and pain are clinical clues to the right diagnosis. Attacks of AHC and epilepsy appear to be two different conditions even in the relatively common cases in which both occur in the same patient. Even though this association implies that cortical involvement may be related or secondary to a disturbance in subcortical structures that seem to be primarily involved in causing the symptoms of AHC.

The course of the paroxysmal features of AHC was variable. A few children, spontaneously or following treatment, had long attack-free periods (up to 2 years) and the rythm of occurrence fluctuated widely. In general, the paroxysmal manifestations associated with the hemiplegias tended to decrease in intensity with time and paralytic episodes. Even pure hemiplegias occurred more purely. After variable periods, delayed development or mental retardation and choreoathetosis or dystonia were present in all patients. At last examination, 8 children were mildly delayed or of borderline intelligence and 21 had moderate to severe cognitive retardation. Only two children of borderline intelligence could attend a normal class with special support. Four patients did not develop communication language and the most severely retarded often had temper tantrums or a hyperkinetic behavior. Thirteen patients had a clearly abnormal development before onset of attacks. However, several children appeared to develop relatively well during their first year only to become retarded later. The clinical impression was that the disorder was progressive during the first year or two, then became relatively stable.

Delay in motor milestones was the rule. Independent walking was acquired at an average age of 44 months (range 14 months to 10 years) in 24 children, and fine motor control remained poor in all. Gross hypotonia was present in all patients and often had existed from onset. They also become ataxic, and choreoathetotic. A dystonic component was added in 12 cases. The onset of abnormal movements was within 2 years of onset in 9 children, between 2 and 3 years in 12 and over 3 years in 8, the longest interval being 5 years.

AHC is such a distinctive disorder that it can be separated easily from vascular disorder such as A-V malformations, multiple emboli or thromboses, Rendu-Osler-Weber disease.

Hemiplegic migraine has often been regarded as including AHC and some of the first reported series were a mixture of cases of AHC and classic hemiplegic migraine [1-9]. In teenagers, a history may be obtained suggestive of a migrainous march but such observations are rare (4 of our cases; LBP Stephenson personal communication, 1991).

However, hemiplegic migraine rarely has its onset before 2 years of age and does not feature tonic attacks, oculomotor abnormalities, or mental retardation. Indeed, we were not able to find an unusually high incidence of familial migraine in our cases and the data in the literature are conflicting.

Mitochondrial diseases, especially mitochondrial encephalopathy with lactic acidosis and stroke-like episodes, share with AHC the occurrence of alternating hemiplegia, seizures, and neurodevelopmental deterioration [10, 11]. However, hemiplegic episodes are more prolonged in this disease and associated signs are different. Atypical forms of mitochondrial disease are known [12] and the hypothesis of such a disorder may be considered. The magnetic resonnance spectroscopic abnormalities [13] suggest the presence of mitochondrial dysfunction. However our patients had normal blood and CSF lactate levels and in three who underwent muscle biopsy with specific search for evidence of mitochondrial disturbance no ragged-red fibers and no PDH deficiency nor mitochondrial respiratory chain deficiency were found. However, PDH-E1 deficiency was observed in a single case reported by Silver [14].

A familial form of AHC has also been reported by Mikati [15]. Two of these patients had a late onset of the disease at 3 years of age and their cognitive development was relatively normal. Karyotype revealed a balanced reciprocal translocation 46, XY, t(3,9)(p26;q34) in the affected patients. It is not clear whether the clinical features in these cases were identical to those in sporadic cases regarding the effect of sleep and the intensity of the dystonic symptoms or whether minor differences might exist between familial as opposed to more common sporadic cases, an important issue for genetic counselling.

Whether vascular phenomena are a cause of deterioration remains uncertain as the few SPECT studies available have given conflicting results with either a moderate decrease [16, 17] or an increase [18] in blood flow. SPECT was normal in 5 of our patients and showed a mild decrease in perfusion on ipsilateral in 2 and controlateral side in one during hemiplegic episode. Such discrepancies may result from different timing of the SPECT with respect to the onset of an attack. PET studies [19] have revealed symmetrical cerebral metabolism.

The neuropathological findings [20] in one case showed extensive bilateral involvement of the hippocampi, these results are consistent with recurrent episodes of hypoxia-ischemia.

Twenty-four patients were treated by flunarizine, who has been shown to reduce the frequency and duration of attacks in many children [21]. Most patients had previously received a large number of antiepileptic and antimigraine drugs to no avail. Some positive effect, mainly shortening and lesser severity of attacks rather than a diminution in frequency, was apparent in 19 children at doses varying between 5 and 10 mg. In one patient, the effect was marked with a considerable reduction of the total time with hemiplegia. A much longer experience will be required before the safety of the drug is proved. Other agents that seemed occasionally effective were clonazepam and phenytoin in two patients each. Haloperidol [22] and niapranazine (E Veneselli, personal communication, 1994) have also been reported to be effective in some cases.

This large series of cases of AHC permits to further delineate the clinical features of the condition. All patients exhibited six major characteristics:
- the onset was before 18 months of age;
- there were repeated attacks of hemiplegia involving either side of the body;
- other paroxysmal disturbances including tonic or dystonic spells, nystagmus or other oculomotor abnormalities, dyspnea and various autonomic phenomena occurred during hemiplegic bouts or in isolation;
- episodes of bilateral hemiplegia were observed either during attacks that started unilaterally at the time hemiplegia shifted to the contralateral side or from the beginning of attacks;
- sleep consistently produced immediate disappearance of all symptoms that reappeared 10 to 20 minutes after awakening in long-lasting bouts;
- there was evidence of developmental delay, mental retardation and neurological abnormalities including choreoathetosis, dystonia or ataxia.

The association of these features does not seem to occur in any other known condition. Because of the current absence of known laboratory marker, we think a complete clinical picture is required at this point if the practical consequences of the diagnosis are to be drawn. The suggestion of an abnormality of energy metabolism and of mitochondrial dysfunction in patients with AHC in the absence of demonstrable structural abnormalities encourages us to continue investigations in that area.

References

1. Verret S, Steele JC. Alternating hemiplegia in childhood: a report of eight patients with complicated migraine beginning in infancy. *Pediatrics* 1971 ; 47 : 675-80.
2. Hosking GP, Cavanagh NPC, Wilson J. Alternating hemiplegia: complicated migraine of infancy. *Arch Dis Child* 1978 ; 53 : 656-9.
3. Dalla Bernardina B, Fontana E, Colamaria V, Zullini E, Darra F, Giardina L, Franco A, Montagnini A. Alternating hemiplegia of childhood: epilepsy and electroencephalographic investigations. In : Andermann F, Aicardi J, Vigevano F, eds. *Alternating hemiplegia of childhood*. New York : Raven Press, 1993 : 75-87.
4. Krägeloh I, Aicardi J. Alternating hemiplegia in infants: report of five cases. *Dev Med Child Neurol* 1980 ; 22 : 784-91.
5. Aicardi J. Alternating hemiplegia of childhood. *Int Pediatr* 1987 ; 2 : 115-9.
6. Aicardi J, Bourgeois M, Goutières F. Alternating hemiplegia of childhood: clinical findings and diagnostic criteria. In : Andermann F, Aicardi J, Vigevano F, eds. *Alternating hemiplegia of childhood*. New York : Raven Press, 1993 : 19-28.
7. Ricci S. Sleep studies of children with alternating hemiplegia of childhood. In : Andermann F, Aicardi J, Vigevano F, eds. *Alternating hemiplegia of childhood*. New York : Raven Press, 1993 : 95-8.
8. Dittrich J, Havlova M, Nevsimalova S. Paroxysmal hemiparesis of childhood. *Dev Med Child Neurol* 1979 ; 21 : 800-7.

9. Golden GS, French JH. Basilar artery migraine in young children. *Pediatrics* 1975 ; 56 : 722-6.
10. Pavlakis SG, Rowland LP, De Vivo DC, Bonilla E, Di Mauro S. Mitochondrial myopathies and encephalomyopathies. In : Plum F, ed. *Advances in contemporary neurology*. Philadelphia : FA Davis, 1988 : 95-123.
11. Montagna P, Galassi R, Medori R. MELAS syndrome: characteristic migrainous and epileptic features and maternal transmission. *Neurology* 1988 ; 30 : 751-4.
12. Dvorkin GS, Andermann F, Carpenter S. Classical migraine, intractable epilepsy and multiple strokes: a syndrome related to mitochondrial encephalomyopathy. In : Andermann F. Lugaresi F, eds. *Migraine and epilepsy*. London : Butterworths, 1987 : 203-32.
13. De Stephano N, Siver K, Andermann F, Arnold DL. Mitochondrial dysfunction in patients with alternating hemiplegia of childhood: fluctuation over time in relation to clinical states. In : Andermann F, Aicardi J, Vigevano F, eds. *Alternating hemiplegia of childhood*. New York : Raven Press, 1993 : 115-22.
14. Silver K, Scriver C, Arnold DL, Robinson B, Andermann F. Alternating hemiplegia of childhood associated with mitochondrial disease: a deficiency of pyruvate deshydrogenase. In : Andermann F, Aicardi J, Vigevano F, eds. *Alternating hemiplegia of childhood*. New York : Raven Press, 1993 : 165-72.
15. Mikati MA, O'Tuama L, Dangond F. Autosomal dominant alternating hemiplegia of childhood. In : Andermann F, Aicardi J, Vigevano F, eds. *Alternating hemiplegia of childhood*. New York : Raven Press, 1993 : 165-72.
16. Zupanc ML, Perlman SB, Rust RS. Single photon emission computed tomography studies in alternating hemiplegia. In : Andermann F, Aicardi J, Vigevano F, eds. *Alternating hemiplegia of childhood*. New York : Raven Press, 1993 : 125-44.
17. Sakuragawa N, Matsuo T, Kihira S, *et al*. Alternating hemiplegia in infancy: two case reports and reduced regional cerebral blood flow in 11CO2 dynasmic positron emission tomography. *Brain Dev* 1985 ; 7, 2 : 207.
18. Kanazawa O, Shirazaka Y, Hattori H, Okuno T, Mikawa H. Ictal 99m Tc-HMPAO SPECT in alternating hemiplegia. *Pediatr Neurol* 1991 ; 7 : 121-4.
19. Mikati MA, Fischman AJ. Positron emission tomography in children alternating hemiplegia of childhood. In : Andermann F, Aicardi J, Vigevano F, eds. *Alternating hemiplegia of childhood*. New York : Raven Press, 1993 : 109-14.
20. Becker LE. Alternating hemiplegia of childhood : a neuropathologic review. In : Andermann F, Aicardi J, Vigevano F, eds. *Alternating hemiplegia of childhood*. New York : Raven Press, 1993 : 57-65.
21. Bourgeois M, Aicardi J. The treatment of alternating hemiplegia of childhood with Flunarizine: experience with 17 patients. In : Andermann F, Aicardi J, Vigevano F, eds. *Alternating hemiplegia of childhood*. New York : Raven Press, 1993 : 191-4.
22. Wilson J. Treatment of alternating hemiplegia of childhood: the effect of Haloperidol. In : Andermann F, Aicardi J, Vigevano F, eds. *Alternating hemiplegia of childhood*. New York : Raven Press, 1993 : 201-2.

20

Peroxisomal disorders

B.T. POLL-THE

University Children's Hospital "Wilhelmina Kinderziekenhuis", Utrecht, The Netherlands.

The peroxisomal disorders constitute a clinically and biochemically heterogeneous group of disease states sharing an impairment of one or more peroxisomal functions [1]. Up to now at least 21 disorders have been found which are linked to peroxisomal dysfunction. Most of them show severe CNS involvement [2].

Clinical presentation

A great clinical heterogeneity exists in the expression of diseases with similar biochemical defects. This variability comprises the type and severity of symptoms as well as the age of onset of symptoms. On the other hand, similar clinical phenotypes may also be associated with different biochemical lesions. This absence of correlation between clinical expression and biochemical defects is illustrated by the classical Zellweger syndrome (CZ) and infantile Refsum's disease (IRD), which have similar multiple enzyme defects; it is also evident in the dissimilar enzyme defects underlying one clinical syndrome, *e.g.* rhizomelic chondrodysplasia punctata (RCDP) [3]. Given the diversity of clinical and biochemical abnormalities, an arbitrary approach has been made to divide peroxisomal disorders into two groups: those with a deficient assembly of peroxisomes, and those with one single deficient peroxisomal enzyme (Table I). However, this biochemical "classification" is not useful for clinicians who are faced with clinical symptoms and not with biochemical phenotypes. In general, the onset of symptoms is not accompanied by an acute metabolic event or abnormal routine laboratory tests indicating metabolic derangement. In most disorders, the presentation is more likely to be associated with chronic encephalopathy from infancy/early childhood or a progressive neurologic manifestation from the school-age period. Peroxisomal disorders should be considered in various clinical conditions which depend on the age of the patient: predominant errors of morphogenesis, predominant neurologic presentation, and predominant hepato-digestive presentation. All these presentations are possible in the neonatal period.

Table I. Classification of peroxisomal disorders.

	Peroxisomes	Enzyme defect
Peroxisome assembly deficiencies		
Classical Zellweger syndrome Neonatal adrenoleukodystrophy Infantile Refsum disease	Absent	Generalized
Pseudo Infantile Refsum disease	Absent	Generalized
Zellweger-like syndrome	Present	VLCFA oxidation, THCA oxidation, DHAPAT, Phytanic acid oxidation
Rhizomelic chondrodysplasia punctata (classical/atypical phenotype)	Abnormal	DHAPAT, alkyl DHAP synthase, Phytanic acid oxidase, Unprocessed peroxisomal thiolase
Atypical Refsum disease		Phytanic acid oxidase Pipecolic acid oxidase
Single peroxisomal enzyme deficiencies		
Rhizomelic chondrodysplasia punctata		Isolated DHAPAT or alkyl DHAP synthase
Rhizomelic chondrodysplasia punctata		Phytanic acid oxidase
X-linked adrenoleukodystrophy	Normal	VLCFA-CoA synthetase transport
Pseudo-neonatal adrenoleuko-dystrophy	Enlarged	Acyl-CoA oxidase
Bifunctional enzyme deficiency	Normal	Bi(tri)functional enzyme
Pseudo-Zellweger syndrome	Enlarged	Peroxisomal thiolase
Trihydroxycholestanoic acidemia		THCA-CoA oxidase
Isolated pipecolic acidemia	Abnormal	Pipecolic acid oxidase
Mevalonic aciduria		Mevalonate kinase
Classical Refsum disease		Phytanic acid oxidase
Glutaric aciduria type III	Normal	Peroxisomal glutaryl-CoA oxidase
Hyperoxaluria type I	Normal	Alanine: glyoxylate amino-transferase
Hyperoxaluria type I		Mistargeting
Acatalasemia	Normal	Catalase

DHAPAT: dihydroxyacetone phosphate acyltransferase;
DHAP: dihydroxyacetone phosphate;
VLCFA: very long chain fatty acids;
THCA: trihydroxycholestanoic acid.

Polymalformative syndrome and dysmorphia

Cranio facial abnormalities including large fontanelles, high forehead, epicanthus, and abnormal ears may be mistaken for chromosomal aberrations such as Down syndrome. They are frequently associated with other abnormalities: rhizomelic shortening of limbs in RCDP, stippled calcifications of epiphyses in RCDP and CZ, renal cysts in CZ, abnormalities in neuronal migration (gyral abnormalities, neuronal heterotopias) and cerebral myelination. These congenital manifestations point to dysmorphogenesis during the prenatal period, as observed in some inborn errors affecting energy-producing pathways of the fetus and in metabolic dysfunctions of the mother during pregnancy [4].

Neurologic dysfunction

At birth, the predominant symptom is often a severe hypotonia with areactivity which can be mistaken for a neuromuscular disorder, a disorder of the CNS and autonomic nervous system, and malformation syndromes. An increasing number of inborn errors of metabolism without evident biochemical abnormalities by routine laboratory screening should also be considered [4]. Severe axial hypotonia may be associated with a neurologic distress with hypertonia of the limbs, and seizures. It may be difficult to differentiate between a mitochondrial respiratory chain disorder and a peroxisomal disease. An important difference is that peroxisomal disorders are not associated with an acute metabolic derangement or abnormal routine laboratory tests, such as metabolic acidosis or lacticacidemia.

Hepatodigestive manifestations

The predominant manifestations may be hepatomegaly, cholestasis, hyperbilirubinemia, and prolonged jaundice especially in isolated di- and trihydroxycholestanoic acidemia.

Specific disorders

Two prototypes of neonatal presentation are CZ, which is the most severe condition, and RCDP. Their phenotypes are distinct from the other disorders and should not cause difficulties in the differential diagnosis.

Classical Zellweger syndrome

CZ is characterized by the association of the following: errors of morphogenesis, severe neurologic dysfunction, sensorineural hearing loss, ocular abnormalities, degenerative changes, hepatodigestive involvement with failure to thrive, absence of recognizable hepatic peroxisomes (presence of peroxisomal "ghosts"), and death usually in the first year. The patients show typical facial dysmorphia, which may become less characteristic if the patient survives beyond the first year of life. Although certain milestones develop, only some "older" CZ patients attain the ability to sit without support and subsequently develop peripheral hypertonia.

Classical rhizomelic chondrodysplasia punctata

Another typical phenotype is the classical RCDP, which is characterized by the presence of shortened proximal limbs, facial dysmorphia, cataracts, psychomotor retardation, coronal clefts of vertebral bodies, and stippled foci of calcification of the epiphyses in infancy, which may disappear after the age of 2 years. The chondrodysplasia punctata is more widespread than in CZ and may involve extraskeletal tissues. Some patients have ichthyosis. Peroxisomal structures appear to be intact in fibroblasts, whereas in liver these organelles may be fewer or absent in some hepatocytes and enlarged in size in others. Patients were described with a new variant of chondrodysplasia punctata associated with the characteristic peroxisomal defects observed in classical RCDP, but without the rhizomelic shortening of the limbs [5, 6]. Conversely, patients were identified with the typical clinical phenotype of classical RCDP, but with a single enzyme deficiency [3]. Classical RCDP and its variants must be distinguished from other forms of chondrodysplasia punctata such as the Conradi-Hünermann syndrome and the X-linked dominant and recessive forms of chondrodysplasia punctata.

Neonatal adrenoleukodystrophy

These patients are somewhat less severely affected than CZ [7]. Facial dysmorphia is not always present, and patients may show some development before their progressive deterioration sets in, followed usually by death before the age of 6 years. Cerebral demyelination is more prominent than dysmyelination and grey matter heterotopia. CT-scan of the brain may show abnormal contrast enhancement around demyelination areas. Chondrodysplasia punctata and renal cysts are absent. Several patients have been described with a single enzyme defect but with clinical manifestations resembling those of neonatal adrenoleukodystrophy (NALD; pseudo-NALD, acyl-CoA oxidase deficiency [8]; bi(tri)functional enzyme deficiency [9] or those of the CZ (pseudo-Zellweger syndrome, peroxisomal thiolase deficiency [10]). Liver peroxisomes were normal (bi-(tri) functional enzyme deficiency) or appeared to be enlarged in size (acyl-CoA oxidase and peroxisomal thiolase deficiency), whereas in the CZ and NALD they are morphologically absent or severely decreased in number.

Hyperpipecolic acidemia

This term was assigned to patients on the basis of the observation of an accumulation of pipecolic acid prior to the discovery of the generalized peroxisomal defects. However, hyperpipecolic acidemia should only be assigned to patients with solely elevated pipecolic acid values in body fluids. Hyperpipecolic acidemia associated with a Joubert syndrome has been observed in three siblings.

Di- and trihydroxycholestanoic acidemia

This has been reported in patients with predominant hepatic manifestations associated with neurologic involvement.

Mevalonic acidura

This is a disorder with dysmorphic features and cataracts and probably should be considered a peroxisomal disorder, since mevalonate kinase is predominantly localized in peroxisomes [11, 12].

First six months of life

During this period of life, the predominant symptoms may be hepatomegaly associated or not with prolonged jaundice, liver failure, and nonspecific digestive problems (anorexia, vomiting, diarrhea) leading to failure to thrive and osteoporosis. Hypocholesterolemia, hypolipoproteinemia, and decreased values of fat-soluble vitamins which resemble a malabsorption syndrome are frequently present. Most CZ patients develop hepatomegaly and seizures and do not survive beyond this period.

Infantile Refsum disease

IRD is similar to CZ biochemically as well as in the absence or with a significantly decreased number of liver peroxisomes [7]. However, IRD patients differ clearly from CZ with respect to age of onset, initial symptoms, degree of CNS involvement and duration of survival. Only minor or no facial dysmorphia is noted in early childhood. Early developmental milestones are usually normal, before slowing sets in between the age of 1 and 3 years. This is followed by completely arrested development associated with autistic behaviour in some patients. Most patients walk independently before the age of 3 years. Recently a patient with pseudo-IRD has been described with clinical similarity to IRD, but with somewhat different biochemical abnormalities [13].

Between six months and four years

In this period of life severe psychomotor retardation becomes evident. Sensorineural hearing loss is associated with abnormal brain stem auditory-evoked responses. Various ocular abnormalities can be observed, including cataract, retinitis pigmentosa, optic nerve atrophy, glaucoma, and brushfield spots. The electroretinogram and visual-evoked responses are frequently disturbed, and this may precede the fundoscopic abnormalities. Retinitis pigmentosa associated with hearing loss, developmental delay, and dysmorphia may be mistaken for other diseases including malformative syndromes [14]. In this respect, it has to be realized that the limits between malformative syndromes and inborn errors are not well delineated. This fact is confirmed by the recent finding of a defective cholesterol biosynthesis in the Smith-Lemli-Opitz syndrome [15]. Most NALD patients do not survive beyond this period.

Beyond four years of age

X-linked adrenoleukodystrophy (ALD)

ALD is the most common peroxisomal disorder. Considerable clinical variability exists even within the same kindred [16]. The childhood form is the most common and the most severe phenotype with onset of neurologic involvement usually between 5-10 years of age, leading to a vegetative state and death in a few years. The affected males may present with school failure, attention deficit disorder, or behaviour changes as first manifestations, followed by visual impairment and quadriplegia, whereas seizures are usually a late symptom. Hypoglycemic episodes and a dark discoloration of the skin may reflect adrenal insufficiency, which may precede, coincide with, or follow the onset of neurologic involvement. Most childhood patients show characteristic symmetric cerebral lesions on CT or MRI involving the periventricular white matter in the posterior and occipital lobes. Following intravenous injection of contrast material, a garland contrast enhancement adjacent to hypodense lesions is shown by CT. The CNS demyelination has a caudorostral progression. Liver peroxisomes are normal.

Behaviour changes associated with visual impairment may initially be mistaken for psychiatric manifestations. Intellectual deterioration in this period of life may be related to various other regressive encephalopathies including Sanfilippo disease, Niemann-Pick type C, Wilson's disease, subacute sclerosing panencephalitis, multiple sclerosis, and ceroid lipofuscinosis.

Classical Refsum's disease

Classical Refsum's disease is another peroxisomal disorder with a clinical onset in the school-age period. Retinitis pigmentosa, peripheral polyneuropathy, cerebellar ataxia, and elevated cerebrospinal fluid protein level are the main features. Less constant are nerve deafness, anosmia, ichthyosis, and skeletal and cardiac abnormalities. Mental retardation, liver dysfunction, and dysmorphia are absent. The onset of clinical manifestations varies from childhood to the fifth decade. The disorder is associated with a deficiency of phytanic acid α-oxidation.

Recently, there has been a report of four related patients, three with classical Refsum disease and the fourth who died from a progressive neurologic disorder with clinical and neuropathologic abnormalities unusual for classical Refsum disease. In addition to increased plasma levels of phytanic acid, those of pipecolic acid were also increased in two of these patients [17].

Metabolic derangements

The most important peroxisomal functions are [18], (Table I):

Plasmalogen biosynthesis

The enzymes acyl-CoA: dihydroxyacetone phosphate acyltransferase (DHAP-AT) and alkyl-dihydroxyacetone phosphate (alkyl-DHAP) synthase are essential in the biosynthesis of ether phospholipids known as plasmalogens. Plasmalogens are present in cell membranes and are particularly abundant in nervous tissue. Their physiological function has not yet been clarified, although they are known to be involved in platelet activation and in the scavenging of free radicals.

Bile acids biosynthesis

The β-oxidation of di-trihydroxy cholestanoic acid, normal intermediates in the biosynthesis of the primary bile acids, is carried out in peroxisomes.

Cholesterol biosynthesis

Peroxisomes are not only involved in cholesterol oxidation (biosynthesis of bile acids), but also in cholesterol biosynthesis. Peroxisomes contain aceto-acetyl-CoA thiolase, 3-hydroxy-3-methylglutaryl-CoA reductase, mevalonate kinase, and the sterol carrier protein-2, at least in rat liver [12].

β–oxidation of fatty acids

The peroxisomal β-oxidation system is involved in the chain-shortening of a distinct group of compounds which includes saturated very long chain fatty acids (VLCFA; 22 carbons or more), long chain dicarboxylic acids, polyunsaturated fatty acids, and branched-chain fatty acids such as pristanic acid [19]. Following activation to their corresponding acyl-CoA esters *via* membrane-bound acyl-CoA synthetases, fatty acyl-CoA esters are degraded in the peroxisomal matrix *via* the β-oxidation cycle, which consists of acyl-CoA oxidase, bi(tri)functional protein, and peroxisomal 3-oxoacyl-CoA thiolase. Human liver peroxisomes contain two acyl-CoA oxidases: a palmitoyl-CoA oxidase and a branched-chain acyl-CoA oxidase which oxidizes pristanoyl-CoA as well as di-and trihydroxycoprostanoyl-CoA. The enzyme known as the bifunctional protein appears to be a trifunctional protein as it also includes an enoyl-CoA isomerase in additon to the hydratase and the dehydrogenase activities.

Phytanic acid α-oxidation

Phytanic acid, which is exclusively of dietary origin, is primarily oxidized to pristanic acid in peroxisomes in humans and in mitochondria in rodents.

Glutaric acid oxidation

Glutaric acid is an intermediate in the catabolism of lysine as well as pipecolic acid. Apart from the mitochondrial glutaryl-CoA dehydrogenase, there probably also exists a peroxisomal glutaryl-CoA oxidase.

Pipecolic acid oxidation

The first step in the degradation of L-pipecolic acid, an intermediate in lysine catabolism, is catalyzed by L-pipecolic acid oxidase present in human liver peroxisomes.

Glyoxylate metabolism

Glyoxylate, the most important precurser of oxalate, can be transaminated to glycine in a reaction catalyzed by alanine: glyoxylate aminotransferase [20].

Diagnostic tests

Independently of the clinical symptoms and age of onset, most peroxisomal disorders can clinically be screened by neurophysiological investigations (electroretinogram, visual-evoked responses, brain auditory-evoked potentials), which are almost constantly abnormal.

Summarizing the possible clinical manifestations, peroxisomal disorders should be considered in patients showing one or more of the following abnormalities:
- craniofacial abnormalities and/or other dysmorphic features;
- skeletal abnormalities, including calcific stippling and shortened proximal limbs;
- neurologic abnormalities, including encephalopathy, hypotonia, seizures, hearing loss, and cerebral abnormalities;
- ocular abnormalities, including retinopathy, cataract, optic nerve dysplasia and abnormal electroretinogram and/or visual-evoked potentials;
- hepatological abnormalities, including hepatomegaly, liver dysfunction, cholestasis, and fibrosis/cirrhosis.

Table II lists a variety of assays which are available for the diagnosis of peroxisomal disorders. Only urinary pipecolic acid excretion, medium- and long- chain dicarboxylic aciduria, hyperoxaluria, and mevalonic aciduria can be detected by an "overall metabolic screening". Nine of the seventeen peroxisomal disorders with neurologic involvement are associated with an accumulation of VLCFA, which suggests that an assay of plasma VLCFA should be used as a primary test. However, assays of plasma phytanic acid and plasma/urine bile acid intermediates should also be performed in view of the recent reports of atypical chondrodysplasia variants (without rhizomelic shortening) and isolated trihydroxycholestanoic aciduria. The clinical presentation of the typical phenotype of RCDP (phytanic acid, plasmalogens) and classical Refsum (phytanic acid) are distinct from the other disorders and should not cause difficulties in their diagnosis. In order to elucidate whether the accumulation of VLCFA in a patient's plasma results from a defect in peroxisome biogenesis or is caused by a defect in one of the peroxisomal β-oxidation enzyme activities, additional assay procedures must be carried out, in particular plasmalogen levels and immunoblotting of peroxisomal β-oxidation proteins.

Table II. Diagnostic assays in peroxisomal disorders.

Disease	Material	Type of assay
Classical ZS Neonatal ALD Infantile Refsum Zellweger-like Pseudo Infantile Refsum	Plasma RBC Fibroblasts	VLCFA, Bile acids, Phytanic acid, Pristanic acid, Pipecolic acid, Polyunsaturated fatty acids Plasmalogens Plasmalogens biosynthesis, DHAPAT, alkyl DHAP synthase, Particle bound catalase, VLCFA β-oxidation, Immunoblotting β-oxidation proteins Phytanic acid oxidation
Rhizomelic chondrodysplasia punctata (classical/atypical phenotypes)	Plasma RBC Fibroblasts	Phytanic acid Plasmalogens DHAPAT, alkyl DHAP synthase, Phytanic acid oxidation
Isolated peroxisomal β-oxidation defects	Plasma Fibroblasts	VLCFA, Bile acids VLCFA β-oxidation, Immunoblotting β-oxidation proteins
Isolated defect of bile acid synthesis	Plasma Liver	Bile acids THCA-CoA oxidase
Isolated pipecolic acidemia	Plasma Liver	Pipecolic acid Pipecolic acid oxidase
Mevalonic aciduria	Plasma Urine Fibroblasts Lymphocytes	Organic acids Mevalonate kinase
Classical Refsum	Plasma Fibroblasts	Phytanic acid Phytanic acid oxidation
Glutaric aciduria type III	Urine Liver	Organic acids Glutaryl-CoA oxidase
Hyperoxaluria type I	Urine Liver	Organic acids AGT
Actalasemia	RBC	Catalase

VLCFA: very long chain fatty acids;
DHAPAT: dihydroxyacetone phosphate acyltransferase;
DHAP: dihydroxyacetone phosphate;
THCA: trihydroxycholestanoic acid;
AGT: alanine: glyoxylate aminotransferase;
RBC: red blood cells

Therefore, it should be stressed that it is no longer possible to screen all peroxisomal disorders only by measuring plasma VLCFA. It would be advisable to carry out assays of plasma bile acid intermediates, phytanic, pristanic, and pipecolic acid, plasmalogens in red blood cells, and DHAPAT and alkyl DHAP synthase in cultured skin fibroblasts. In some patients with variant forms, the enzymatic deficit(s) are only expressed in liver and not in cultured fibroblasts. Extensive peroxisomal investigations are necessary (even when the clinical phenotype is very typical), since some disorders may be associated with very atypical biochemical phenotypes.

For some disorders, a retrospective diagnosis can be obtained by analyzing stored blood spots collected during neonatal screening [21].

Histological detection of peroxisomes is facilitated by using the diaminobenzidine staining procedure, which reacts with the peroxisomal marker enzyme catalase, and by immunochemical techniques with antibodies against matrix and membrane peroxisomal proteins [22]. The abundance, size, and structure of liver peroxisomes should be studied. When peroxisomes are lacking, virtually all of the catalase is present in the cytosolic fraction, instead of the particulate fraction.

As for prenatal diagnosis, a variety of techniques are available. Almost all the peroxisomal disorders can be identified prenatally, either by using (cultured) chorion villous samples or amniocytes or by direct analysis of levels of VLCFA and bile acid intermediates in amniotic fluid. Measurement of VLCFA and/or assay of plasmalogen synthesis are the most useful methods today, except in the case of THCA-CoA oxidase deficiency, isolated pipecolic acidemia, glutaric aciduria type III and hyperoxaluria type I (fetal liver biopsy). Another approach is the cytochemical staining of peroxisomes in chorion villus samples.

Heterozygote identification is only available for X-linked ALD using VLCFA analysis or restriction fragment polymorphism [23].

Abbreviations

ALD: adrenoleukodystrophy
CZ: classical Zellweger syndrome
IRD: infantile Refsum's disease
NALD: neonatal adrenoleukodystrophy
RCPD: rhizomelic chondrodysplasia punctata

References

1. Fournier B, Smeitink JAM, Dorland L, Berger R, Saudubray JM, Poll-The BT. Peroxisomal disorders: a review. *J Inher Metab Dis* 1994 ; 17 : 470-86.
2. Wanders RJA, Heymans HSA, Schutgens RBH, Barth PG, van den Bosch H, Tager JM. Peroxisomal disorders in neurology. *J Neurol Sci* 1988 ; 88 : 1-39.

3. Wanders RJA, Schumacher H, Heikoop J, Schutgens RBH, Tager JM. Human dihydroxy-acetonephosphate acyltransferase deficiency: a new peroxisomal disorder. *J Inher Metab Dis* 1992 ; 15 : 389-91.
4. Poll-The BT, Saudubray JM, Ogier H, Lombes A, Munnich A, Frézal J. Clinical approach to inherited peroxisomal disorders. In : Vogel F, Sperling, eds. *Human genetics*. Heidelberg : Springer-Verlag, 1987 : 345-51.
5. Poll-The BT, Maroteaux P, Narcy C, Quetin P, Guesnu M, Wanders RJA, Schutgens RBH, Saudubray JM. A new type of chondrodysplasia punctata associated with peroxisomal dysfunction. *J Inher Metab Dis* 1991 ; 14 : 361-3.
6. Smeitink JAM, Beemer FA, Espeel M, Donckerwolcke RAMG, Jakobs C, Wanders RJA, Schutgens RBH, Roels F, Duran M, Dorland L, Berger R, Poll-The BT. Bone dysplasia associated with phytanic acid accumulation and deficient plasmalogen synthesis: a peroxisomal entity amenable to plasmapheresis. *J Inher Metab Dis* 1992 ; 15 : 377-80.
7. Poll-The BT, Saudubray JM, Ogier HAM, Odièvre M, Scotto JM, Monnens L, et al. Infantile Refsum disease: an inherited peroxisomal disorder. Comparison with Zellweger syndrome and neonatal adrenoleukodystrophy. *Eur J Pediatr* 1987 ; 146 : 477-83.
8. Poll-The BT, Roels F, Ogier H, Scotto J, Vamecq J, Schutgens RBH, Wanders RJA, van Roermund CWT, van Wijland MJA, Schram AW, Tager JM, Saudubray JM. A new peroxisomal disorder with enlarged peroxisomes and a specific deficiency of acyl-CoA oxidase (pseudo-neonatal adrenoleukodystrophy). *Am J Hum Genet* 1988 ; 42 : 422-34.
9. Watkins PA, Chen WN, Harris CJ, Hoefler G, Hoefler S, Blake DC, Balfe A, Kelley RI, Moser AB, Beard ME, Moser HW. Peroxisomal bifunctional enzyme deficiency. *J Clin Invest* 1989 ; 83 : 771-7.
10. Schram AW, Golfischer S, van Roermund CWT, Brouwer-Kelder EM, Collins J, Hashimoto T, Heymans HSA, van den Bosch H, Schutgens RBH, Tager JM, Wanders RJA. Human peroxisomal 3-oxoacyl-coenzyme A thiolase deficiency. *Proc Natl Acad Sci USA* 1987 ; 84 : 2494-6.
11. Hoffmann G, Gibson KM, Brandt IK, Bader PI, Wappner RS, Sweetman L. Mevalonic aciduria - an inborn error of cholesterol and nonsterol isoprene biosynthesis. *N Engl J Med* 1986 ; 314 : 1610-4.
12. Biardi L, Sreedhar A, Zokaei A, Vertak NB, Bozaet RL Shackelford JE, Keller GA, Krisans SK. Mevalonate kinase is predominantly localized in peroxisomes and is defective in patients with peroxisome deficiency disorders. *J Biol Chem* 1994 ; 269 : 1197-205.
13. Aubourg P, Kremser K, Roland MO, Rocchiccioli F, Singh I. Pseudo infantile Refsum's disease: catalase-deficient peroxisomal particles with partial deficiency of plasmalogen synthesis and oxidation of fatty acids. *Pediatr Res* 1993 ; 34 : 270-6.
14. Poll-The BT, Billette de Villemeur T, Abitbol M, Dufier JL, Saudubray JM. Metabolic pigmentary retinopathies: diagnosis and therapeutic attempts. *Eur J Pediatr* 1992 ; 151 : 2-11.
15. Irons M, Elias ER, Salen G, Tint GS, Batta AK. Defective cholesterol biosynthesis in Smith-Lemli-Opitz syndrome. *Lancet* 1993 ; 341 : 1414.
16. Moser HW, Moser AB, Smith KD, Bergin A, Borel J, Sankroff J, Stine OC, Merette C, Ott J, Krivit W, Shapiro E. Adrenoleukodystrophy: phenotype variability and implications for therapy. *J Inher Metab Dis* 1992 ; 15 : 645-64.
17. Tranchant C, Aubourg P, Mohr M, Rocchiccioli F, Zaenker C, Warter JM. A new peroxisomal disease with impaired phytanic and pipecolic acid oxidation. *Neurology* 1993 ; 43 : 2044-8.
18. Van den Bosch H, Schutgens RBH, Wanders RJA, Tager JG. Biochemistry of peroxisomes. *Annu Rev Biochem* 1992 ; 61 : 157-97.

19. Vanhove S, Eyssen HJ, Wanders RJA, Mannaerts GP. The CoA esters of 2-methyl-branched chain fatty acids and of the bile acid intermediates di- and trihydroxycopro-stanic acids are oxidized by one single peroxisomal branched chain acyl-CoA oxidase in human liver and kidney. *J Biol Chem* 1993 ; 268 : 10335-44.
20. Danpure CJ, Copper PJ, Wise PJ, Jennings PR. An enzyme trafficking defect in two patients with primary hyperoxaluria type 1: peroxisomal alanine: glyoxylate aminotransferase rerouted to mitochondria. *J Cell Biol* 1989 ; 108 : 1345-52.
21. Jakobs C, van den Heuvel CMM, Stellaard F, Largillière, Skovby F, Christensen E. Diagnosis of Zellweger syndrome by analysis of very long-chain fatty acids in stored blood spots collected at neonatal screening. *J Inher Metab Dis* 1993 ; 16 : 63-6.
22. Roels F, Espeel M, De Craemer D. Liver pathology and immunocytochemistry in congenital peroxisomal diseases: a review. *J Inher Metab Dis* 1991 ; 14 : 853-75.
23. Aubourg PR, Sack GH, Meyers DA, Lease JJ, Moser HW. Linkage of adrenoleukodystrophy to a polymorphic DNA probe. *Ann Neurol* 1987 ; 21 : 349-52.

21

Diagnosis of basal ganglia lesions; additional aspects from proton spectroscopy

I. KRÄGELOH-MANN [1], W. GRODD [2], D. AUER [3], P. TOFT [4]

1. Division of Child Neurology, Pediatric Hospital, University of Munchen (TU), Germany.
2. Department of Neuroradiology, University of Tübingen, Germany.
3. Max Planck Institute for Psychiatry, München, Germany.
4. Magnetic Resonance Research Center, Hvidovre Hospital, Copenhagen, Denmark.

Progress in neuro-imaging, especially the advent of MRI, has shown increasing evidence for involvement of basal ganglia in a variety of disease processes, which are etiologically very different. The question is, whether morphology and localisation of basal ganglia abnormalities can give specific hints for etiology. Biochemical investigation with 1H-MR-spectroscopy may give additional information.

Patients and methods

Findings from 24 children (2 to 18 years of age) with bilateral signal abnormalities in the basal ganglia on MRI were compared to the literature. Fourteen also had 1H-MRS of basal ganglia, and were compared to 12 normal children (3 to 14 years of age) and 10 children (2 to 8 years of age) with normal basal ganglia but other brain pathology. Children with basal ganglia calcifications without signal abnormalities on MRI were excluded.

MRI was performed on a 1.5T Magnetom Siemens (in four children on a 1.5T Signa GE), T1w images (TR 600ms, TR 15ms) in axial and sagittal orientation and T2w images (TR 2100ms, TE 45, 90ms) in axial and coronal orientation were obtained.

1H-MRS was done with a spin-echo technique (TR 1.5s, TE 135 and 270 ms) or a STEAM sequence (TR 6s and TE 20 and 272ms), and a VOI of 2x2x2cm was placed in the region of the caudate head and lentiformis.

Normal morphology

Basal ganglia undergo changes during maturation which are represented by MRI on T2w images especially. During the first year of life, the pallidum is hyperintense in comparison to the putamen, then isointense during the second year, thereafter hypointense (iron deposition), hypointensity in the thalamus starts in the lateral and rostral parts, and is homogeneous in the adult, the posterior part of the capsula interna only is slightly hyperintense in comparison to the surrounding tissue [1].

Aetiological groups

Hypoxic-ischemic and thrombembolic

Term born or mildly preterm born children with severe birth asphyxia may show basal ganglia signal abnormalities which are very characteristic in localisation, they affect the posterior striatum and the medio-lateral thalamus and are seen on T2w images only (hyperintense). They may occur isolated or in combination with other hypoxic-ischemic lesions (parasagittal, cortical) and are associated to athetotic or spastic CP [2, 3]. In preterm infants with lower gestational ages severe periventricular leukomalacia may be associated with basal ganglia signal abnormalities in the latero-dorsal thalamus on T2w images (hyperintense) (Figure 1).

Thrombembolic defects, seen on T1, T2w images, can occasionly occur in the basal ganglia.

Toxic

Intoxication with carbonmonoxid or methanol affects the pallidum [4].

Infectious, parainfectious

Bacterial meningitis complicated by periarteriitis may cause thalamic infarctions. Viral encephalitis may be accompagnied by signal hyperintensities in the thalamus on T2w images [5]. Infantile bilateral striatal necrosis, which is supposed to be a parainfectious process, typically affects the putamen bilaterally, seen on T1,2w images [4].

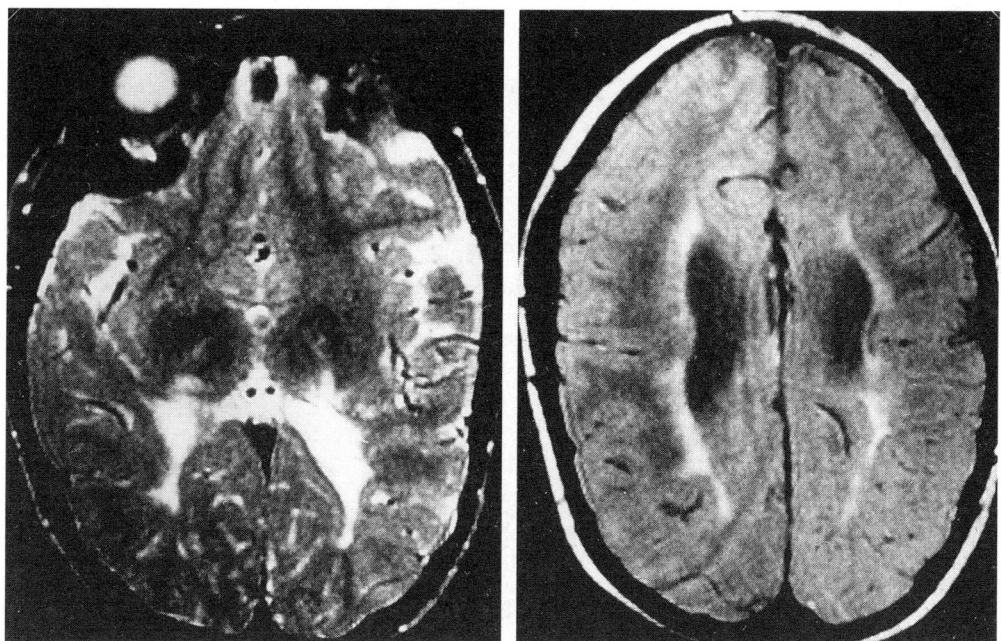

Figure 1. Thalamic hyperintensities (latero-dorsal, arrow) (left, TR 2.1s, TE 90ms) and periventricular leukomalacia (right, arrow, TR 2.1s, TE 45ms) in a 6 year old boy, born at a gestational age of 33 weeks, with spastic tetraplegia.

Neurometabolic

- Aminoacid disturbances: maplesirup urine disease typically is associated with hyperintensity on T2w images of the pallidum bilaterally.
- Organic acid diseases: methymalonacidemia is also characterised by signal abnormalities of the pallida, but seen on T1w and T2w images [6].
- Mitochondrial enzyme deficiencies associated with a symptomatology of Leigh's disease and also Leber's hereditary optic atrophy show characteristic lesions of both caudate heads and putamina, seen on T1w and T2w images [7]. MELAS may show similar abnormalities in the putamina, but usually is associated with white matter lesions, whereas Kearns-Sayre disease more typically has evidence for signal hyperintensities of the pallida on T2w images only [8].
- In Wilson's disease, caudate heads and putamina are also typically involved, seen essentially on T2w images.
- The juvenile form of Canavan's disease does not show the white matter abnormalities of the infantile form, but signal hyperintensity of putamina and caudate heads on T2w images only [9].
- Infantile progressive striatal degeneration is described with signal hyperintensities of the putamen and caudate head on T2w images only [10].

- M. Sandhoff is characterized by bilateral thalamus hypointensities on T2w images [11].
- Hallervorden-Spatz disease by signal hypointensity of the pallida on T2w images [12].

Miscellaneous

In Recklinghausen's disease, NF1, hyperintensity on T2w images is often seen in the posterior part of the capsula interna without any clinical correlate. Haemolytic uremic syndrome may particularly involve the striatum [13].

1H MRS-results

Results were analysed especially concerning the presence of lactate. Basal ganglia lesions of the caudate and putamen seem to be rather characteristic for mitochondrial enzyme deficiencies which may present with a mainly encephalopathic clinical picture. The question was, whether lactate in a chronic lesion indicates a mitochondrial enzyme deficiency even in the presence or normal serum and CSF lactate.

Basal ganglia of normal children did not show any evidence for elevated lactate, neither did normal basal ganglia of children with other brain pathology (with the exception of a child with infantile neuroaxonal dystrophy which had elevated lactate twice in its otherwise normal basal ganglia). Children with mitochondrial enzyme deficiencies associated with a symptomatology of M. Leigh (three with PDHc and two with COX defect) and Leber's hereditary optic atrophy (one with a NADH defect) had elevated lactate, also during the non-acute stage of the disease (Figure 2).

This was true with only one exception for a child with PDHc defect, where the lactate peak disappeared during therapy with a ketogenic diet [14]. Serum lactate was normal or moderately elevated and CSF lactate in 4 was mildly elevated. Children with basal ganglia lesions or signal abnormalities of other origin (ischemic during the non acute stage in two children, M. Wilson in two (Figure 3), maple sirup disease in one (Figure 4), lactacidimia of unknown origin in one, infantile progressive striatal degeneration in one) did not show elevated lactate (see also [15, 7]).

Conclusion

Analysis of morphology, localisation and signal characteristics of basal ganglia abnormalities seen by MRI can help to differentiate between disease entities. 1H-MRS can detect elevated lactate in mitochondrial diseases restricted to the brain. This seems to be rather specific especially during the non-acute stage of the disease. Then unspecifically elevated lactate due to ischemia does not play a role.

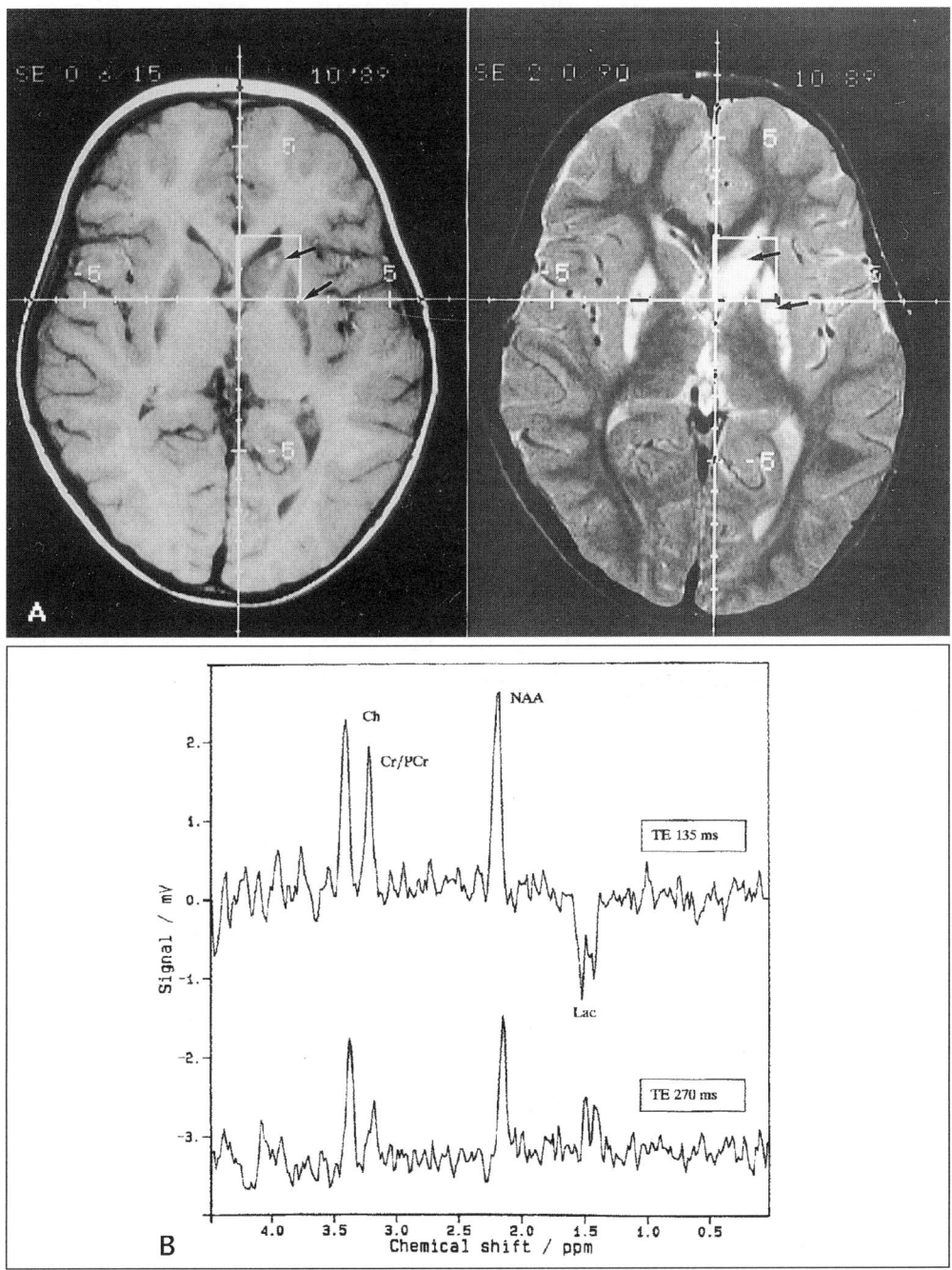

Figure 2. A. Defects of the putamina and of the left caudate head (right on the image), hypointense on T1w (left, arrows) and hyperintense on T2w (right, arrows) images in a 4 year old boy with Leigh's disease and PDHc defect. **B.** Spectroscopy (VOI indicated in A) shows elevated lactate (negative with a TE of 135ms and positive with a TE of 270ms, spin-echo technique).

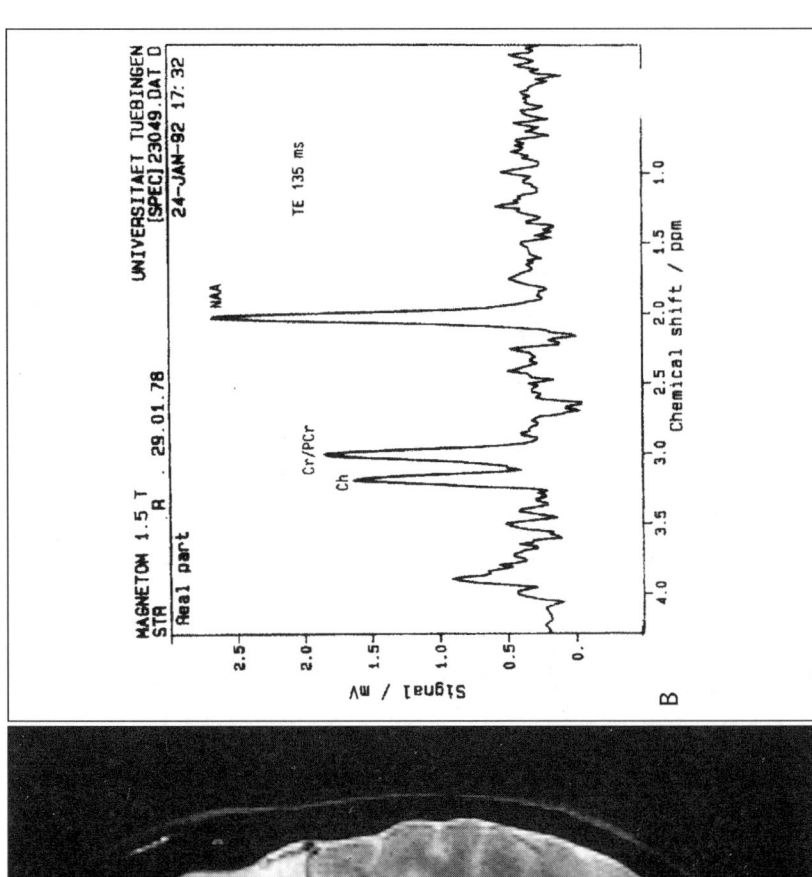
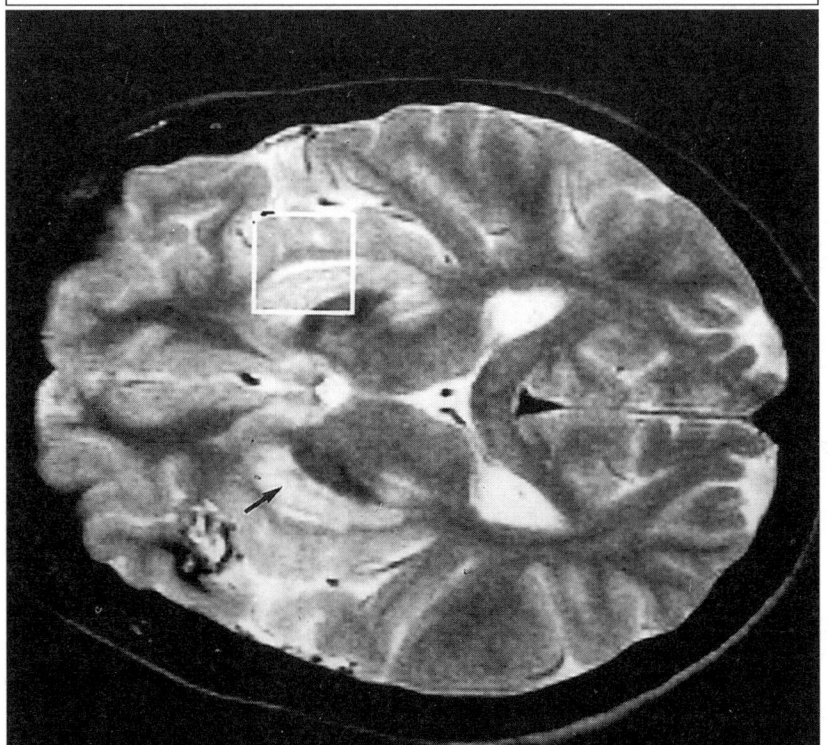

Figure 3. A. Signal hyperintensities of the putamina (arrow) and to a lesser degree of caudate heads on a T2w image of a 12 year old girl with Wilson's disease. B. Spectroscopy does not show definite abnormalities, especially no lactate increase.

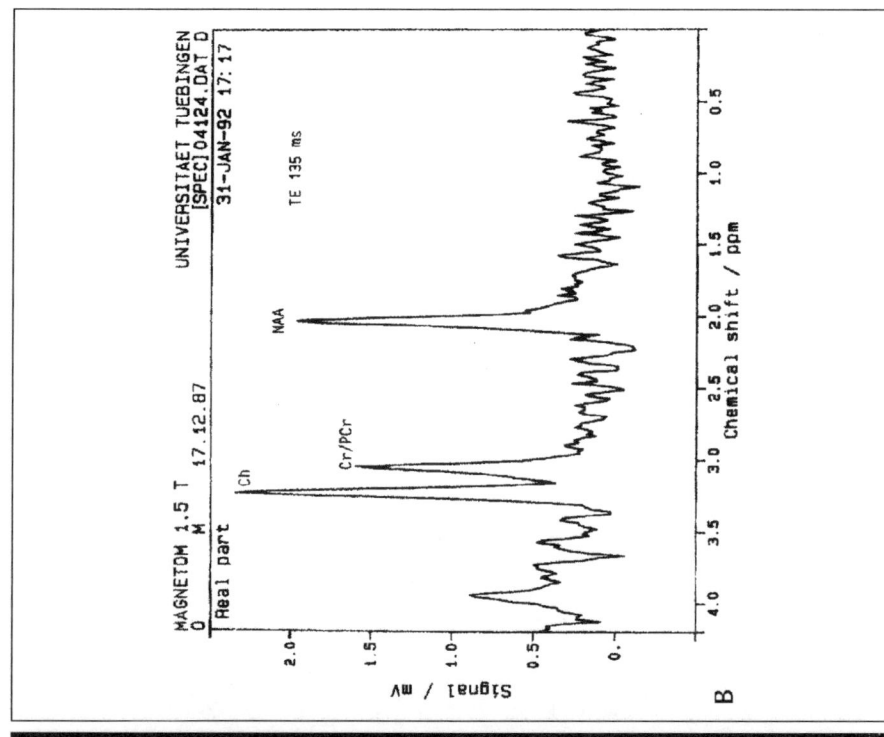
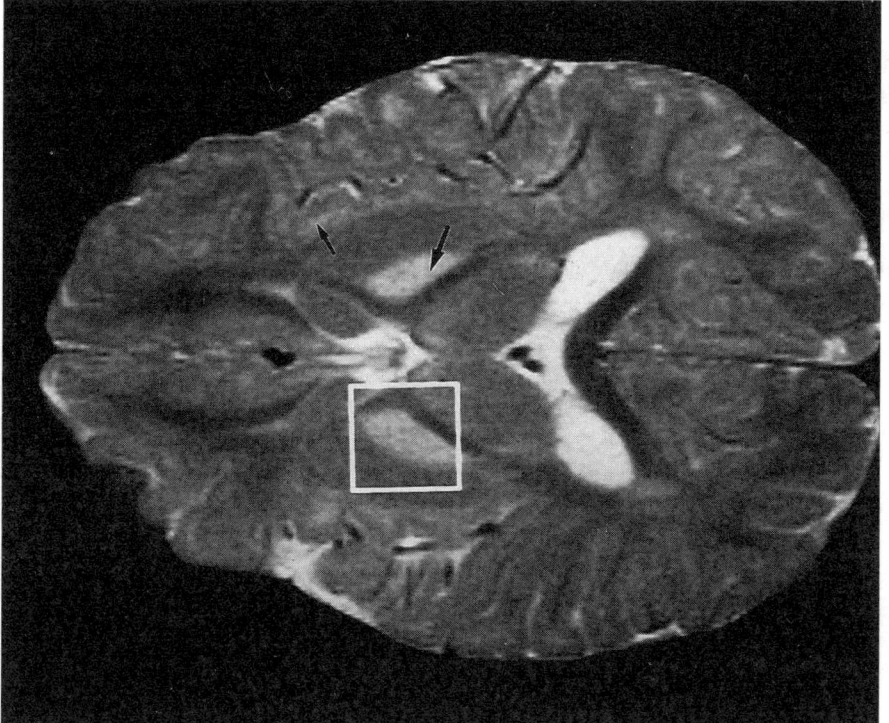

Figure 4. A. Signal hyperintensities of the pallida (big arrow) and subcortical dysmyelination (small arrow) on a T2w image of a 4 year old boy with maple sirup urine disease. **B.** Spectroscopy shows a choline increase and a NAA decrease, but no lactate increase.

References

1. Grodd W. Kernspintomographie neuropadiatrischer Erkrankungen. Normale Reifung des kindlichen Gehirns. *Neuroradiol* 1993 ; 3 : 13-27.
2. Yokochi K, Aiba K, Kodama M, Fujimoto S. Magnetic resonance imaging in athetotic cerebral palsied children. *Acta Paediatr Scand* 1991 ; 80 : 818-23.
3. Krägeloh-Mann I, Petersen D, Hagberg G, Vollmer B, Hagberg B, Michaelis R. Bilateral spastic cerebral palsy - MRI pathology and origin. Analysis from a representative series of 56 cases. *Dev Med Child Neurol* 1995 ; 38 : 379-97.
4. Aicardi J. *Diseases of the nervous system in childhood.* New York, Oxford : Mac Keith Press, 1992.
5. Barkovich AJ. *Pediatric neuroimaging* 2nd edition. New York : Raven Press, 1995.
6. Andreula CF, De Blasi R, Carella A. CT and MR studies of methylmalonic acidernia. *AJNR* 1991 ; 12 : 410-2.
7. Krägeloh-Mann I, Grodd W, Schoning M, Marquard K, Nagele T, Ruitenbeek W. Elevated basal ganglia lactate assessed *in vivo* by 1H-MRS in Leigh disease with mitochondrial enzyme deficiency. *Dev Med Child Neurol* 1993 ; 35 : 769-76.
8. Barkovich AJ, Good WV, Koch TK, Berg BO. Mitochondrial disorders: analysis of their clinical and imaging characteristics. *AJNR* 1993 ; 14 : 1119-37.
9. Toft P, Geiß-Holtorff R, Rolland MO, Pryds O, Muller-Forell W, Christensen E, Lehnert W, Lou HC, Ott D, Henning J, Henriksen O. Magnetic imaging in juvenile Canavan disease. *Eur J Pediatr* 1993 ; 152 : 750-3.
10. Gieron MA, Gilbert-Barnes E, Vonsattel JP, Korthals JK. Infantile progressive striato-thalamic degeneration in two siblings: a new syndrome. *Pediatr Neurol* 1995 ; 12 : 260-3.
11. Caliskan M, Ozmen M, Beck M, Apak S. Thalamic hyperdensity - is it a diagnostic marker of Sandhoff disease? *Brain Dev* 1993 ; 15 : 387-8.
12. Angelini L, Nardocci N, Rumi V, Zorci C, Strada L, Savoiardo M. Hallervorden-Spatz disease: clinical and MRI study of 11 cases diagnosed in life. *J Neurol* 1992 ; 239 : 417-25.
13. Barnett NDP, Kapllan AM, Bernes SM, Cohen ML. Hemolytic uremic syndrome with particular involvement of basal gganglia and favorable outome. *Pediatr Neurol* 1995 ; 12 : 155-8.
14. Krägeloh-Mann I, Grodd W, Niemann G, Haas G, Ruitenbeek W. Assessment and therapy - monitoring of Leigh disease by MR imaging and proton spectroscopy. *Pediatr Neurol* 1992 ; 8 : 60-4.
15. Grodd W, Krägeloh-Mann I, Klose U, Sauter R. Metabolic and destructive brain disorders in children: findings with localized proton MR spectroscopy. *Radiology* 1991 ; 181 : 173-81.

22

Pelizaeus Merzbacher disease and X-linked dysmyelinating diseases

O. BOESPFLUG-TANGUY [1], C. MIMAULT [1], G. GIRAUD [1],
F. CAILLOUX [1], D. PHAM DINH [2], B. DASTUGUE [1], A. DAUTIGNY [2]

1. INSERM U. 384, Faculté de Médecine, Clermont-Ferrand, France.
2. URA CNRS 1488 Université Paris VI, Paris, France.

Among the numerous leucodystrophies without biochemical markers, the distinction between inherited defects of myelin formation (dysmyelinating diseases) and genetic diseases leading to myelin destruction (demyelinating diseases) has been introduced at the beginning of the century by Pelizaeus (1885) and Merzbacher (1910). They defined this disease in terms of (1) a clinical presentation which is characterized by an early onset of motor development impairment and the X-linked mode of transmission and (2) the neuropathological finding of severe hypomyelination that is strictly limited to the central nervous system (CNS), with no nerve-cell or axon involvement, without inflammation, and with preserved myelin islets around blood vessels. When normal neutral lipid material was demonstrated in white matter areas by sudan black staining, the disease was classified as a "sudanophilic leukodystrophy". Using these neuropathological characteristics, Seitelberger subdivided Pelizaeus-Merzbacher Disease (PMD) into seven forms, taking into account the mode of transmission and age of onset [1] but as suggested by Jean Aicardi, the term PMD should only be used for the first two forms of CNS dysmyelination defined by early onset and X-linked mode of inheritance: type I corresponding to the slow progressive "classical" form, described by Pelizaeus, and the more severe type II (described by Seitelberger as the "connatal" form) with rapid progression and death occurring during the first ten years of life.

Diagnostic criteria of PMD

By including electrophysiological and magnetic resonance imaging (MRI) studies to demonstrate the abnormal formation of CNS myelin, Boulloche and Aicardi [2] redefined the diagnostic criteria of PMD, which we used to select 68 PMD affected families (130 affected patients) in which 24 were familial forms. The main clinical characteristic was an impairment of normal motor development, present very early and throughout the life of affected patients. We chose nystagmus as a clinical selection criterion for our first 34 index cases. In fact this sign was present in only 88% of the affected males analysed in all of our 34 families. The observed neurological signs were gradually modified by the maturating nervous system: bobbing movements of the head and trunk and choreoathetosic movements of the limbs were reported between 6 and 18 months, limb joint spasticity with pyramidal tract signs involvement was distingly present in all cases around 4 years.

Motor handicaps were greater than the impairments of psycho-intellectual development, and a rapid degradation of CNS functions was never observed. In four families, 100% of the affected males had the rapid progressive form with an almost total absence of psychomotor development and death ensuing before 10 years. In the remaining 64 families, 10% of the affected males had the same rapid progression, whereas 90% demonstrated a classical slow progression with an improvement in performance up to 10-12 years. The level of performance reached varied from one family to another and, to a lesser extent, between affected males of the same family: 85% acquired a head control between 2 and 5 years, 43% were able to sit down without support and only 15% were able to walk with support between 5 and 10 years. After a plateau, a slow deterioration was noticed after ages 15-20 and death occurred on average at 40 years (± 11 years).

Abnormal central conduction, analysed by central evoked potentials, contrasted in all cases with normal peripheral nerve conduction velocities. Cerebral computer tomography (CT) scan analysis demonstrated an almost normal density of white matter in striking contrast to the abnormal hypersignal observed on T2 weighted MRI after the age of 2.

These strict diagnostic criteria, which can be applied at any time during the life of the patient, have allowed to select an extended group of PMD-affected families and to study the disease-causing gene.

Proteolipoprotein (PLP) gene mutations in PMD

Three lines of evidence thus led to consider the involvement of the PLP gene in PMD (see for references [3]):
- it has been assigned to the X chromosome at the Xq2 1.3-q22 position,

- it codes in the oligodendrocytes for two proteolipids (PLP and DM20) which are the main proteins of the CNS myelin, mimicking the CNS restricted distribution of the myelin abnormalities found in PMD,
- different mutations of PLP exons have been described in different myelin-deficient animal mutants as presumed animal models for PMD.

Despite extensive analysis with PCR amplification and sequencing of the 7 coding regions, exon/intron junctions and the splicing site of the PLP gene, we found only one mutation among the first 15 families analysed [4]. However, using linkage analysis, we demonstrated a tight, homogeneous linkage between PMD and the PLP locus [5], leading us to pursue the identification of the molecular defects in the PLP genomic region.

Among the total of 67 index cases we analysed, 3 missense base substitutions in the coding sequence of the PLP gene were found. A good correlation was observed between the severity of the disease and the fact that mutations led to the substitution of a highly conserved amino acid (when aligned to other members of the "DM family", using the sequence data of Kitagawa *et al.* [6]).

In addition, we found a frameshift mutation due to a deletion/insertion event in exon IV of the PLP gene in a family where the 2 affected patients were able to walk and expressed a mild form of the disease [7].

Different arguments led to search for PLP gene duplications in PMD. Among the 64 PMD index cases without obvious PLP gene mutation we investigated, a quantitative Southern analysis suggested PLP gene duplications in 25 cases: 12 cases were familial and 13 sporadic cases, and all had a typical classical form of PMD [8].

More recently, analysing PLP transcripts from the peripheral nerve biopsy of 6 PMD affected patients without obvious PLP exon mutations, we found abnormalities in two cases.

Despite extensive molecular analysis, neither PLP gene abnormalities have been found in 34% of our familial cases of PMD patients nor 66% of sporadic forms.

X-linked spastic paraplegia and the PLP gene

Clinical observations gave us arguments to consider X-linked spastic paraplegia (SPG2) as a milder form of dysmyelinating disease and to test PLP gene involvement (for references see [9]).

In a large SPG2 pedigree, a point mutation was identified in the alternatively spliced exon IIIB of the gene, predicting a mutant form of PLP but, interestingly, a normal DM20 protein [9]. Among the 11 affected males in this family, 10 expressed the complicated form and one a pure form of SPG. In contrast to PMD patients, nystagmus was markedly delayed in the course of this disease (onset after 6 months), the age of first walking was delayed in 7 out of 11 patients. Moreover, hypotonia, choreoathetosis or bobbing movements of the head and trunk were not observed in the first few years of life. All SPG2 patients could walk unaided for a long period (over 20 years), and most of them were able to attend school. In two patients, electrophysiological studies demonstrated abnormal CNS conduction velocities, and MRI scans demonstrated a moderate myelin-deficiency of the temporo-occipital lobes. Interestingly, four obligate carrier mothers expressed a "tardive", mild form of spastic paraplegia. This involvement of also adult female heterozygotes (who are mosaics with respect to this mutation) is best explained by a demyelinating component of this disease. In a large SPG2 family with a very similar phenotype, Kobayashi *et al.* [10] found the same PLP mutation that defines the rumpshaker mutation in the mouse [11]. Among 14 index cases of spastic paraplegia affected males in our study, all had an early onset (2-5 years), a very slow progression, and CNS myelin abnormalities by electrophysiological criteria and MRI scans. The relatedness of PMD and SPG2, in fact a clinical continuum, has now been demonstrated directly in a two-generation family in which the PLP gene is partially deleted (the deletion includes the promoter, exon I, and most of the intron I). In this family, the index case expressed a mild (classical) form of PMD, his maternal uncle an early onset spastic paraplegia and the two obligate female carriers a late onset spastic paraplegia.

Conclusion

Pelizaeus-Merzbacher disease (PMD) and spastic paraplegia (SPG2) are two alternative phenotypes of a human dysmyelinating disease, caused by mutations in the gene for myelin proteolipid proteins (PLP/DM-20). PMD is characterized by an impairment of motor development, the severity of the disease being related to the level of motor functions acquired before adolescence. In contrast, SPG2 is characterized by progressive gait abnormalities, occurring after an almost normal motor development during the first 2 years of age. However, a clinical continuum exists between the two phenotypes with mild forms of PMD disease closed to complicated forms of SPG2. Point mutations in highly conserved regions of PLP/DM20, truncations of the proteins, or duplications of the entire gene are responsible for severe forms of PMD, whereas substitutions of less conserved amino acids or complete deletions of the PLP gene cause relatively mild forms of PMD or SPG2. Spontaneous mutants and PLP-transgenic mice provide accurate animal models for the human diseases. Their detailed analysis has revealed that dysmyelination in PMD/jimpy mutant mice is largely the result of abnormal oligodendrocyte maturation and cell death. In SPG2/rumpshaker, in contrast, oligodendrocytes are not reduced. Here, the PLP/DM20-dependent defect prevents myelination despite that mutant PLP is incorporated into myelin.

We conclude that the PLP gene is highly susceptible to mutations and that the clinically most severe and less severe associated diseases (PMD type II and pure SPG2, respectively) define a continuum of disease expression.

References

1. Seitelberger F. Pelizaeus Merzbacher disease. In : Vinken PJ, Bruyn GW, eds. *Handbook of clinical neurology*. North Holland, Amsterdam 1970 ; 10 : 150-202.
2. Boulloche J, Aicardi J. Pelizaeus-Merzbacher disease: clinical and nosological study. *J Child Neurol* 1986 ; 1 : 233-9.
3. Pham-Dinh D, Nussbaum JL, Popot JL, Boespflug-Tanguy O, Landrieu P, Dautigny A. Mutations du gène codant pour les protéolipides de la myéline (PLP et DM20) et dysmyélinisations liées au chromosome X. *Médecine/Sciences* 1992 ; 8 : 664-72.
4. Pham-Dinh D, Popot JL, Boespflug-Tanguy O, Landrieu P, Boue J, Deleuze JF, Jolles P, Dautigny A. Pelizaeus Merzbacher disease: a valine to phenylalanine point mutation in a putative extracellular loop of myelin proteolipid. *Proc Natl Acad Sci USA* 1991 ; 88 : 7562-6.
5. Boespflug-Tanguy O, Mimault C, Melki J, Cavagna A, Giraud G, Pham Dinh D, Dastugue B, Dautigny A and the PMD Clinical Group Genetic Homogeneity of Pelizaeus Merzbacher Disease (PMD). Tight linkage to the proteolipoprotein (PLP) locus in 16 affected families. *Am J Hum Genet* 1994 ; 55 : 461-7.
6. Kitagawa K, Sinoway MP, Yang C, Gould RM, Colman DR. A proteolipid protein gene family: expression in sharks and rays and possible evolution from an ancestral gene encoding a pore-forming polypetide. *Neuron* 1993 ; 11 : 433-48.
7. Pham-Dinh D, Boespflug-Tanguy O, Mimault C, Cavagna A, Giraud G, Leberre G, Lemarec B, Dautigny A. Pelizaeus Merzbacher disease: a frameshift deletion/insertion event in the myelin proteolipid gene. *Hum Mol Genet* 1993 ; 4 : 465-7.
8. Boespflug-Tanguy O, Mimault C, Giraud G, Cailloux F, Pham Dinh D, Dastugue B, Dautigny A. PLP gene mutations in human X-linked dysmyelinating diseases: correlation between phenotype and genotype. *Dev Neurosc* 1995 (in press).
9. Saugier-Veber P, Munnich A, Bonneau D, Rozet JM, Le Merrer M, Gil R, Boespflug-Tanguy O. X-linked spastic paraplegia and Pelizaeus Merzbacher disease are allelic disorders at the proteolipid protein locus. *Nature Genet* 1994 ; 6 : 257-61.
10. Kobayashi H, Hoffman E, Marks H. The rumpshaker mutation in spastic paraplegia. *Nature Genet* 1994 ; 7 : 351-2.
11. Schneider A, Montague P, Griffiths IR, Fanarraga M, Kennedy P, Brophy P, Nave K-A. Uncoupling of hypomyelination and glial cell death by a mutation in the proteolipid protein gene. *Nature* 1992 ; 358 : 758-61.

23

Schilder's myelinoclastic diffuse sclerosis and other multifocal leukoencephalopathies

A. LEVY-GOMES

Pediatric Unit Neurology, Hospital Santa Maria, University of Lisbon, Portugal.

H.C., a 11 year-old white girl was admitted to our hospital in Lisbon with a history of rapidly evolving left hemiplegia, central facial palsy and dysartria; she also complained of headache. Her previous medical history was unremarkable. Her mother's pregnancy and delivery had been normal; the family history was entirely normal. She was the youngest of eight siblings.

On admission she was alert and oriented, with intact comprehension and a dysartric speech. She had a almost complete left hemiplegia. Her reflexes were very active at left side with Babinski sign; the ophtalmoscopic examination was normal.

Unenhanced head CT scan revealed six bilateral hypodense lesions. On left hemisphere the lesions were located in occipital region and on right hemisphere the lesions were located in frontal and parietal region (Figure 1). Contrast enhancement revealed a very dense ring surrounding all hypodense lesions.

On magnetic resonance imaging (MRI) (Figure 2) T1-weighted images revealed lesions of low signal intensity in previous described locations. The lesions measured between 0,5 and 4 cm. T2-weighted images revealed increased signal intensity within the lesions.

No significant oedema was present around the lesions on either CT or MRI.

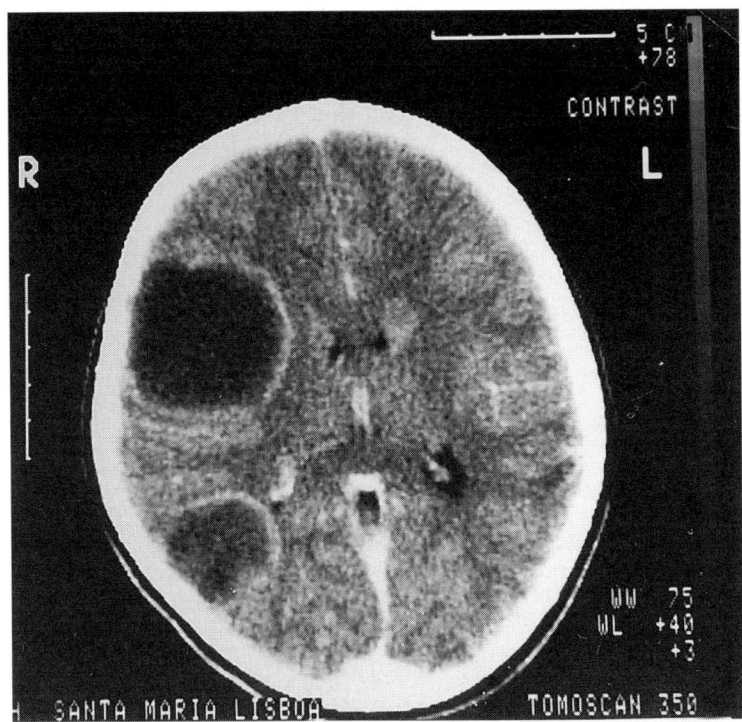

Figure 1. CT scan shows hypodense lesions.

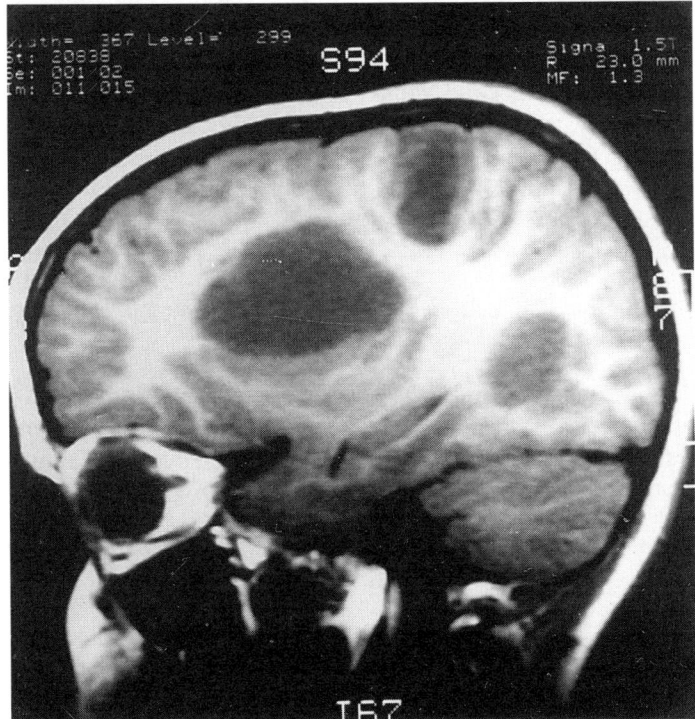

Figure 2. MRI T1-weighted low signal lesions.

The original diagnosis was that of a neoplasm; surgical exploration was carried out for biopsy of the lesions. The pathologist believed it was a gemistocytic astrocytoma and, consequently, radiotherapy and corticosteroids were begun.

Two months later there was a massive shrinking of the lesion (Figure 3), with small size increased signal in T2-weighted images. At this moment the patient was present to our Unit and the diagnosis of Schilder's myelinoclastic diffuse sclerosis was retained.

Complete blood count, liver function tests, total serum protein, very long chain fatty acids, virus titers were normal. A spinal tap was said normal.

Nine months later the patient was re-admitted because of progressing vomiting, headache, ataxia and decreased visual acuity. She had right-sided hemiparesis and Babinski sign. She didn't carry simple commands. The optic fundi revealed bilateral papilledema.

CT scan showed hypodense bilateral lesions with ring enhancement in different localisations.

She received immediately corticosteroids with a dramatic recovery: in 10 days the lesions were of smaller size without ring enhancement.

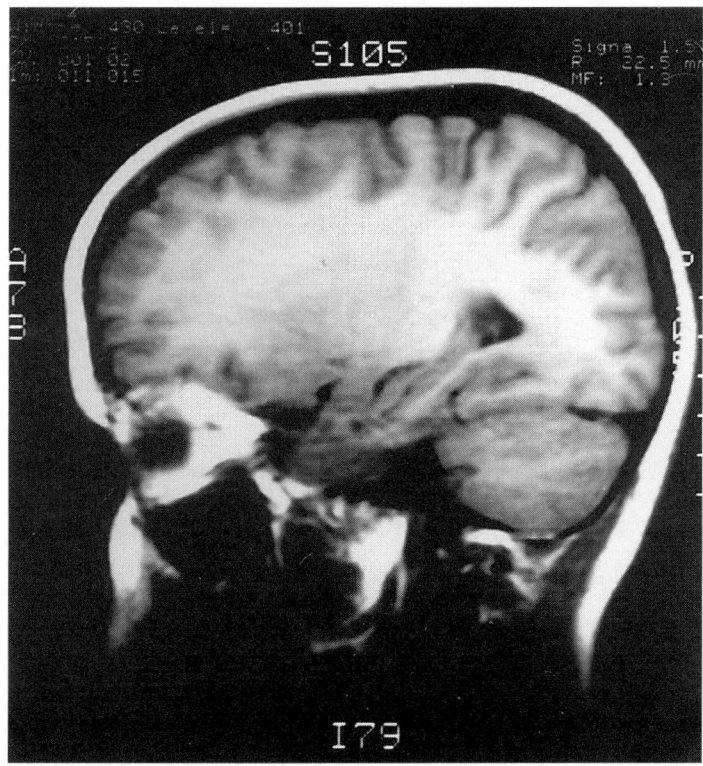

Figure 3. MRI T1-weighted almost disappearance of previous lesions.

We stopped corticosteroids after 3 months with complete recovery.

There were no recurrences since then (15 months).

The clinical picture, as well as the neuroimaging and biochemical findings in our patient are consistent with the diagnosis of true Schilder's disease (myelinoclastic diffuse sclerosis). There are frequent mis-diagnosis of gemistocytic astrocytoma. In most reported patients the disease was a single episode although recurrences have been reported (2 in 11 cases). In our patient the recurrence occurred with new demyelinating lesions with contralateral hemiplegia and optic neuritis.

In our Paediatric Unit we have admitted 6 patients with subacute disorders with variable clinical features like headaches, somnolence, hyperreflexia, Babinski signs or seizures. Cerebral fluid showed either pleocytosis or significant elevation of protein or both. CT scan was normal or showed multiple low-density lesions. The lesions never presented ring enhancement after contrast as we observed in Schilder disease. Magnetic resonance more readily demonstrated the high signal intensity abnormality on both the T2 and spin density-weighted studies. Lesions of the brainstem and internal capsule were most common. The diagnosis of acute disseminated encephalomyelitis (ADEM) was made in these patients. Some cases followed common childhood infections.

Both diseases show multiple low-density white matter lesions, but their size, location and type are different. On the contrary, both respond to steroid therapy. In ADEM patients have marked improvement within 24 to 48 hours.

In our patient with Schilder disease contrast enhancement disappeared ten days after glucocorticosteroid treatment was initiated.

ADEM are syndromes caused by the host's immune response to an infectious agent. The same mechanism against central nervous system myelin could be responsible for Schilder's disease.

24

Schilder's myelinoclastic diffuse sclerosis

C.M. POSER

Department of Neurology, Harvard Medical School and Beth Israel Hospital, Boston, USA.

In 1986, Poser *et al.* [1] redefined Schilder's myelinoclastic diffuse sclerosis (SMDS) as a subacute or chronic illness characterized by the presence of two roughly symmetrical plaques of demyelination measuring at least 3 x 2 cm, in two dimensions, involving the centrum semi-ovale, in the absence of other lesions demonstrated either by clinical or paraclinical testing. Progression was an obligatory component of the illness. It also required normal adrenal function or that the cholesterol esters of serum fatty acids contained carbon chains of normal length.

It was clearly shown that this was a disease which occurred almost exclusively in children. In a previous analysis Poser and van Bogaert [2] showed that many of the case reports in the literature under the term Schilder's disease not only consisted of other entities among which post-infectious encephalomyelitis and adrenoleukodystrophy were prominent, but that in many cases additional scattered lesions were found indicating a transitional phase to multiple sclerosis (MS). These cases were termed diffuse-disseminated sclerosis [3]. This classification was established on the basis of pathological findings. The areas of demyelination are not only much larger than those seen in MS, but they are characterized by sharply defined borders, elegantly described by van Bogaert as *découpés à l'emporte-pièce*, just as they are in MS.

The advent of brain imaging, both computer assisted tomography (CT) and magnetic resonance imaging (MRI), have led to a need to re-evaluate the diagnostic criteria for this entity. Another factor contributing to this problem is the increasing use of corticosteroids in the treatment of demyelinating conditions, such as acute disseminated encephalomyelitis and MS.

In the case discussed by Poser *et al.* [1], contrast-enhanced CT revealed two large frontal lesions (Figure 1). Very similar abnormalities were seen in another case also believed to be one of SMDS (Figure 2). Neither were confirmed by *post-mortem* examination. However, the same kind of images were demonstrated in a patient in whom the diagnosis of MS was established at autopsy (Figure 3). MRI has shown that large, bilateral, fairly symmetrical demyelinating lesions of the centrum semi-ovale

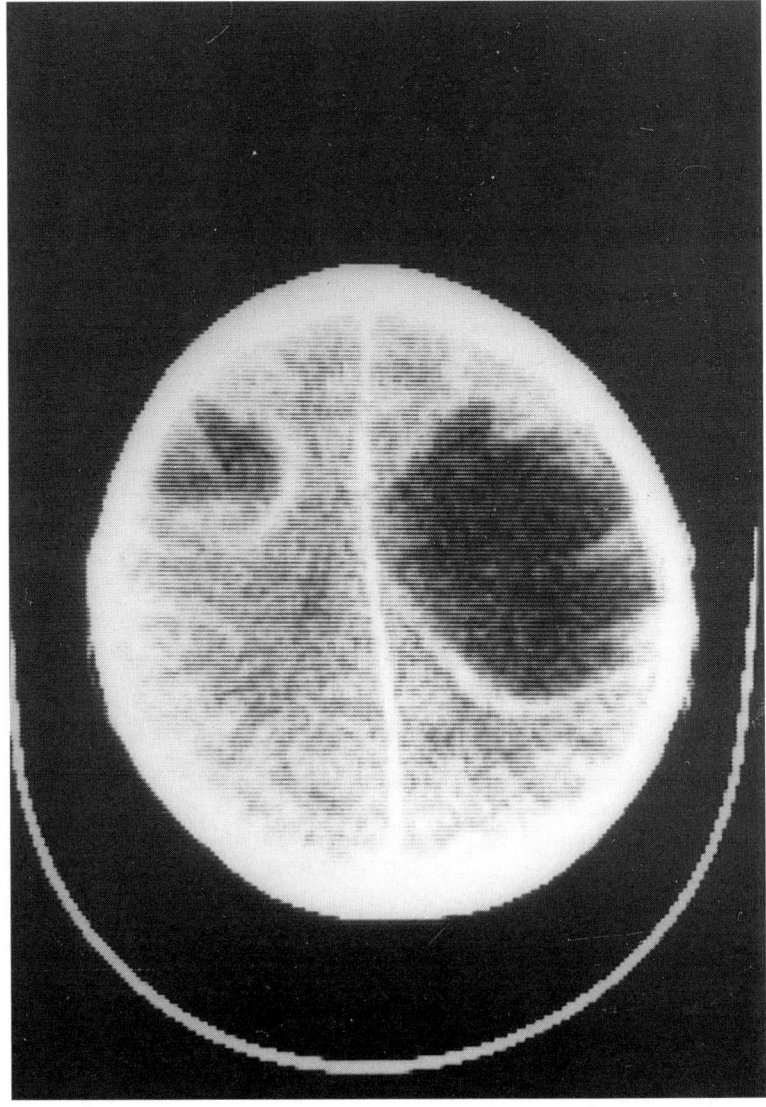

Figure 1. Contrast-enhanced CT scan: five-year-old boy with expressive aphasia and right hemiplegia [1].

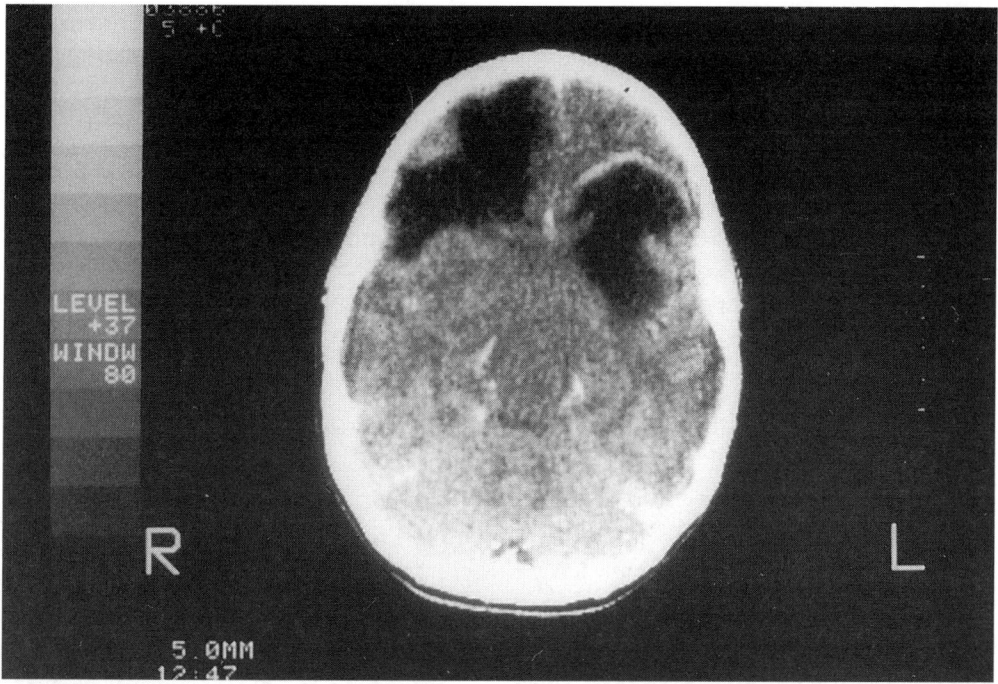

Figure 2. Contrast-enhanced CT scan: eight-year-old boy with expressive aphasia and bilateral spastic paraparesis.

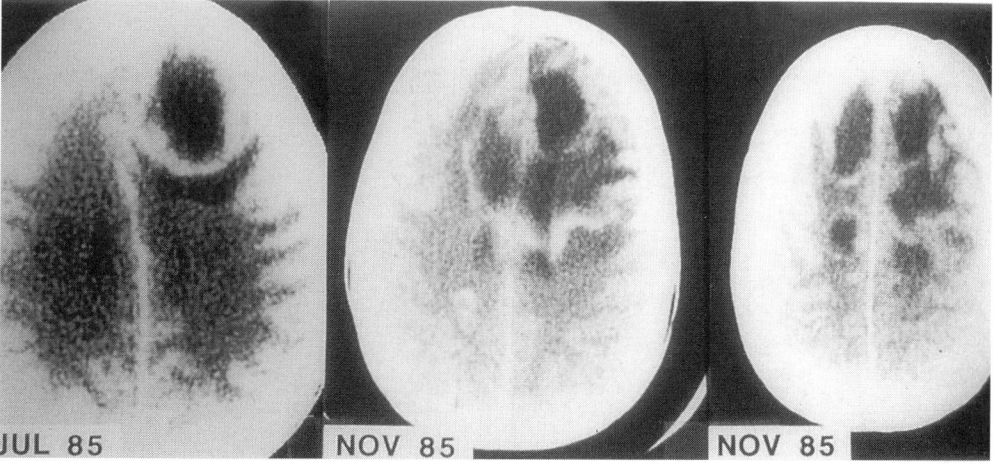

Figure 3. Contrast-enhanced CT scan: 28-year-old man with progressive dementia and severe ataxic quadriparesis. Autopsy-proven multiple sclerosis.

may result from classical postinfectious or post-vaccinal encephalomyelitis (Figures 4 and 5). Although the latter conditions are usually monophasic, multiphasic disseminated encephalomyelitis (MDEM) [4, 5] clinically fulfills the generally accepted diagnostic criteria for MS [6].

The major criterion of progression as a characteristic of SMDS is often modified by vigorous treatment with corticosteroids and occasionally by immunosuppressive drugs. Thus, the progression becomes modified into a remitting-relapsing course closely mimicking that of MS; as the effects of the corticosteroids abate, and steroid-dependency develops, recurrences may occur as it happens in the condition known as recurrent disseminated encephalomyelitis (RDEM) [4].

It is, of course, not possible to deny treatment of an acute demyelinating condition at the onset, thus leading to the extreme difficulty of differentiating between SMDS and RDEM.

Brain biopsy is of little value since the findings in both SMDS and RDEM are identical. As in MS, it is the topography of the lesion and, in particular, the sharply defined edges of the lesion which allow differentiation from MDEM and RDEM. In

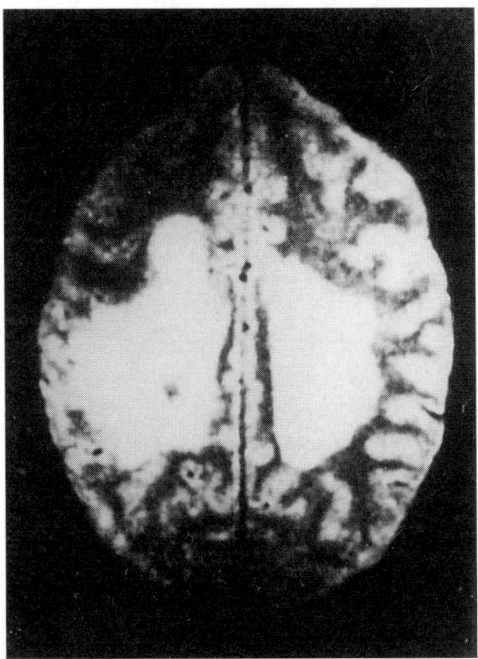 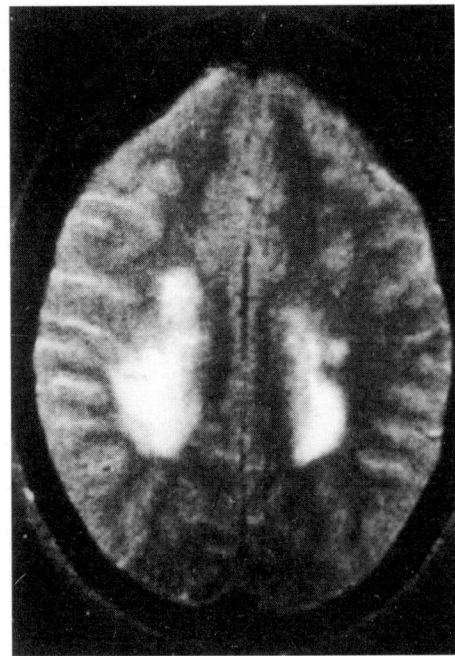

Figure 4. MRI. Left: 32-year-old man with acute postinfectious encephalomyelitis presenting with a *grand mal* seizure, lethargy and spastic paraparesis. Right: one year later after corticosteroid treatment. Patient had become completely asymptomatic.

most instances it is impossible to determine these crucial characteristics in tissue fragments obtained by needle biopsy.

In conclusion, it would appear that it is no longer possible to establish the diagnosis of SMDS short of pathological examination of the brain.

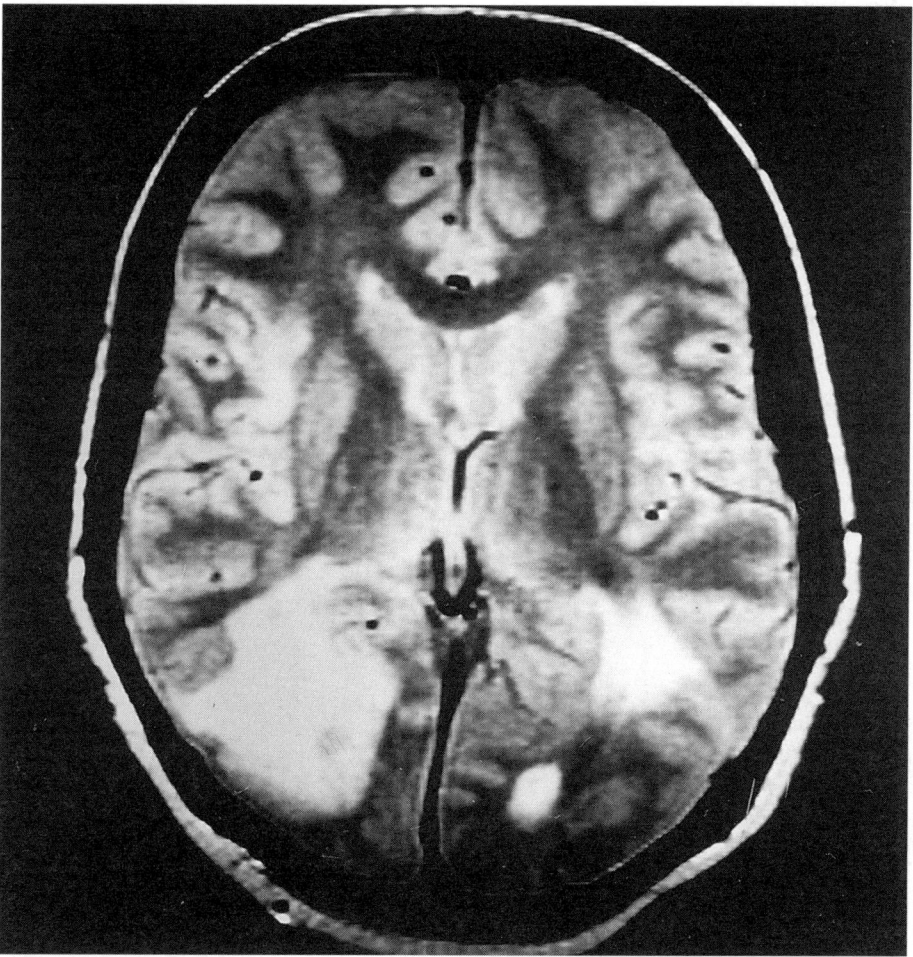

Figure 5. MRI: 39-year old woman with left homonymous hemianopsia and mild left hemiparesis.

Abbreviations

MDEM: multiphasic disseminated encephalomyelitis
MS: multiple sclerosis
RDEM: recurrent disseminated encephalomyelitis
SMDS: Schilder's myelinoclastic diffuse sclerosis

References

1. Poser C, Goutières F, Carpentier M. Aicardi J. Schilder's myelinoclastic diffuse sclerosis. *Pediatrics* 1986 ; 77 : 107-12.
2. Poser C, van Bogaert L. Natural history and evolution of the concept of Schilder's diffuse sclerosis. *Acta Neurol Psychiat Scand* 1956 ; 31 : 285-331.
3. Poser C. Diffuse-disseminated sclerosis in the adult. *J Neuropathol Exper Neurol* 1957 ; 16 : 61-78.
4. Poser C. The epidemiology of multiple sclerosis. A general overview. *Ann Neurol* 1994 ; 36 (S2) : S231-43.
5. Khan S, Yaqub B, Poser C, Al Deeb S, *et al.* Multiphasic disseminated encephalomyelitis presenting as alternating hemiplegia. *J Neurol Neurosurg Psychiatry* 1995 ; 50 : 467-70.
6. Poser C, Paty D, Scheinberg L. McDonald I, *et al.* New diagnostic criteria for multiple sclerosis. *Ann Neurol* 1983 ; 13 : 227-31.

25

X-linked adrenoleukodystrophy

P. AUBOURG

*Medical School University of Paris V-René-Descartes,
Inserm U342 and Hôpital Saint-Vincent-de-Paul, Paris, France.*

Clinical aspects of X-ALD

X-ALD affects 1/15 000 males and its phenotype is extremely varied [1]. The frequencies of ALD clinical phenotypes observed actually in France (Table I) differ markedly from previous reports in which 53% to 57% of ALD patients were reported to develop cerebral ALD [2-4]. The numbers are however much similar to results from a recent survey made in the Netherlands. Among 77 phenotyped male patients, 46% had AMN and 31% cerebral ALD [5]. This reflects likely that AMN was underdiagnosed in the past. A *de novo* mutation occurs in 7.8% of ALD cases and the first recognized mutation occur in the mother of 42% of index cases [6].

Table I. Clinical phenotypes of X-ALD among 363 French patients.

Cerebral ALD	- between 5-14 years	38.29 %
	- "chronic" forms	5.23 %
	- adult forms	4.40 %
Adrenomyeloneuropathy	- without cerebral involvement	19.28 %
	- with cerebral involvement	15.15 %
	- preclinical	4.68 %
Symptomatic women as index cases		3.06 %
Isolated Addison's disease		5.78 %
Asymptomatic		4.13 %

Patients with the cerebral form develop between 5-12 years neuropsychological and neurological symptoms from cerebral demyelination leading inexorably to a vegetative state or death within 2-5 years. Ninety percent of patients with cerebral ALD have adrenal insufficiency. The onset and evolution of cerebral and adrenal clinical symptoms are however independant.

In cerebral ALD, brain MRI demonstrates demyelination earlier than CT scan. The MR signal changes of affected white matter result in prolongation of T_1 and T_2 relaxation times. Early involvement of corpus callosum, pyramidal tracts within brain stem or internal capsules can be detected with this technique and the localization of the demyelinating lesions within the parieto-occipital junctions and the frontal lobes can be more easily evaluated. Multislice proton magnetic resonance spectroscopy (MRSI) shows a reduction in N-acetyl aspartate (NAA) and an increase in choline-containing compounds (Cho) in ALD white matter [7-9]. These abnormalities are not specific of ALD and their significance remains unclear. They are however more widespread than those detected by conventional MRI. An elevated content of Cho can also be detected in white matter apparently normal at MRI. Thus, MRSI may help to identify patients with early neurologic involvement.

With the advent of brain MRI and identification of biochemically affected patients in X-ALD families, it has been possible to diagnose cerebral ALD when clinical symptoms are restricted to neuropsychological deficits. Although sharing some resemblance with other genetic (metachromatic leukodystrophy) or acquired (multiple sclerosis) disorders of myelin, the neuropsychologic deficits observed in X-ALD are distinct and relatively well correlated with the topography of the demyelinating lesions within the cerebral hemispheres.

In the posterior cerebral forms, neuropsychological deficits involve the visuo-spatial functions. The motion and spatial processing of objects is early affected but recognition processing is intact. This correlates with the fact that the demyelinating lesions of ALD involve initially the myelinated fibers of dorsal stream pathway which is mainly involved in the analysis of spatial relationships of objects ("where things are"). When the lesions extend further into posterior parietal lobes, it is not unusual to observe deficits of working memory and subtle abnormalities in the executive functions. When executive functions and visuo-spatial perception deteriorate, the patients experience difficulties in solving problems, while oral and writtten langage learning remains preserved. In the frontal forms, the patients early develop impaired flexibility in problem solving strategies and difficulties in anticipatory processing and decision-making. In contrast with the "occipital forms", the cognitive impairments due to frontal demyelinating lesions have an early impact on school performances. These difficulties are often interpretated as "psychologic". At a later stage, patients show decreased verbal fluency, immediate memory impairment and marked difficulties in complex visual constructive tasks.

The stage of isolated cognitive dysfunction lasts 1 to 5 years. As a rule, the earlier the disease starts, the shorter is the inital period of isolated neuropsychologic impairment. The initial topography of demyelinating lesions influences markedly the progression of the disease. The occipital forms progress much more rapidly than the frontal forms. The later forms are more frequently observed in adolescents whereas the fulminating occipital forms are seen mainly in 4-6 year-old boys. Approximately 15% of occipital or frontal cerebral forms occuring in boys older than 10 years have a very slow progression ("chronic form") during the first 5 years of evolution, and sometimes longer. The vast majority of these chronic forms have in a second phase a rapid and devastating progression, similar to classical cerebral ALD.

Early symptoms of adrenomyeloneuropathy (AMN) usually appear when patients are between 20-30 years [1, 10]. Men present stiffness and clumsiness in their legs. Neurologic examination reveals a mild to moderate spastic paraparesis, impaired vibration sense and graphesthesia disturbances in the distal lower limbs, urinary disturbances and mild signs of peripheral neuropathy. MRI shows spinal cord atrophy which is not correlated to neurological disability [10]. Alterations of nerve conduction velocity, brain-stem auditory and somatosensory evoked potentials are consistently present but visual evoked potentials are normal. Addison's disease is diagnosed prior to the neurologic deficit in one third of AMN patients. Another third of patients have clinical or biological evidence of adrenal insufficiency at time of diagnosis. Fifteen percent of AMN patients will never develop Addison's disease.

In two-third of AMN patients, gait disturbance becomes severe within 10-15 years requiring the use of a cane or a wheelchair. The long tract signs involves progressively the upper limbs and it is common to observe at MRI on T2-weighted images an hypertensity of the pyramidal tracts within the pons that reaches the internal capsules. Thirty-five percent of patients with AMN have however a marked progression of their disease within 3 years of diagnosis. In these patients, brain MRI shows a characteristic ascending involvement of the pyramidal tracts through the pons to the internal capsules. In addition, approximately one third of AMN patients develop cerebral demyelinating lesions five to ten years after the onset of spinal cord symptoms. The cognitive deficits presented by these adults with cerebral involvement are very similar to those observed in boys or adolescents with cerebral ALD. Later on, a rapid and devastating evolution occur in a large fraction of these AMN patients.

A recent systematic clinical survey demonstrated that up to 55% of heterozygous women have clinical signs of spinal cord involvement that consist of mild pyramidal signs and urinary disturbances (Naidu and Moser, 1994, unpublished). It is likely that electrophysiologic tests are abnormal in a greater proportion of heterozygous ALD women. The clinical progression of the disease is variable. Most of these women have minimal complaint and do not consult a neurologist. Twenty percent will develop at age 30-40 years severe neurologic disability like adult males with AMN [11]. These abnormalities resemble AMN, but are generally milder and frequently without peripheral neuropathy manifestations. Unlike AMN, adrenal function is almost intact and demyelinating cerebral lesions occur rarely.

Among children with Addison's, 30 percent of them have ALD, regardless of sex [3]. ALD is therefore the most frequent cause of Addison's in children. At least 35% of adult males with primitive Addison's disease have ALD. Adrenal insufficiency affects first the glucocorticoid function but the mineralocorticoid function is ultimately deficient in approximately half of ALD patients. Isolated Addison's disease accounts for less 10% of the clinical forms of ALD. It must be emphasized that the great majority of these patients are at risk to develop cerebral or spinal cord involvement and that no tests are able to predict such evolution.

Biochemistry of ALD

Myelin and adrenal glands

The initial key to the biochemistry of ALD was the obervation that adrenal glands and white matter contain characteristic lipid inclusions, followed by the demonstration that these inclusions consist of cholesterol ester with a striking excess of saturated VLCFA [1]. The greatest excess of VLCFA is observed in cholesterol ester fractions in actively demyelinating lesions or adrenal cortex [12], then in phosphatidylcholine and glycerophosphatide fractions [13, 14]. In contrast to these abnormalities, VLCFA are only slightly increased in lipid fractions of intact myelin of ALD patients.

Cultured skin fibroblasts, plasma, erythrocytes, amniocytes and chorionic villus cells

Saturated VLCFA are moderately increased (by 3 fold) in cultured skin fibroblasts and plasma of affected ALD males [15, 16]. This biochemical abnormality is however sufficient to diagnose unambiguously affected ALD males and 85% to 95% of heterozygous women. Plasma VLCFA levels of affected males show little or no variation from the neonatal period. There is unfortunately no correlation between the clinical phenotype and the VLCFA levels in plasma or fibroblasts [1]. Prenatal diagnosis has been achieved by demonstrating similar accumulation of saturated VLCFA in cultured chorionic villus samples (9-11 weeks of gestation) or cultured amniocytes (15-18 weeks of gestation) [1].

Enzyme deficiency associated with ALD in cultured fibroblasts

VLCFA are derived both from the diet and from endogenous synthesis by a microsomal system that elongates long chain fatty acids [17]. Endogenous synthesis appears to be more prominent than diet as a source of VLCFA in human [1]. Although the activity of the microsomal fatty acid elongation system is increased by 50% to 80% in ALD fibroblasts [18], the accumulation of VLCFA seems essentially to be due to an impaired capacity to β-oxidize these fatty acids in peroxisomes [19]. The oxidation rate of $(1-^{14}C)$ C24:0 or $(1-^{14}C)$ C26:0 is reduced by 60% to 80 % in ALD fibroblasts.

Similar impairment is observed in white blood cells and in amniotic or chorionic villus cells. From the observation that ALD fibroblasts are able to oxidize the CoA-ester of VLCFA normally, it was concluded that the primary defect of ALD was a deficient VLCFA-CoA synthetase activity [20]. The activation of VLCFA to VLCFA-CoA occurs both in peroxisomes and in endoplasmic reticulum [21]. Two laboratories demonstrated independently that only the peroxisomal VLCFA-CoA synthetase activity is deficient in ALD fibroblasts [22, 23]. As for oxidation of VLCFA, 20% to 30% of VLCFA-CoA synthetase residual activity is found in purified peroxisomal fraction from ALD fibroblasts. This residual activity may be accounted by the activity of the peroxisomal long-chain-fatty acid-CoA synthetase towards VLCFA. All these data were taken as a strong indication that the gene coding for the peroxisomal VLCFA-CoA synthetase was the ALD. The identification of the ALD gene by positional cloning [24] has led to a rather different conclusion, making the situation much more complicated.

The ALD gene and its product

Localization and structure

The ALD locus is closely linked to the glucose-6-phosphate dehydrogenase (G6PD) gene and to the DXS52 marker locus in the Xq28 region [25]. The ALD gene is 625 kb distal from DXS52 and 1350 kb proximal from F8C. In addition, the ALD gene is 720 kb proximal from R/GCP genes and at least two other genes (L1CAM, AVPR2) lie between the ALD and R/GCP genes. The occurence of color vision abnormalities in ALD initially thought to represent a contiguous gene syndrome [26, 27] is in fact a secondary manifestation of ALD. The ALD gene is 21 kb long and contains 10 exons [28]. Putative regulatory sequences in the 5' end include numerous Sp1 site typical for housekeeping gene but no peroxisomal proliferator activated receptor (PPAR) responsive elements, TATA, CAAT boxes or regulatory sequences (SCIP and MyT1) implicated in the expression of myelin basic protein, proteolipid and P0 genes. Homologous sequences to the ALD genes have been identified in all species tested, including *S. cerevisiae* and *C. elegans*. Two yeast genes showing significant homology with the ALD and the 70 kDa peroxisomal membrane protein (PMP70) gene have recently been indentified in yeast [29, 30].

ALD mRNA expression

A 3.7 kb transcript is present in all tissues, including liver, skeletal muscle, testis, adrenal gland, brain, retina and fibroblasts. The expression of ALD transcript is high in adrenal glands and low in liver. Expression of ALD mRNA does not increase in cerebral regions that myelinate during the post-natal period (P14-P21) in rat [31]. This suggests that ALD gene function may be not essential to myelogenesis. In contrast to the genes of the β-peroxisomal enzymes (acyl-CoA oxidase, bifunctional protein and β-ketothiolase) and the 70 kDa PMP in rat or mouse liver, the expression of the

ALD gene is not inducible by fenofibrate in mouse liver (Bugeaut *et al.*, 1995 unpublished).

ALD protein

The ALD gene encodes a 75 kDa protein [24, 32] that shows 38.8% identity with the human or rat 70 kDa peroxisomal membrane protein (PMP) [33, 34] and 66% identity with a mouse ALD related protein recently identified [35]. The three proteins have 6 potential transmembrane α-helical segments and a hydrophobic amino terminal region that includes two nucleotide binding fold (NBF) consensus sequences characteristic of ATP-binding cassette (ABC) protein [36]. Although ALD protein and the 70 kDa PMP show significant homology, the organization of their genes is markedly different suggesting that these genes have diverged long time ago. The mouse ALD cDNA nucleotide sequences exhibit 84% identity to human cDNA within the protein coding sequence [37]. There is no indication that ALDP can be phosphorylated or post-translationally modified. Monoclonal antibodies raised against part of ALDP detect a 75-kDa band in normal fibroblasts, lymphocytes or lymphoblasts [33]. Using indirect immuno-fluorescence, ALDP shows a punctate pattern similar to that observed with catalase, peroxisomal β-ketothiolase or the 70 kDa PMP. Co-localization studies, electron microscopy and Western blot analysis of human peroxisomes purified by density gradient centrifugation have confirmed that ALD protein is an integral component of the peroxisomal membrane [33, 38]. In human liver, ALD protein represents however a minor fraction of all peroxisomal membrane proteins. Recently, retro-viral mediated transfer of the ALD gene was shown to restore the oxidation of VLCFA in ALD fibroblasts following expression and appropriate targeting of the vector-encoded ALD protein in peroxisomes [39]. This confirmed definitively that the gene identified by positional cloning is the ALD gene. Immunohistochemical analysis of brain, adrenal gland and testis with ALDP antibodies shows that ALD expression pattern is correlated with the major site of ALD pathology. ALDP is markedly expressed in adrenocortical cells but not in the medulla, in Leydig cells but not in Sertoli or germinal cells. In the brain, ALDP is markedly expressed in astrocytes and microglia but not in oligodendrocytes or in neurons. ALDP is relatively more expressed in human cultured oligodendrocytes than in oligodendrocytes *in vivo* where its presence is hardly detectable, even during post-natal period of myelination (Fouquet *et al.*, in preparation). In contrast to ALDP, catalase and acyl-CoA oxidase are expressed at the same level in neurons, astrocytes and oligodendrocytes (Fouquet *et al.*, in preparation and [40]). Interestingly, peroxisome content of astrocytes is heterogenous. Some peroxisomes contain both ALDP, catalase and acyl-CoA oxidase, while other peroxisomes contain only ALDP. This may reflect difference in import of peroxisomal proteins or difference in function.

Putative function (s) of the ALD protein

Although these is definitive evidence that the gene identified by positional cloning is the ALD gene, the function of ALD protein remains unknown. Alike the 70 kDa PMP,

ALDP is an integral protein of the peroxisomal membrane. The two NBF consensus sequences of ALD protein are highly homologous to the NBFs of other ABC proteins that are involved in transport events. Transport of VLCFA across the peroxisomal membrane is normal in ALD fibroblasts [41]. It is unclear yet whether ALDP controls the import of a factor necessary for the activation of the VLCFA-CoA synthetase or transport the activated VLCFA-CoA esters into peroxisomes. The recent identification of a fatty acid binding domain in ALDP gives support to the latter hypothesis [30]. Another yet unsolved issue is whether ALD protein associates with a related PMP to form a functional hetero-dimer transporter. PMP70 was proposed as a candidate partner for ALDP. PMP70 and ALDP mRNAs have however different temporal and spatial expression in the brain [31]. The absence of coordinated expression between ALDP and PMP70 makes unlikely that ALDP and PMP70 function as obligate partners, at least in the brain. Depending of the expression of ALDP and of its partner, ALDP might have functions that could be cell-specific. As mentioned previously, ALDP is much more expressed in astrocytes and microglia than in oligodendrocytes and neurons, unlike acyl-CoA oxidase and catalase that show similar expression in these cells. This raises the possiblity that ALDP may have a specific function not obligatory related to the β-oxidation of VLCFA.

Mutations of the ALD gene

Approximately 5-7% of ALD patients have partial deletions of the ALD gene. No deletion of the entire gene has been reported. Using RT-PCR, SCCP or DGGE, more than 120 mutations have now been identified in ALD kindred over the world [6, 42-49]. They include missense, nonsense, splice mutations and deletion of 1-3 base pairs. Except one "hot spot" of mutations (delAG 1801-1802: ~ 10% of all mutations), nearly every ALD family has a different mutation. As expected, there is no correlation between ALD mutations and clinical phenotypes. Mutations (nonsense mutations, deletion of 1-3 bp, deletion affecting multiple exons or splice acceptor site mutations) leading theorically to a truncated and possibly labile protein are detected in 50% of ALD kindred. In fact, Western blot and immunofluorescence analysis show that all these mutations lead to a complete absence of ALD protein. In the remaining kindred (50%), the mutation affects a single amino acid residue. Many of these non polymorphic amino acid changes occur in the transmembrane domains and in the ATP-binding domain of the ALD protein. Surprisingly, most of these missense mutation (60%) lead to a complete absence of the ALD protein. This includes many missense mutations of the ATP-binding domain which were expected to abolish the binding or hydrolysis of ATP. Up to now, no abnormal acummulation or mis-localization of the ALD protein have been indentified in ALD fibroblasts. Taken together, these data suggest that minimal change of ALD protein leads to a labile protein which is rapidly destroyed in the cytoplasm. Whether or not some of these mutations can affect the targeting of the ALD protein to the peroxisomal membrane is not known.

Identification of heterozygous women can now be performed with molecular methods when the ALD gene mutation has been characterized in the family. This diagnostic procedure is however time-consuming because nearly each ALD family has a different mutation. Since eighty percent of ALD hemizygotes have a complete absence of ALDP, study of ALDP can be performed in fibroblasts or peripheral white cells of women at risk to be carrier to determine their status. Because of X-inactivation, fibroblasts of ALD hemizygotes will have a double population of fibroblast cells. One which is not mutated and expresses normal ALDP and one which is mutated with a complete absence of ALDP. Molecular methods (mutation analysis and/or study of ALD protein) can also now be proposed in families with identified ALD gene mutation to perform prenatal diagnosis [6].

Therapeutic approaches

Diet therapy

Despite uncertainties on causal relationship between accumulation of saturated VLCFA and demyelination, it seemed logical to expect clinical improvement from therapeutic approaches aimed at reducing their concentrations. Lorenzo's oil that normalize plasma VLCFA of ALD patients within 2 months has unfortunately no detectable effect on the rate of demyelinating lesions in the cerebral form of the disease and do not prevent neurologic deterioration in patients [50-54]. Patients with AMN, the less severe neurologic form of ALD, were expected to benefit from the dietary approach. Recent reports document however various degrees of progression in preexisting myelopathy, cerebral lesions seen at MRI and electrophysiological tests in a large fraction of them [52-55]. This also occurs in symptomatic heterozygous women and in pre-clinical AMN patients despite normalization of plasma VLCFA. The only clear benefit of Lorenzo's oil is a slight improvement of peripheral nerve conduction that did not modify the disability of patients. Preliminary studies indicate that one third of true asymptomatic ALD patients (*i.e.* children less than 12 years with normal MRI) develop demyelination at MRI within 3 years of diet treatment. Some of them have already developed aggravation similar to untreated patients during this interval. To interpret these data, one should keep in mind that at most 30-40 % of chidren are at risk to develop cerebral ALD before 14 years of age. It also discouraging to observe that a significant number of children that do not develop cerebral ALD under Lorenzo's oil develop AMN in their fifteen. Two different groups were recently unable to detect any increased of erucic acid in brain of treated patients indicating that little erucic acid cross the blood-brain barrier [56, 57]. Altogether, these results do not discard the possibility that Lorenzo's oil might help slow the disease in asymptomatic patients but clearly indicate that the dietary approach is not fully preventive.

Bone marrow transplantation

The rationale for proposing bone marrow transplantation in neurodegenerative diseases is based on the fact that brain microglia cells are derived from bone marrow hematopoietic system [58]. Although the origin of microglia is not totally elucidated, there is no doubt that microglia resembles the macrophages of the liver (Kupffer cells) and that microglia cells comprise up to 20% of all glial cells in cerebral white matter. Apart from contributing to immune response, microglial cells contribute to chemical signalling network by interaction with other cells, especially astrocytes. Several groups have now clearly demonstrated in mice that there is significant turn-over of resident microglia cells 3 to 6 months after bone marrow transplantation (reviewed in [59]). This normal mechanism of microglia turnover offers therefore a mechanism to express therapeutic genes in the brain by genetic manipulation or allogenic transplantation of bone marrow cells.

The first attempts to use bone marrow transplantation in ALD patients with advanced form of the disease were unsuccesful and there was concern that the treatment may accelerate neurologic deterioration [60]. This procedure was reevaluated in an 8-year old boy who had early neurologic involvement. Two years after the transplant, there was a complete disappearance of the neuropsychological, and neurologic deficits and the MRI scan normalized [61]. Complete reversal of neurologic manifestations are still maintained 8 years later in this patient. Similar encouraging results have been obtained in 24 other ALD patients (Krivit, Moser and Aubourg, unpublished).When bone marrow transplantation is performed at a stage of minimal MRI lesions, a complete reversal is obtained. When it is attempted at a stage when MRI lesions are more marked but still moderate, a stabilization is obtained. In both cases, significant neuropsychological improvement is observed. Importantly, some patients continue to show neuropsychological and neuroradiological improvement 5 years after the BMT, indicating that spontaneous remyelination occurs and is clinically effective. Considering that no other therapeutic approaches have proven any effect in the severe cerebral form of the disease, the mortality risk of bone marrow transplantation, although high (10%), remains acceptable. Bone marrow transplantation has however serious limitations. It is effective only at an early stage of the disease: 18 ALD patients had CNS deterioration when BMT was performed at advanced stage of the disease. In addition BMT requires a perfectly HLA matched donor and the morbidity and mortality risk of the procedure increases sharply (25-30%) when the donor is unrelated. In this situation the risk to benefit ratio of bone marrow transplantation must be balanced, considering the probability of aggravation during the following 3-5 years.

Towards gene therapy

While there is no doubt that there is an association between ALD and VLCFA accumulation, it remains uncertain whether the fatty acid abnormality is the direct cause of pathology. There is circumstancial evidence that saturated VLCFAs increase the microviscosity of red cell membranes [62] and that human adrenocortical cells cultured in the presence of C26:0 excess show decreased basal and ACTH-stimulated cortisol release compared with cells cultured with exogenous fatty acids [63]. It is therefore conceivable that an alteration in myelin lipid properties results in destabilization of myelin membranes with subsequent demyelination. However, the putative toxic action of these fatty acids on myelin sheaths has not been evaluated, for example by studying their effects on cultured oligodendrocytes. As mentioned previously, it is possible that ALD protein has in fact several functions, only one of them being related to VLCFA oxidation.

Abnormal immune response is likely involved in the cerebral form of the disease [1]. Based on MRI imaging (gadolinium enhancement reflecting abnormal blood-brain barrier), this abnormal immune response occurs however several years after the demyelination process has started in the cerebral hemispheres, in fact when the disease is already markedly advanced. CSF lymphocytes of ALD patients express a restricted repertoire of T cell receptor Vβ chains. The oligoclonal expansion of these CSF T cells suggests that they may react against a limited set of antigens (Picard *et al.*, submitted). There is however no clear correlation between Vβ restricted expression and the phenotype. Candidate antigens include gangliosides and proteolipid protein (PLP) whose acylation profile is modified by VLCFA accumulation [64]. Other antigens may be revealed when an animal model of ALD will be available. Thus, it will be necessary to clarify the sequence of events that are associated with initial demyelination and the secondary production or action of cytokines. A recent observation has demonstrated that TNF-α, a cytokine which is particularly toxic for oligodendrocytes [65,] is secreted by reactive astrocytes in ALD brain [66]. Overexpression of cytokines has also been reported in multiple sclerosis and in experimental allergic encephalomyelitis and is thought to contribute to the pathogenesis of these two disorders [67]. Thus, modification of cytokine synthesis or action might prove a valuable area for future therapeutic interventions in advanced form of cerebral ALD.

ALD is characterized by a wide phenotypical expression, a situation which is shared by many genetic disorders. Two causes can be suspected: stochastic variation or the requirement of additional predisposing genes. That identical genotypes can be phenotypically discordant might be due to purely stochastic variation and the marked phenotypic heterogeneity found in monozygotic ALD twin supports the importance of non genetic factors [68]. Additional cellular events under the control of modifier genes may also be necessary to result in demyelination [69]. The identification of these putative modifier genes will remain difficult, but one may hypothesize that mouse genetics will bring significant breakthrough in this search.

An ALD murine model obtained by homologous recombination should help to decipher many of these unresolved issues. This animal model should also be valuable to evaluate the efficacy of new therapeutic approaches. At present, bone marrow transplantation is the only therapeutic intervention with proven efficacy in the lethal cerebral form of ALD. Retroviral mediated transfer of ALD cDNA normalizes VLCFA oxidation and content in ALD fibroblasts [39] and work is already in progress to target the normal ALD gene in hematopoietic stem cells, *i.e.* CD34$^+$ cells. The insertion of the normal gene followed by autologous bone marrow transplantation would circumvent the need for a histocompatible donor and decreases the morbidity and mortality risk of the procedure. This approach may provide the most suitable gene therapy approach before attempting to deliver the ALD gene directly in the central nervous system. Microglia cells comprise up to 10-20% of all glial cells and genetically modified microglial cells might induce metabolic cooperation or other cell-contact-dependant mechanisms by which corrective metabolites could be transferred to oligodendrocytes and astrocytes.

In a near future, gene therapy will be combined with the administration of growth factors and/or transplantation of glial cells into brain to promote myelin repair. The growth and survival factor requirements of oligodendrocyte progenitors and their progeny are now better understood [70]. Although gaps in knowledge remain to be filled, there is a prospect for strategies that seek to enhance endogenous repair by growth factors therapy (IGF-1, CNTF). Many issues remain to be resolved before attempting to graft glial cells in ALD patients [71]. One is to define what cell type should be transplanted: oligodendrocytes, Schwann cells or neurospheres; another concerns the quality of the myelin formed by transplanted glial cells. At present, Schwann cells appear to be the best candidate. Schwann cell engrafting promotes remyelination in the central nervous system of animal models with chemical or genetic demyelination [72]. Schwann cells can be obtained by sural nerve biopsy of ALD patients, expanded *in vitro* [73] and genetically corrected before transplantation. The advantage of this approach is of course that rejection and immunosupressive treatment would be avoided. These and other exciting therapeutic approaches will be soon tested in animal models.

References

1. Moser HW, Smith KD, Moser AB. X-linked adrenoleukodystrophy. In : Scriver CR, Beaudet AL, Sly WS, Valle D, eds. *The metabolic basis of inherited disease*. New York : McGraw-Hill, 1995 : 2325-50.
2. Moser HW, Moser AB, O'Neill BP. Adrenoleukodystrophy. Survey of 303 cases: biochemistry, diagnosis and therapy. *Ann Neurol* 1984 ; 16 : 628-41.
3. Aubourg P, Chaussain JL. Adrenoleukodystrophy presenting as Addison's disease in children and adults. *Trends Endocrinol Metab* 1991 ; 2 : 49-52.
4. Moser HW, Moser AB, Smith KD, Bergin A, Borel J, Shankroff J, Stine OC, Merette C, Ott J, Krivit W, Shapiro E. Adrenoleukodystrophy: phenotypic variability and implications for therapy. *J Inherited Metab Dis* 1992 ; 15 : 645-64.
5. Van Geel BM, Assies J, Weverling GJ, Barth PG. Predominance of the adrenomyeloneuropathy phenotype of X-linked adrenoleukodystrophy in the Netherlands: a survey of 30 kindreds. *Neurology* 1994 ; 44 : 2343-6.
6. Fanen P, Guidoux S, Sarde C-O, Mandel J-L, Goossens M, Aubourg P. Identification of mutations in the putative ATP-binding domain of the adrenoleukodystrophy gene. *J Clin Invest* 1994 ; 94 : 516-20.
7. Tzika AA, Ball WS, Vigneron DB, Scott Dunn R, Nelson SJ, Kirks DR. Childhood adrenoleukodystrophy: assessment with proton MR spectroscopy. *Radiology* 1993 ; 189 : 467-80.
8. Kruse B, Barker PB, Van Zijl PCM, Duyn JH, Moonen CTW, Moser HW. Multislice proton magnetic resonance spectroscopic imaging in X-linked adrenoleukodystrophy. *Ann Neurol* 1994 ; 36 : 595-608.

9. Confort-Gouny S, Vion-Dury J, Chabrol B, Nicoli F, Cozzone PJ. Localized proton NMR spectroscopy in X-linked adrenoleukodystrophy. *Neuroradiology* 1995 (in press).
10. Aubourg P, Adamsbaum C, Lavallard Rousseau MC, Lemaitre A, Boureau F, Mayer M, Kalifa G. Brain MRI and electrophysiologic abnormalities in preclinical and clinical adrenomyeloneuropathy. *Neurology* 1992 ; 42 : 85-91.
11. O'Neill BP, Moser HW, Saxena KM, Marmion LC. Adrenoleukodystrophy: clinical and biochemical manifestations in carriers. *Neurology* 1984 ; 34 : 789-801.
12. Kishimoto Y, Moser HW, Suzuki K. Adrenoleukodystrophy. In : Lajtha A, ed. *Handbook of neurochemistry* Vol 10. Plenum Publishing Corp, 1985 : 125-51.
13. Sharp P, Johnson D, Poulos A. Molecular species of phosphatidylcholine containing very long chain fatty acids in human brain: enrichment in X-linked adrenoleukodystrophy brain and diseases of peroxisome biogenesis. *J Neurochem* 1991 ; 56 : 30-7.
14. Theda C, Moser AB, Powers JM, Moser HW. Phospholipids in X-linked adrenoleukodystrophy white matter: fatty acid abnormalities before the onset of demyelination. *J Neurol Sci* 1992 ; 110 : 195-204.
15. Moser HW, Moser AB, Kawamura N, Murphy J, Suzuki K, Schaumburg HH, Kishimoto Y, Milunsky A. Adrenoleukodystrophy: elevated C26 fatty acid in cultured skin fibroblasts. *Ann Neurol* 1980 ; 7 : 542-9.
16. Moser HW, Moser AB, Frayer KK, Chen W, Sailman JC, O'Neill BP, Kishimoto Y. Adrenoleukodystrophy: increased plasma content of saturated very long chain fatty acids. *Neurology* 1981 ; 31 : 1241-9.
17. Bourre JM, Daudu O, Baumann N. Nervonic acid biosynthesis by erucyl-CoA elongation in normal and quaking mouse brain microsomes. Elongation of other unsaturated fatty acyl-CoAs (mono and polyunsaturated). *Biochim Biophys Acta* 1976 ; 424 : 1-7.
18. Koike R, Tsuji S, Ohno T, Suzuki Y, Orii T, Miyatake T. Physiological significance of fatty acid elongation system in adrenoleukodystrophy. *J Neurol Sci* 1991 ; 103 : 188-94.
19. Singh I, Moser AB, Moser HW, Kishimoto Y. Adrenoleukodystrophy: impaired oxidation of very long chain fatty acids in white blood cells, cultured skin fibroblasts and amniocytes. *Pediatr Res* 1984 ; 18 : 286-90.
20. Hashmi M, Stanley W, Singh I. Lignoceroyl CoASH ligase: enzyme defect in fatty acid β-oxidation in X-linked adrenoleukodystrophy. *FEBS Lett* 1986 ; 196 : 247-50.
21. Lazo O, Contreras M, Yoshida Y, Singh AK, Stanley W, Weise M, Singh I. Cellular oxidation of lignoceric acid is regulated by the cellular localization of lignoceroyl-CoA ligases. *J Lipid Res* 1990 ; 31 : 583-95.
22. Lazo O, Contreras M, Hashmi M, Stanley W, Irazu C, Singh I. Peroxisomal lignoceroyl-CoA ligase deficiency in childhood adrenoleukodystrophy and adrenomyeloneuropathy. *Proc Natl Acad Sci USA* 1988 ; 85 : 7647-51.
23. Wanders RJA, Van Roermund CWT, Wijland MJA, Schutgens RBH, Schram AW, Tager JM, Van den Bosch H, Schalkwijk C. X-linked adrenoleukodystrophy: identification of the primary defect at the level of a deficient peroxisomal very long chain fatty acyl-CoA synthetase using a newly developed method for the isolation of peroxisomes from skin fibroblasts. *J Inher Metab Dis* 1988 ; 11,2 : 173-7.
24. Mosser J, Douar A-M, Sarde C-O, Kioschis P, Feil R, Moser H, Poustka A-M, Mandel J-L, Aubourg P. Putative X-linked adrenoleukodystrophy gene shares unexpected homology with ABC transporters. *Nature* 1993 ; 361 : 726-30.
25. Aubourg P, Sack GHJ, Meyers DA, Lease JJ, Moser HW. Linkage of adrenoleukodystrophy to a polymorphic DNA probe. *Ann Neurol* 1987 ; 21 : 349-52.
26. Aubourg P, Sack GH Jr, Moser HW. Frequent alterations of visual pigment genes in adrenoleukodystrophy. *Am J Hum Genet* 1988 ; 42 : 408-13.

27. Aubourg P, Feil R, Guidoux S, Kaplan JC, Moser H, Kahn A, Mandel JL. The red-green visual pigment gene region in adrenoleukodystrophy. *Am J Hum Genet* 1990 ; 46 : 459-69.
28. Sarde C-0, Mosser J, Kioshis P, Kretz C, Vicaire S, Aubourg P, Poutska A-M, Mandel J-L. Genomic organization of the adrenoleukodystrophy gene. *Genomics* 1994 ; 22 : 13-20.
29. Bossier P, Fernandes L, Vilela C, Rodrigues-Pousada C. The yeast YKL 741 gene situated on the left arm of chromosome XI codes for a homologue of the human ALD protein. *Yeast* 1994 ; 10 : 681-6.
30. Shani N, Watkins PA, Valle D. PXA1, a possible *S. cerevisiae* ortholog of the human adrenoleukodystrophy gene. *Proc Natl Acad Sci USA* 1994 ; 92 : 6012-6.
31. Pollard H, Moreau J, Aubourg P. Localization of mRNAs for adrenoleukodystrophy and the 70 kDa peroxisomal (PMP70) proteins in the rat braun during post-natal development. *J Neurosci Res* 1995 ; 42 : 433-7.
32. Mosser J, Lutz Y, Stoeckel ME, Sarde CO, Kretz C, Douar AM, Lopez J, Aubourg P, Mandel JL. The gene responsible for adrenoleukodystrophy encodes a peroxisomal membrane protein. *Hum Mol Genet* 1994 ; 3 : 265-71.
33. Kamijo K, Taketani S, Yokota S, Osumi T, Hashimoto T. The 70-kDa peroxisomal membrane protein is a member of the Mdr (P-glycoprotein)-related ATP-binding protein superfamily. *J Biol Chem* 1990 ; 265 : 4534-40.
34. Gärtner J, Moser HW, Valle D. Mutations in the 70K peroxisomal membrane protein gene in Zellweger syndrome. *Nature Genet* 1992 ; 1 : 16-23.
35. Lombard-Platet G, Savary S, Sarde C-O, Mandel J-L, Chimini G. A close relative of the adrenoleukodystrophy (ALD) gene codes for a peroxisomal protein with a specific expression pattern. *Proc Natl Acad Sci* 1996 ; 93 : 1265-9.
36. Higgins CF. ABC transporters: from microorganisms to man. *Annu Rev Cell Biol* 1992 ; 8 : 67-113.
37. Sarde C-0, Thomas J, Sadoulet H, Garnier J-M, Mandel J-L. cDNA sequence of the mouse homologue of the X-linked adrenoleukodystrophy gene. *Mammalina Genome* 1994 ; 5 : 810-3.
38. Contreras M, Mosser J, Mandel JL, Aubourg P, Singh I. The protein coded by the X-adrenoleukodystrophy gene is a peroxisomal integral membrane protein. *FEBS Lett* 1994 ; 344 : 211-5.
39. Cartier N, Lopez J, Moullier P, Rocchiccioli F, Rolland M-O, Jorge P, Mosser J, Mandel J-L, Bougnères P-F, Danos O, Aubourg P. Retroviral-mediated gene transfer corrects very-long-chain fatty acid metabolism in adrenoleukodystrophy fibroblasts. *Proc Natl Acad Sci USA* 1995 ; 92 : 1674-8.
40. Houdou S, Takashima S, Suzuki Y. Immunohistochemical expression of peroxisomal enzymes in developing human brain. *Mol Chem Neuropathol* 1993 ; 19 : 235-48.
41. Singh I, Lazo O, Dhaunsi GS , Contreras M. Transport of fatty acids into human and rat peroxisomes. Differential transport of palmitic and lignoceric acids and its implication to X-adrenoleukodystrophy. *J Biol Chem* 1992 ; 267 : 13306-13.
42. Cartier N, Sarde C-O, Douar A-M, Mosser J, Mandel J-L, Aubourg P. Abnormal messenger RNA expression and a missense mutation in patients with X-linked adrenoleukodystrophy. *Hum Mol Genet* 1993 ; 2 : 1949-51.
43. Uchiyama A, Suzuki Y, Song X-Q, Fukao T, Imamura A, Tomatsu S, Shimozawa N, Kondo N, Orii T. Identification of a nonsense mutation in ALD protein cDNA from a patient with adrenoleukodystrophy. *Biochem Biophys Res Commun* 1994 ; 198 : 632-6.
44. Fuchs S, Sarde CO, Wedemann H, Schwinger E, Mandel JL, Gal A. Missense mutations are frequent in the gene for X-chromosomal adrenoleukodystrophy (ALD). *Hum Mol Genet* 1994 ; 3 : 1903-5.

45. Kemp S, Ligtenberg MJL, Van Geel BM, Barth PG, Wolterman RA, Schoute F, Sarde C-O, Mandel J-L, Van Oost BA, Bolhuis PA. Identification of a two base pair deletion in five unrelated families with adrenoleukodystrophy: a possible hot spot for mutations. *Biochem Biophys Res Commun* 1994 ; 202 : 647-53.
46. Barcelo A, Giros M, Sarde C-O, Martinez-Bermejo A, Mandel J-L, Pampols T, Estivil XL. Identification of a new frameshift mutation (1801delAG) in the ALD gene. *Hum Mol Genet* 1994 ; 3 : 1889-90.
47. Berger J, Molzer B, Faé I, Bernheimer H. X-linked adrenoleuko-dystrophy (ALD): a novel mutation of the ALD hene in 6 members of a family presenting with 5 different phenotypes. *Biochem Biophys Res Commun* 1994 ; 205 : 1638-43.
48. Ligtenberg MJL, Kemp S, Sarde C-O, Van Geel BM, Barth PG, Mandel J-L, Van Oost BA, Bolhuis PA. Spectrum of mutations in the gene encoding the adrenoleukodystrophy protein. *Am J Human Genet* 1995 ; 56 : 44-50.
49. Braun A, Ambach H, Kammerer S, Rolinski B, Stöckler S, Rabl W, Gärtner J, Ziere S, Roscher AA. Mutations in the gene for X-linked adrenoleukodystrophy in patients with different clinical phenotypes. *Am J Hum Genet* 1995 ; 56 : 854-61.
50. Rizzo WB, Leshner RT, Odone A, Dammann AL, Craft DA, Jensone ME, Jenningd SS, Davis S, Jaitly R, Sgro JA. Dietary erucic acid therapy for X-linked adrenoleukodystrophy. *Neurology* 1989 ; 39 : 1415-22.
51. Uziel G, Bertini E, Bardelli P, Rimoldi M, Gambetti M. Experience on therapy of adrenoleukodystrophy and adrenomyeloneuropathy. *Dev Neurosci* 1991 ; 13 : 274-9.
52. Aubourg P, Adamsbaum C, Lavallard-Rousseau MC, Rocchiccioli F, Cartier N, Jambaqué I, Jakobezak C, Lemaitre A, Boureau F, Wolf C, Bougnères PF. A two-year trial of oleic and erucic acids (Lorenzo's oil) as treatment for adrenomyeloneuropathy. *N Engl J Med* 1993 ; 329 : 745-52.
53. Asano J, Suzuki Y, Yajima S, Inoue K, Shimozawa N, Kondo N, Murase M, Orii T. Effects of erucic acid therapy on Japanese patients with X-linked adrenoleukodystrophy. *Brain Dev* 1994 ; 16 : 454-8.
54. Korenke GC, Hunneman DH, Kohler J, Stöckler S, Landmark K, Hanefeld F. Glyceroltrioleate/ glyceroltrierucate therapy in 16 patients with X-chromosomal adrenoleukodystrophy/ adrenomyeloneuropathy: effect on clinical, biochemical and neurophysiological parameters. *Eur J Pediatr* 1995 ; 154 : 64-70.
55. Kaplan PW, Tusa RJ, Shankroff J, Heller J, Moser HW. Visual evoked potentials in adrenoleukodystrophy: a trial swith glycerol trioleate and Lorenzo oil. *Ann Neurol* 1993 ; 34 : 169-74.
56. Rasmussen M, Moser AB, Borel J, Khangoora S, Moser HW. Brain, liver, and adipose tissue erucic and very long chain fatty acid levels in adrenoleukodystrophy patients treated with glyceryl trierucate and trioleate oils (Lorenzo's oil). *Neurochem Res* 1994 ; 19 : 1073-82.
57. Poulos A, Gibson R, Sharp P, Beckman K, Grattan-Smith P. Very long chain fatty acids in X-linked adrenoleukodystrophy brain after treatment with Lorenzo's oil. *Ann Neurol* 1994 ; 36 : 741-6.
58. Perry VH, Gordon S. Macrophages and microglia in the nervous system. *Trends Neurosci* 1988 ; 11 : 273-7.
59 Kriwit W, Shapiro E. Bone marrow transplantation for storage diseases. In : Desnick RJ, ed. *Treatment of genetic diseases.* New York : Churchill Livingstone, 1991 : 203-21.
60. Moser HW, Tutschka PJ, Brown III FR, Moser AB, Yeager AM, Singh I, Mark SA, Kumar AJ, McDonnell JM, White CL, Maumenee IH, Green WR, Power JM, Santos GW. Bone marrow transplant in adrenoleukodystrophy. *Neurology* 1984 ; 34 : 1410-7.

61. Aubourg P, Blanche S, Jambaque I, Rocchiccioli F, Kalifa G, Naud-Saudreau C, Rolland MO, Debre M, Chaussain JL, Griscelli C, Fischer A, Bougnères PF. Reversal of early neurologic and neuroradiologic manifestations of X-linked adrenoleukodystrophy by bone marrow transplantation. *N Engl J Med* 1990 ; 322 : 1860-6.
62. Knazek RA, Rizzo WB, Schulman JD, Dave JR. Membrane microviscosity is increased in the erythrocytes of patients with adrenoleukodystrophy and adrenomyeloneuropathy. *J Clin Invest* 1983 ; 72 : 245-8.
63. Whitcomb RW, Linehan WR, Knazek RA. Effects of long-chain, saturated fatty acids on membrane microviscosity and adrenocorticotropin responsiveness of human adrenocortical cells *in vitro*. *J Clin Invest* 1988 ; 81 : 185-8.
64. Bizzozero OA, Zuñiga G, Lees MB. Fatty acid composition of human myelin proteolipid protein in peroxisomal disorders. *J Neurochem* 1991 ; 56 : 872-8.
65. Selmaj K, Raine C. Tumor necrosis factor mediates myelin and oligodendrocyte damage *in vitro*. *Ann Neurol* 1988 ; 23 : 339-46.
66. Powers JM, Liu Y, Moser AB, Moser HW. The inflammatory myelinopathy of adreno-leukodystrophy: cells, effector molecules, and pathogenic implications. *J Neuropathol Exp Neurol* 1992 ; 51 : 630-43.
67. Rothwell NJ, Hopkins SJ. Cytokines and the nervous system II: actions and mechanisms of action. *Trends Neurosci* 1995 ; 18 : 130-6.
68. Sobue G, Ueno-Natsukari I, Okamoto H, Connell TA, Aizawa I, Mizoguchi K, Honma M, Ishikawa G, Mitsuma T, Natsukari N. Phenotypic heterogeneity of an adult form of adrenoleukodystrophy in monozygotic twins. *Ann Neurol* 1994 ; 36 : 912-5.
69. Maestri NE, Beaty TH. Predictions of a 2-locus model for disease heterogeneity: application to adrenoleukodystrophy. *Am J Med Genet* 1992 ; 44 : 576-82.
70. McKinnon R, Dubois-Dalcq M. Growth factors in the development and regeration of oligodendrocytes. In : Benveniste E, Ransohoff RM, eds. *Cytokines and the CNS development, health and disease*. Boca Raton, Florida : CRC Press, 1995.
71. Franklin RJM, Blakemore WF. Glial-cell transplantation and plasticity in the O-2A lineage-implications for CNS repair. *Trends Neurosci* 1995 ; 18 : 151-6.
72. Fischer LJ, Gage FH. Grafting in the mammalian central nervous system. *Physiol Rev* 1993 ; 73 : 583-616.
73. Rutkowski JL, Kirk CJ, Lerner MA, Tennekoon GI. Purification and expansion of human Schwann cells *in vitro*. *Nature Med* 1995 ; 1 : 80-3.

26

Genetic and environmental determinants of neocortical development

P. EVRARD

Service de Neurologie Pédiatrique et Laboratoire de Neurologie du Développement,
Hôpital Robert-Debré, Paris, France.

This lecture is a review of conceptual and methodological tools permitting to analyze the influences of genetic, epigenetic and environmental determinants on developing neural tissue, including on developing neocortex, during early life. A special attention is paid to the different types of neocortical units (Table I) and to the excitotoxic cascade during neocortical development.

During the period of preparation of the neural germinative epithelium, the environmental influences, including the nutritional, circulatory, maternal and placental factors, can interfere with the genetic program in a very complex way. Whole postimplantation mouse embryo cultures are a powerful tool for the study of environmental, nutritional, hypoxic, and genetic factors at this developmental phase. At this step, we shall especially review the role of recently recognized growth factors (as vasointestinal peptide -VIP) on brain growth, a new avenue to explore microcephaly and intrauterine growth retardation. At the step of neuronal migration, we shall review mainly the alcohol and cocaine-induced disturbances of corticogenesis. Alcohol and cocaine interfere with development of the human fetal brain. The teratogenic mechanisms of these drugs on neurogenesis were recently explored on animal models. Cocaine severely disturbs neocortical architecture, disrupting horizontal and vertical lamination, and inducing abnormal array of the axonal-dendritic bundles. Cocaine also alters several steps of gliogenesis. The severity of malformations is variable, but evident

Table I. Possible ontogenic and phylogenic links between the germinative zone, the angiogenetic corridors, the synaptic stabilization, and the cortical architecture.

Perivascular neuronal units (Kuban and Gilles, Bar)
Neuronal unit supported by a radial vessel and its horizontal branches: possible role on morphogenesis through metabolic gradients within the perivascular units.

Neuronal domains coupled by gap junctions (Yuste)
Early coupling of postmigrational neurons by gap junctions define cortical domains of spontaneously active neurons. This early coupling could «inform neurons that they are members of a distinct radial group».

Protomap of cytoarchitectonic areas (Rakic)
Radially arranged glial guides keep a topographical correspondance between the proliferative units of the germinative zone and the cortical vertical columns. Recent studies showing an early regional specification of neuronal precursors in the absence of extrinsic stimuli support the protomap hypothesis.

Dispersed clonally-related neurons (Austin, Walsh, and Cepko; Fishell; O'Rourke)
Cortical spatial dispersion of clonally-related neurons: temporary horizontal migration independent from RGCs and vertical migration along the non-perfectly radially arranged glial guides.

Radially and tangentially distributed neurons (Tan and Breen)
Based on early random labelling of half the neural progenitors, two thirds of neurons seem to be radially distributed while the remaining neurons are tangentially dispersed.

The pyramidal cell and its local-circuit interneurons (Marin-Padilla)
A constant structural and functional unit throughout the mammalian species. It suggests to us a developmental mechanism based on migratory units and/or upon mechanisms of synaptic stabilization.

Glial fascicles (Evrard, Gadisseux, Kadhim, and Gressens)
Neuronal migration along regularly spaced and early formed glial fascicles: guiding role, energy corridors during neuronal anaerobiosis, and organization of cortical neurons. This unit is constant throughout the mammalian species.

Vertical physiological column (Mountcastle)
Radially organized basic module of a constant amount of neurons responsive to a specific modality of stimulation. It has been suggested that this unit developed from neurons that have migrated along a radial glial cell.

Neuropsychological unit (Changeux and Danchin; Edelman)
Functionally but not structurally redundant cortical units; the function is produced by the association of units according to their final connections shaped by synaptic stabilization.

---

in all animals exposed to doses comparable to the doses used by human cocaine-abusers. The cocaine-induced cortical pattern seems the result of dyschronologic mitoses and of a defect of the radial glial cells. This pattern may represent the pathological basis of the neuropsychological modifications described in *in utero* cocaine exposed children. Immediate early genes — IEGs — (*c-fos, c-jun,* and *zif-268*) are disturbed by cocaine during development. As transcription factors, IEGs can directly dysregulate target genes. Ethanol locally enhances cell death in the primitive neuroepithelium. During neuronal migration, ethanol induces a premature transformation of the radial glial guides into astrocytes. Ethanol also inhibits the late gliogenesis.The resulting postmigratory neocortex displays an abnormal neuronal pattern almost completely deprived of vertical columnization. These glial-neuronal disturbances can explain neuropathological and clinical features of the fetal alcohol syndrome. At the end and after neuronal migration, the infragranular layers are a sensitive target for perfusion failures/hypoxias around mid gestation. During the second half of pregnancy, the transformation of radial glial cells into astrocytic precursors is a target for environmental disturbances, among which nutritional factors and hypoxia/ischemia are candidates. Several residual neuronal migrations or displacements occurring after mid gestation have complex pathophysiological relationships with ischemia/hypoxia and with circulatory events. The late germinative zone produces migrating astrocytic precursors for the upper neocortex. It confirms the dual origin of astrocytic precursors and it suggests the transitory existence of a late astroglial protomap destined to the upper cortex, which could explain cortical consequences of periventricular leucomalacias — PVLs — and intraventricular hemorrhages — IVHs.

The developing brain is weltering in a complex mixture including excitotoxic substances, cytokins, and growth factors. These substances are sometimes environmental friends like maternal VIP which could prevent brain intrauterine growth retardation. They are sometimes excellent endogenous friends like neurotrophic excitatory agents in physiological conditions. They become often dangerous killers triggered by environmental signals, like hypoxias/ischemias and toxins produced by intrauterine infections launching the excitotoxic cascade. The deviant neopallial architectural patterns produced by excitotoxins at the successive steps of early life reproduce the whole spectrum of migration disorders and of posthypoxic developmental lesions. Using ibotenate, a competitive glutamatergic agonist, it is possible to reproduce in mammals most patterns of fetal and neonatal dysmorphogenetic and destructive lesions encountered in human developmental neuropathology. This model can be used also to assess scavengers and excitotoxin antidotes, as magnesium and neurotrophic factors.

Bibliography

1. Barkovich J, Gressens P, Evrard P. Formation, maturation, and disorders of brain neocortex. *Am J Neuroradiol* 1992 ; 13 : 423-46.
2. Ben Ari Y, Gaiarsa JL, Ravira C, Pollard H, Khrestchatisky M. Developmental changes in the properties of glutamatergic and GABAergic receptors in the hippocampus. *Epilepsia* 1993 ; 34 : 196.
3. Caviness VS, Pinto-Lord MC, Evrard P. The development of laminated pattern in the mammalian neocortex. In : Connelly PG, et al., eds. *Morphogenesis and pattern formation.* New York : Raven Press, 1981 : 103-26.
4. Evrard P, Gressens P, Volpe JJ. New concepts to understand the neurological consequences of subcortical lesions in premature brain. *Biol Neonate* 1992 ; 61 : 1-3.

5. Evrard P, Marret S, Gressens P. Environmental determinants of brain development. In : *Genetic versus environmental determination of human behaviour and health*. Nobel Symposium 1996, in press.
6. Evrard P, Miladi N, Bonnier C, Gressens P. Normal and abnormal development of the brain. In : Rapin I, Segalowitz SJ, eds. *Handbook of neuropsychology*. Amsterdam : Elsevier Publ, 1992 : 15-44.
7. Evrard P, Minkowski A. *Developmental neurobiology*. New York : Raven Press, 1989.
8. Gressens P, Cilio MR, Schlogel X, Evrard P. Les mécanismes de l'hypoxie pendant la vie fœtale et néonatale. *Progr Neonatol* 1991 ; 11 : 203-26.
9. Gressens P, Kosofsky B, Evrard P. Cocaine-induced disturbances of neurogenesis in the developing murine brain. *Neurosci Lett* 1992 ; 140 : 113-6.
10. Gressens P, Lammens M, Picard JJ, Evrard P. Ethanol-induced disturbances of gliogenesis and neuronogenesis in the developing murine brain. *Alcohol and Alcoholism* 1992 ; 27 : 219-26.
11. Innocenti G, Berbel P. Analysis of an experimental cortical network: i) Architectonics of visual areas 17 and 18 after neonatal injections of ibotenic acid: similarities with human microgyria. *J Neural Transpl* 1991 ; 2 : 1-28.
12. Marret S, Mukendi R, Gadisseux JF, Gressens P, Evrard P. Effect of ibotenate on brain development: an excitotoxic mouse model of microgyria and posthypoxic-like lesions. *J Neuropathol Exp Neurol* 1995 ; 54 : 358-70.
13. Marret S, Gressens P, Gadisseux JF, Evrard P. Prevention by magnesium of excitotoxic neuronal death in the developing brain: an animal model for clinical intervention studies. *Dev Med Child Neurol* 1995 ; 37 : 473-84.

Achevé d'imprimer par Corlet, Imprimeur, S.A.
14110 Condé-sur-Noireau (France)
N° d'Imprimeur : 19588 - Dépôt légal : octobre 1996

Imprimé en C.E.E.